JAUNDICE

HEPATOLOGY

Research and Clinical Issues

Volume 1 • Viral Hepatitis

Edited by M. M. Fisher and J. W. Steiner
Canadian Medical Association Journal
(Vol. 106, Special Issue, pp. 417 – 528, 1972)

Volume 2 • Jaundice

Edited by C. A. Goresky and M. M. Fisher

A Continuation Order Plan is available for this series. A continuation order will bring delivery of each new volume immediately upon publication. Volumes are billed only upon actual shipment. For further information please contact the publisher.

Library of Congress Cataloging in Publication Data

Main entry under title:

Jaundice: [proceedings of the second international symposium of the Canadian Hepatic Foundation, held in Montreal, May 31 and June 1, 1974]

(Hepatology–research and clinical issues; v. 2)
Includes bibliographical references and index.
1. Jaundice–Congresses. I. Goresky, C. A., 1932- II. Fisher, Murray M., 1934- III. Canadian Hepatic Foundation. [DNLM: 1. Jaundice–Congresses. W1 HE913 v. 2 / WI703 J41 1974]
RC851.J38 616.3'625 75-8782
ISBN-13: 978-1-4684-2651-9 e-ISBN-13: 978-1-4684-2649-6
DOI: 10.1007/ 978-1-4684-2649-6

Proceedings of the Second International Symposium of the Canadian Hepatic Foundation, held in Montreal, May 31 and June 1, 1974

Softcover reprint of the hardcover 1st edition 1975
A Division of Plenum Publishing Corporation
227 West 17th Street, New York, N.Y. 10011

United Kingdom edition published by Plenum Press, London
A Division of Plenum Publishing Company, Ltd.
House (4th Floor), 8 Scrubs Lane, Harlesden, London, NW10 6SE, England

JAUNDICE

Edited by

C. A. GORESKY
McGill University

and

M. M. FISHER
University of Toronto

CANADIAN
FOUN

Davis

PLENUM PR

Preface

Jaundice is much more than a clinical sign of liver disease. It is also a pathophysiological disorder. Through studying it we have come to a much better understanding of how the liver functions under normal and abnormal circumstances. In spite of several important advances in this field, it has not recently been the subject of a comprehensive and interdisciplinary review.

This Symposium was held in Montreal on May 31 and June 1, 1974, and the experts who participated in it came together for the purpose of reviewing the current status of Jaundice. The Editors sincerely appreciate the outstanding contribution which these experts made to the Second International Symposium of the Canadian Hepatic Foundation. They are also particularly indebted to Valerie M. Price, Executive Director, Canadian Hepatic Foundation, for her invaluable role in the preparation of this publication.

Carl A. Goresky
Murray M. Fisher

Contents

BILIRUBIN THROUGHPUT

BILIARY SECRETION

DISORDERS OF BILIRUBIN METABOLISM

EXTRAHEPATIC BILIARY OBSTRUCTION

INTRAHEPATIC CHOLESTASIS

AN OVERVIEW OF BILIRUBIN CHEMISTRY

Antony F. McDonagh

University of California, San Francisco

San Francisco, California 94143

"From gall disease, that is from the yellow jaundice cometh great evil; it is of all disease most powerful, when there wax within a man, unmeasured humors; these are the tokens; that the patient's body all becometh bitter and as yellow as good silk; and under the root of his tongue there be swart veins and pernicious, and his urine is yellow"(1). The yellow pigment referred to in this vivid eleventh-century Anglo-Saxon description of cirrhosis was first isolated in crystalline form by Virchow in 1847(2), and named bilirubin by Stadeler in 1864(3). Its structure was determined by Siedel and Fischer in 1933(4) and confirmed by total synthesis by Fischer and Plieninger in 1943(5) and more recently by Plieninger et al(6). Much of the basic chemistry of the pigment was elucidated more than two decades ago, principally by the Fischer school. And today, despite the fact that bilirubin is a metabolic waste-product of no practical utility other than its diagnostic value, scientific interest in the pigment continues unabated. In the past two to three years alone bilirubin has been mentioned in over 1600 publications, and of these about 400 specifically with some aspect of the chemistry or biochemistry of the molecule. The areas of bilirubin chemistry and biochemistry which appear to have received the most attention in recent years are the mechanism of bilirubin formation, the mechanism of bilirubin conjugation and excretion, the nature of bilirubin conjugates, bilirubin-protein complexes, and the photochemistry of bilirubin. In addition there has been a steady flow of new, or improved, methods for the estimation of bilirubin and its conjugates in biological fluids.

In the brief account of bilirubin chemistry which follows, no attempt has been made to provide a comprehensive review of the subject. Instead, some of the basic chemical properties of the molecule are outlined with particular emphasis on recent work.

GENERAL PROPERTIES

The chemical formula of bilirubin is shown in Figure 1. Inspection of this structure shows that by interchanging the substituents on the pyrrole rings a number of structural isomers of bilirubin would be formed which could, in theory, exist. Few of these bilirubin isomers have in fact been made, and the only one which occurs naturally is the isomer shown. This is designated bilirubin IX-α because it is derived from the natural IX isomer of ferriprotoporphyrin by cleavage of the porphyrin ring at the α bridge position.

Bilirubin IX-α is a stable crystalline solid which crystallizes readily from chloroform-methanol solutions. Commercial preparations of the pigment, which are obtained from animal bile or gallstones, may contain isomers of bilirubin (see below)(7) or non-bilirubin material as impurities(8). Samples which are isomerically homogeneous are easy to purify(9,10), but the removal of unwanted isomers can only be accomplished on a small scale using thin-layer chromatography(7,10). The pure pigment is soluble in a number of organic solvents (e.g. chloroform, methylene chloride, pyridine, dimethyl sulfoxide), but is essentially insoluble in petroleum ether, methanol, or water. Its solubility in water is very low at pH 7.4 but increases with increasing pH (11,12), giving solutions which tend to be unstable in the presence of air even in the dark(13). Metastable supersaturated solutions of bilirubin in water at physiological pH containing about 9 x 10^{-5} moles/l (5 mg%) of the pigment are easy to prepare by addition of a concentrated solution in 0.1M NaOH or dimethyl sulfoxide to excess pH 7.4 buffer. However, the pigment slowly precipitates from these solutions on standing or on agitation.

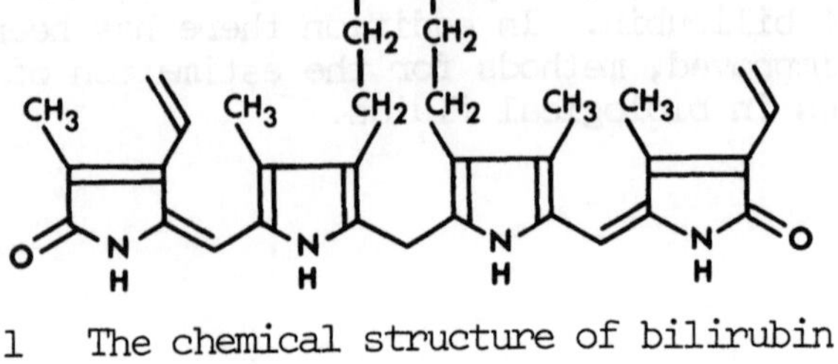

Fig. 1 The chemical structure of bilirubin IX-α

By the use of cationic or neutral detergents such as cetyltrimethylammonium bromide or Tween 20, bilirubin can be solubilized in water over a wide range of acidic and basic pH values(14,15).

Much of the chemistry of bilirubin is readily predictable from its structure. As shown in Figure 2, the molecule contains two carboxylic acid side-chains which should readily form esters and are weakly acidic, and on the lactam positions of the end rings there is a further pair of very weakly acidic protons which should also ionize in strong alkali. The central pyrrole rings, on the other hand, would be expected to be weakly basic and become protonated in strong acids. The molecule has a number of double bonds which should be reducible, especially those in the side-chains and the end rings. However, the more stable double bonds of the aromatic central pyrrole rings would be expected to be more resistant to reduction.

If bilirubin is drawn in the form of the hydroxypyrrole tautomer rather than the lactam tautomer shown in Figure 1, it can be seen that its structure is a hybrid of a pair of dipyrrylmethenes and a dipyrrylmethane (Fig. 3). The dipyrrylmethene portions, with their extended system of conjugated double bonds, are responsible for the yellow color of the molecule and are relatively stable. But the dipyrrylmethane segment is much less stable and may be regarded as the Achilles heel of the molecule. Dipyrrylmethanes are attacked by electrophiles and tend to undergo cleavage about the central $-CH_2-$ bridge in the presence of strong acids. They are also prone to oxidative dehydrogenation to the corresponding, more fully conjugated, dipyrrylmethenes. It is not surprising, therefore, to find that bilirubin undergoes similar reactions.

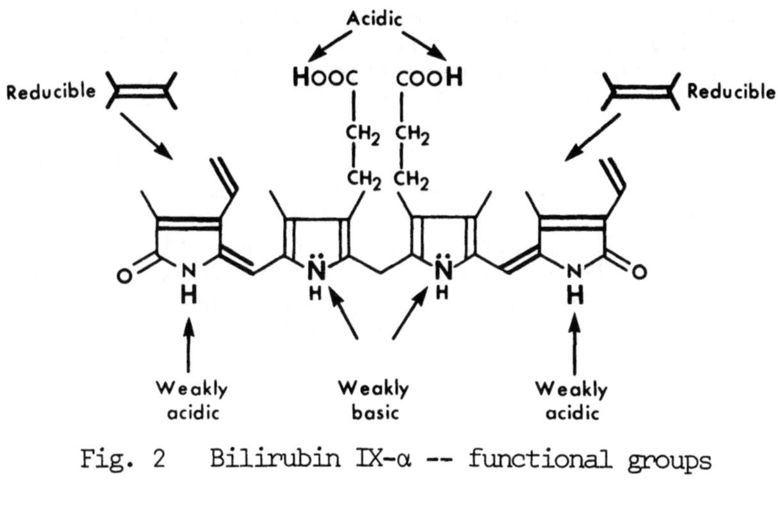

Fig. 2 Bilirubin IX-α -- functional groups

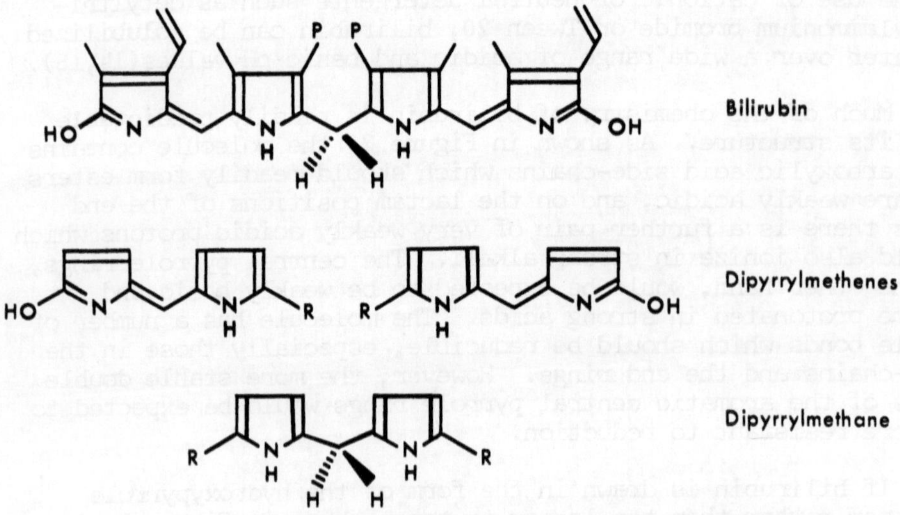

Fig. 3 Bilirubin IX-α -- a hybrid structure

SPECIFIC REACTIONS

1. Esterification

In mammals the water-solubility of bilirubin is enhanced and its excretion facilitated by enzymatic esterification with the polar sugar glucuronic acid. Non-enzymatic esterification of bilirubin with glucuronic acid has not been achieved, but methyl, ethyl and other alkyl esters of the molecule are easily prepared by treating bilirubin with the corresponding commercially-available 1-alkyl-3-p-tolyltriazene (Fig.4)(16). Diazomethane has also been used to prepare bilirubin dimethyl ester, but with this reagent methylation of the lactam oxygen atoms also occurs and several products are obtained(17). Acid-catalyzed esterification with alcohols cannot be used because of the instability of the molecule towards acid (see below). The esters of bilirubin, including bilirubin diglucuronide, are more susceptible to autoxidation than bilirubin itself. This has been attributed to a stabilizing effect of intermolecular hydrogen-bonds in the free acid which is destroyed by esterification(18).

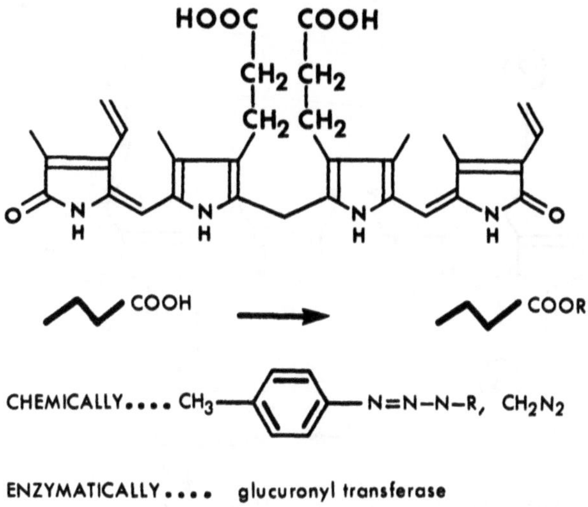

Fig. 4 Bilirubin IX-α -- esterification

2. Reduction

Bilirubin can be readily reduced using sodium amalgam or catalytically hydrogenated using palladium on charcoal (Fig. 5) (19). The hydrogens add on two by two, first at the exo-vinyl group (site 1) and then at the endo-vinyl group (site 2) to give mesobilirubin. Further reduction (sites 3) yields the colorless urobilinogen and finally (sites 4) stercobilinogen. A similar series of reactions takes place in the gut, catalyzed by bacterial enzymes of the gut flora (19).

3. Oxidation

Bilirubin undergoes a variety of oxidative reactions, some of which are summarized in Figure 6. On treatment with strong oxidizing agents such as chromic acid or potassium permanganate the molecule is rapidly cleaved to monopyrrolic units (20).

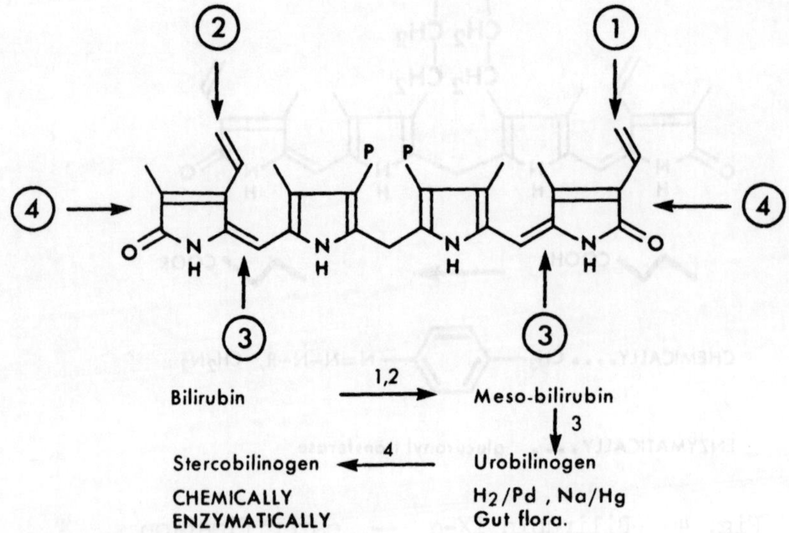

Fig. 5 Reduction (hydrogenation) of bilirubin IX-α

Less powerfull oxidizing agents, for example ferric chloride (21), smoothly dehydrogenate the pigment at the central bridge to give the fully conjugated biliverdin IX-α. This reaction has practical utility for preparing biliverdin, and perhaps the best reagent to use is benzoquinone in the presence of acetic acid with dimethyl sulfoxide as solvent (22).

Even in the dark and in the absence of adding oxidizing agents, bilirubin undergoes spontaneous oxidation in solution by reaction with atmospheric oxygen (23). This auto-oxidation occurs at a negligible rate in chloroform, but is significant in alkaline aqueous solutions, particularly if the concentration of bilirubin is low (15) and transition metal ions are present as trace contaminants (13). The nature of the auto-oxidation products has not been determined but they are probably the colorless water-soluble dipyrrolic compounds called water-propentdyopents (23,24). The autoxidation, which is frequently a nuisance in practical work, can be inhibited by addition of EDTA or ascorbic acid(25), but is most easily obviated by purging the solvent with an inert gas such as argon.

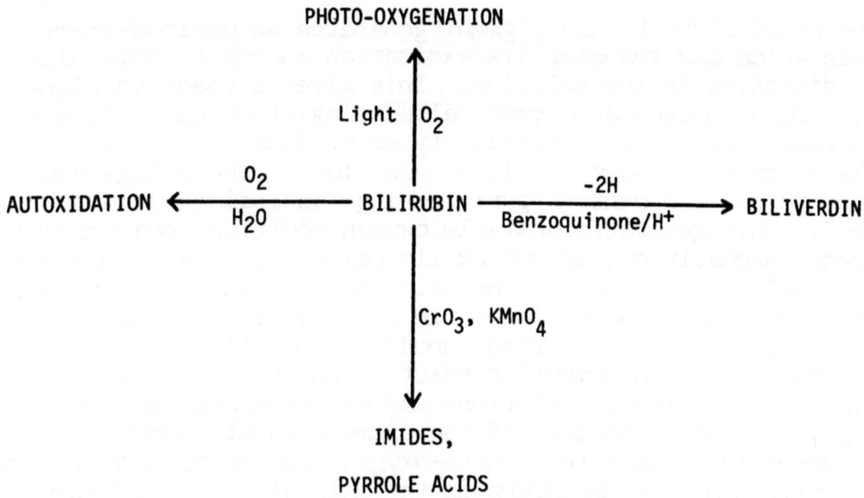

Fig. 6 Some oxidative reactions of bilirubin IX-α

The oxidative reaction of bilirubin which has drawn most attention recently because of its probable significance in phototherapy is photo-oxidation. This reaction is responsible for the familiar photo-degradation of the pigment which occurs when solutions of it are exposed to visible light with wavelengths of about 420-450 nm. The mechanism and products of bilirubin photo-oxidation vary somewhat with the nature of the solvent, but the predominant reaction in most solvents seems to be a photo-oxygenation process in which bilirubin acts as a photosensitizer of its own destruction(26-28). The overall mechanism is as follows:

$$\text{Bilirubin} + \text{Light} \longrightarrow \text{Bilirubin}^*$$

$$\text{Bilirubin}^* + O_2 \longrightarrow \text{Bilirubin} + O_2^*$$

$$\text{Bilirubin} + O_2^* \longrightarrow [\text{Bilirubin} \,.\, O_2] \longrightarrow \text{Products}$$

Absorption of light by the pigment generates an excited-state molecule which can transfer its excitation energy to molecular oxygen dissolved in the solution. This gives a reactive high-energy form of molecular oxygen called singlet oxygen. Singlet oxygen reacts avidly with certain types of double bonds and attacks bilirubin predominantly by addition to the bridge double bonds or across the central pyrrole rings as indicated in Figure 7. This generates unstable oxygen addition products which decompose thermally or, in hydroxylic solvents, undergo secondary reactions with the solvent. The main products which are formed on photo-oxygenation of bilirubin in ammoniacal methanol are shown in Figure 8(28-32). These products are all soluble in water and are colorless. A competing reaction which also occurs on irradiation of bilirubin solutions and may be marked in some solvents, is photo-oxidation of the pigment to biliverdin(31,33,34). It is currently thought that photo-oxygenation of bilirubin by a singlet oxygen mechanism occurs in the skin of jaundiced infants during phototherapy(35,36).

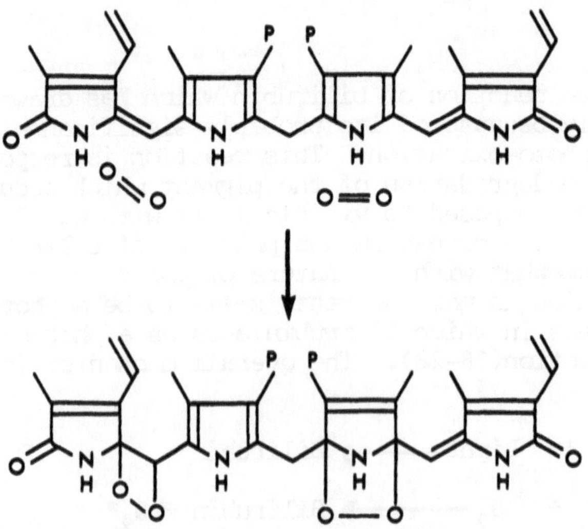

Fig. 7 Predominant modes of addition of singlet oxygen to bilirubin IX-α

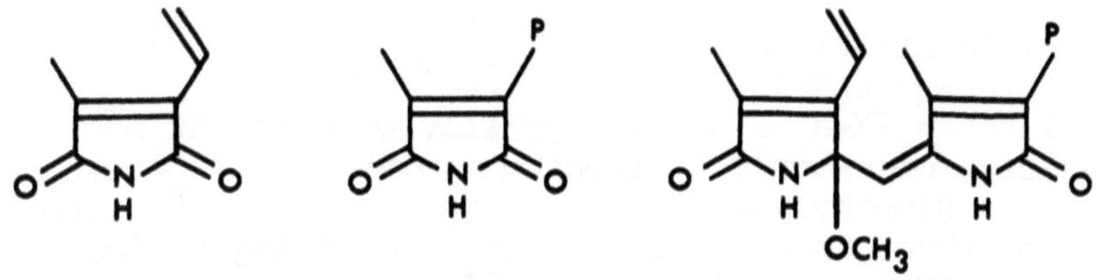

Fig. 8 Major products of the photo-oxygenation of bilirubin IX-α in methanol. L. to R. Methylvinylmaleimide, hematinic acid imide, methanol-propentdyopent (2 other positional isomers of methanol-propentdyopent are also formed).

4. Addition

It was pointed out above that the *exo*-vinyl group of bilirubin can be reduced more readily than the *endo*-vinyl group. The *exo*-vinyl group is also more reactive in other ways. By treatment of bilirubin with alcohol or thiols in the presence of an acid catalyst such as *p*-toluene sulfonic acid, addition occurs preferentially to the exo-vinyl group (Fig.9)(37). A similar reaction also occurs photochemically(38-40), and it has been suggested recently that photochemical addition of naturally-occurring alcohols or thiols to bilirubin might occur *in vivo* during phototherapy(40).

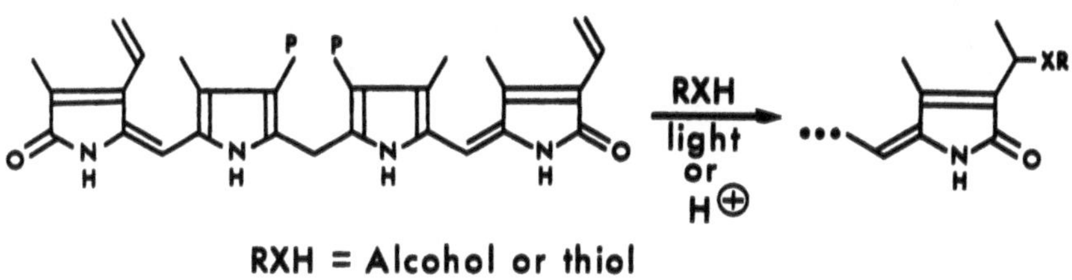

Fig. 9 Addition of alcohols and thiols to bilirubin IX-α

5. Electrophilic Attack

When bilirubin IX-α is treated briefly with strong non-oxidizing acids, for example on treatment with HCl or p-toluene sulfonic acid in dimethyl sulfoxide, it is converted efficiently to a mixture of three isomeric bilirubins containing bilirubin III-α, bilirubin IX-α, and bilirubin XIII-α in the approximate ratio of 1:2:1(27,37,41). The overall reaction, which is reversible, is shown in Figure 10. It is useful for preparing small quantities of the unnatural III- and XIII-α isomers. The mechanism of the reaction is outlined in Figure 11. Electrophilic attack of H^+ at either side of the central methylene bridge causes reversible cleavage of the unsymmetrical IX-α isomer into non-identical pairs of dipyrrylmethene units. Recombination of these dipyrroles then leads to a statistically random mixture of the isomers.

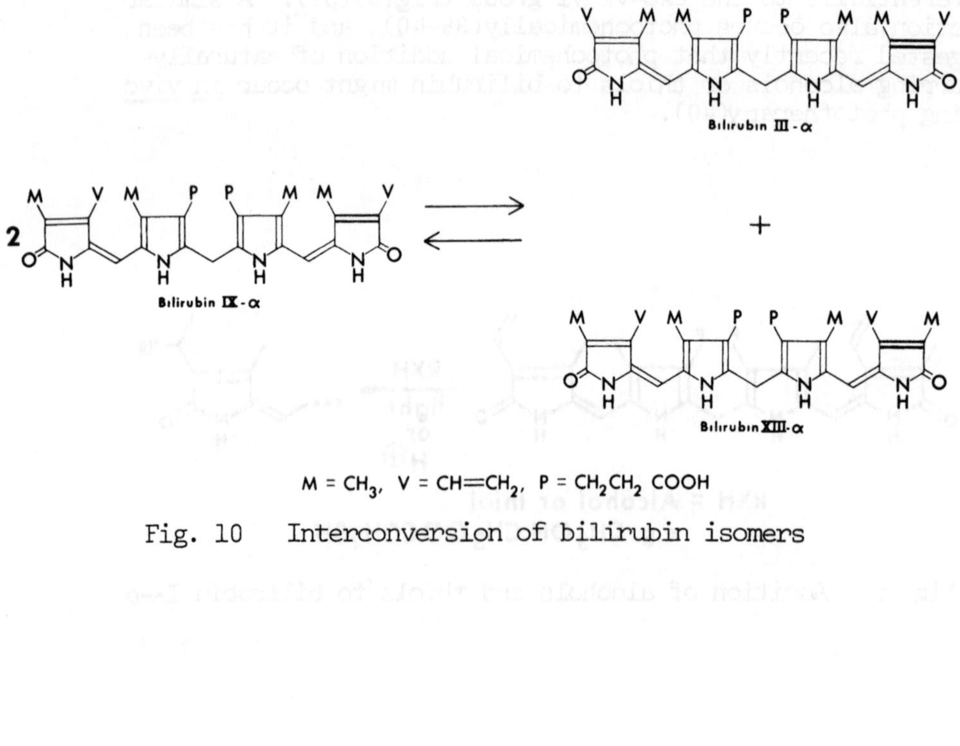

Fig. 10 Interconversion of bilirubin isomers

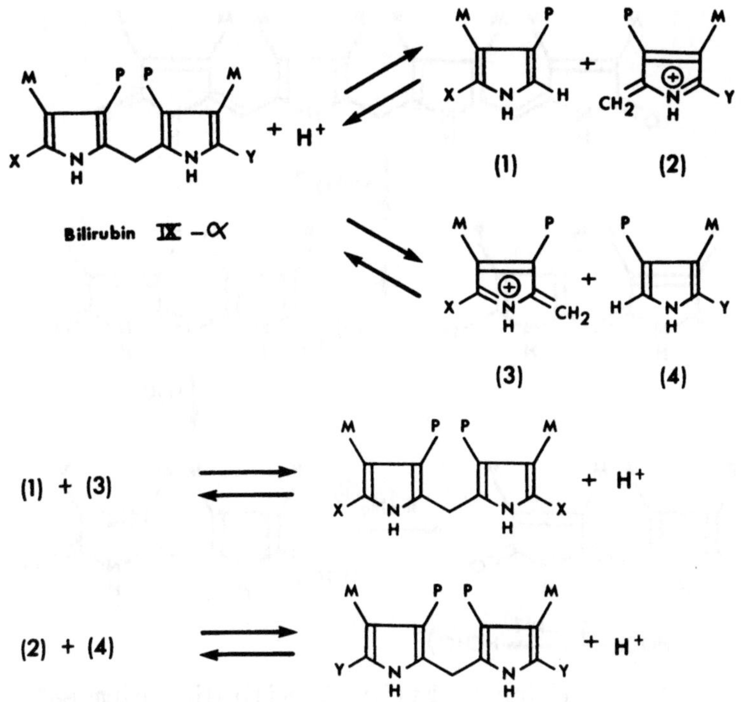

Fig. 11 Mechanism of the acid-catalyzed isomerization of bilirubin IX-α

The acid-catalyzed isomerization reaction of bilirubin is mechanistically reminiscent of the familiar diazo-reaction of bilirubin (Fig. 12). In the diazo-reaction the electrophilic diazonium ion attacks the substrate at either side of the methylene bridge causing rupture of the molecule. But in this case, because a stronger conjugated covalent bond is formed with the diazonium nitrogen atom, the reaction is not reversible and one-half of the bilirubin molecule becomes trapped. The remaining dipyrrole can then react with a second diazonium ion, and the carbon atom which was originally the methylene bridge of bilirubin is eliminated as formaldehyde(42).

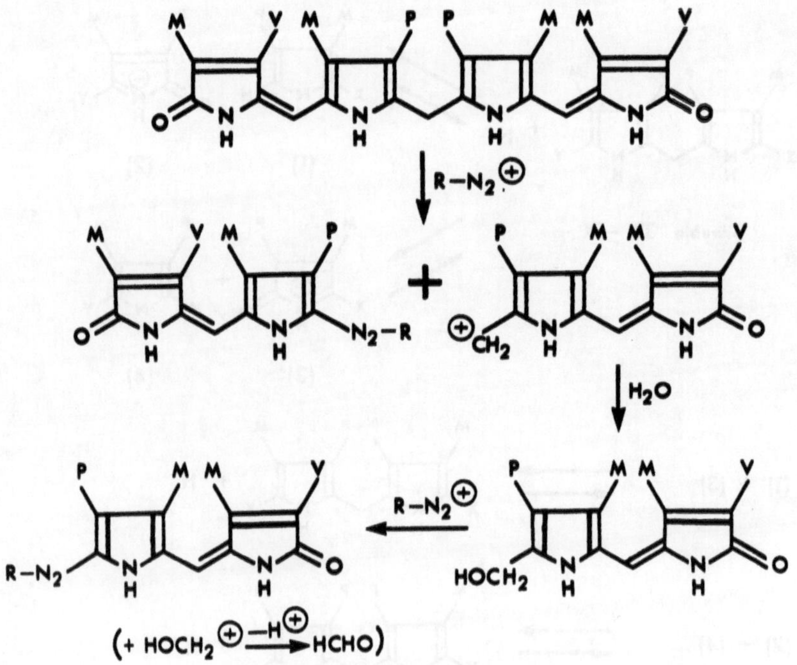

Fig. 12 The reaction of bilirubin with diazonium salts

6. Radical Isomerization

Reversible scrambling of bilirubin IX-α to give a randomized mixture of bilirubin III-, IX-, and XIII-α isomers also occurs when solutions of the pigment in water at pH 7.4-12 are incubated aerobically in the dark(10) or are irradiated with visible light under anaerobic conditions(36). Although the overall reaction in each case is identical to the acid-catalyzed isomerization (Fig. 10), a different mechanism applies. In these reactions randomization occurs via a free radical chain process as follows ($A\text{-}CH_2\text{-}B$ represents bilirubin IX-α):

$$A\text{-}CH_2\text{-}B + R. \longrightarrow AR + .CH_2\text{-}B$$

$$A\text{-}CH_2\text{-}B + R. \longrightarrow A\text{-}CH_2. + RB$$

$$A\text{-}CH_2\text{-}B + .CH_2\text{-}B \rightleftharpoons B\text{-}CH_2\text{-}B + A\text{-}CH_2.$$

$$A\text{-}CH_2\text{-}B + .CH_2\text{-}A \rightleftharpoons A\text{-}CH_2\text{-}A + B\text{-}CH_2.$$

In one case the initiating radical (R.) is molecular oxygen(15,36), whereas in the other it is some photochemically generated radical. Bilirubin monoglucuronide undergoes a similar isomerization in water and is converted to bilirubin diglucuronide and free bilirubin(43). The oxygen-catalyzed radical isomerization has some practical significance since it is probably responsible for the presence of "unnatural" bilirubin isomers in commercial samples of bilirubin which have been prepared by hydrolysis of bilirubin glucuronide from animal bile(7,10).

AREAS OF IGNORANCE

To conclude this overview of bilirubin chemistry, I would like to note briefly some aspects of bilirubin chemistry which are unclear and merit further investigation.

1. pK_a. To my knowledge no reliable pK_a values for the ionization of the four weakly acidic protons of bilirubin have been published. Consequently it is uncertain whether bilirubin exists as a di-, tri-, or even tetra-anion at physiological pH values.

2. Structure. The three-dimensional structure of bilirubin and the way in which the molecule is internally hydrogen-bonded are still controversial. Nor is it clear to what extent bilirubin exists as a monomer, dimer, or polymer in water at physiological pH values. Curiously, x-ray analysis of the crystal structure of bilirubin (or any other bile pigment) does not appear to have been carried out.

3. Nature of protein binding. The two previous points are obviously relevant to the protein-binding of bilirubin, which is another incompletely understood area. Particular questions which require elucidation here are the nature of the bilirubin-albumin bond, whether there is a <u>specific</u> binding-site for bilirubin on albumin, whether unbound unconjugated bilirubin ever really exists in serum and if so, what is its role in kernicterus and how can it be measured reliably.

4. Mechanism of phototherapy. One effect of phototherapy is destruction of bilirubin(44), and this probably is due largely to photo-oxygenation of the pigment. But phototherapy also stimulates biliary excretion of unconjugated bilirubin(44). The photochemical mechanism which leads to this intriguing effect is quite obscure at present.

5. Chemical basis for toxicity. It is well known that bilirubin is neuro-toxic(45). However, the chemical basis for the toxicity of the compound is not so clear. Is it a general effect caused by non-specific absorption of bilirubin onto cell membranes, or is it due to a specific chemical reaction of the pigment?

6. Bilirubin conjugates. Once upon a time it was simple. There was bilirubin monoglucuronide and bilirubin diglucuronide. But recent findings have shown that the situation may be considerably more complex. This area of bilirubin chemistry will be reviewed and clarified in the paper which follows.

SUMMARY

The basic chemistry of bilirubin was reviewed, with emphasis on recent work. A description of the general properties of the molecule was followed by more detailed discussion of specific reactions including esterification, reduction, oxidation, addition, and isomerization. Aspects of bilirubin chemistry which are poorly understood were summarized.

ACKNOWLEDGEMENTS

This work was aided by grants from the Duro-Test Corporation, North Bergen, New Jersey, and the United Cerebral Palsy Research and Education Foundation.

REFERENCES

1. COCKAYNE TO: Leechdoms, Wartcunning and Starcraft of Early England, The Holland Press, 1961, v II, P 107

2. VIRCHOW R: Die pathologischen pigmente. Arch Pathol Anat Physiol Klin Med 1: 379-486, 1847

3. STADELER G: Ueber die Farbstoffe der Galle. Justus Liebigs Ann Chem 132: 323-354, 1864

4. SIEDEL W, FISCHER H: Uber die Konstitution des Bilirubins, Synthesen der neo- und der iso-neoxanthobilirubinsäure. Hoppe Seylers Z Physiol Chem. 214: 145-172, 1933

5. FISCHER H, PLIENINGER H: Synthese des Biliverdins (Uteroverdins) und Bilirubins, der Biliverdine XIIIα und IIIα, sowie der Vinyl-neoxanthosäure. Hoppe Seylers Z Physiol Chem. 274: 231-260, 1942

6. PLIENINGER H, EL-BARKAWI F, EHL K, et al: Neue Synthese und ^{14}C- Markierung von Bilirubin IX-α. Justus Liebigs Ann Chem 758: 195-201, 1972

7. MCDONAGH AF, ASSISI F: Commercial bilirubin: A trinity of isomers. FEBS Lett 18: 315-317, 1971

8. NEWBOLD BT, LEBLANC G: Physical properties of commercial bilirubins. Can J Biochem 42: 1697-1702, 1964

9. FOG J: Bilirubin - purification - purity. Scand J Clin Lab Invest 16: 49-54, 1964

10. MCDONAGH AF, ASSISI F: The ready isomerization of bilirubin IX-α in aqueous solution. Biochem J 129: 797-800, 1972

11. OVERBEEK JTG, VINK CLJ, DEENSTRA H: The solubility of bilirubin. Rec Trav Chim 74: 81-84, 1955

12. BURNSTINE RC, SCHMID R: Solubility of bilirubin in aqueous solutions. Proc Soc Exp Biol Med 109: 356-358, 1962

13. FOG J, BUGGE-ASPERHEIM B: Stability of bilirubin. Nature (Lond) 203: 756-757, 1964

14. JIRSA M, SPONAR J: Das absorptionsspektrum, der physikalische zustand und die geschwindigkeit der diazoreaktion des bilirubins. Zeit gesamte Inn Med 11: 519-522, 1956

15. MCDONAGH AF, PALMA LA: Unpublished observations

16. HUTCHINSON DW, JOHNSON B, KNELL AJ: The synthesis of esters of bilirubin. Biochem J. 133: 493-498, 1973

17. KUENZLE CC, WEIBEL MH, PELLONI RR: The reaction of bilirubin with diazomethane. Biochem J 133: 357-368, 1973

18. FOG J, JELLUM E: Structure of bilirubin. Nature (Lond) 198: 88-89, 1963

19. PETRYKA Z: Variations in hydrogenation of bile pigments depending upon type of solvent and other factors. Ann NY Acad Sci 206: 701-710, 1973

20. RUDIGER W: Gallenfarbstoffe und Biliproteide. Fortschr Chem Org Naturst 29: 60-139, 1971

21. NICHOL AW, MORELL DB: Tautomerism and hydrogen bonding in bilirubin and biliverdin. Biochim Biophys Acta 177: 599-609, 1969

22. BONNETT R, MCDONAGH AF: The isomeric heterogeneity of biliverdin dimethyl ester derived from bilirubin. J Chem Soc D (Chem Commun): 238-239, 1970

23. BINGOLD K: Weitere Untersuchunger zur Formulierung eines biologisch-chemischen Blutkreislaufes. Klin Wochenshr 14: 1287-1289, 1935

24. OSTROW JD, HAMMAKER L, SCHMID R: The preparation of crystalline bilirubin-C^{14}. J Clin Invest. 40: 1442-1452, 1961

25. WITH TK: Bile Pigments. New York, Academic Press, 1968, p 25

26. MCDONAGH AF: The role of singlet oxygen in bilirubin photooxidation. Biochem Biophys Res. Commun 44: 1306-1311, 1971

27. BONNETT R, STEWART JCM: Singlet oxygen in the photo-oxidation of bilirubin in hydroxylic solvents. Biochem J 130: 895-897, 1972

28. LIGHTNER DA, QUISTAD GB: Imide products from photo-oxidation of bilirubin and mesobilirubin. Nature (New Biol) 236: 203-205, 1972.

29. LIGHTNER DA, QUISTAD GB: Hematinic acid and propentdyopents from bilirubin photo-oxidation in vitro. FEBS Lett 25: 94-96, 1972

30. BONNETT R: Recent advances in tetrapyrrole chemistry. Ann NY Acad Sci 206: 722-733, 1973

31. BONNETT R, STEWART JCM: Photo-oxidation of bilirubin in hydroxylic solvents: propentdyopent adducts as major products. J Chem Soc Chem Commun: 596-597, 1972

32. BONNETT R, STEWART, JCM: Personal communication.

33. MCDONAGH AF: Evidence for singlet oxygen quenching by biliverdin IX-α dimethyl ester and its relevance to bilirubin photo-oxidation. Biochem Biophys Res Commun 48: 408-415, 1972

34. LIGHTNER DA, CRANDALL DC, GERTLER S, et al: On the formation of biliverdin during photooxygenation of bilirubin in vitro. FEBS Lett 30: 309-312, 1973

35. MCDONAGH AF: Phototherapy of neonatal jaundice: photochemistry and photometabolism of bilirubin, in Phototherapy: An Overview, Washington, National Academy of Sciences, In Press

36. MCDONAGH AF: Thermal and photochemical reactions of bilirubin IX-α. Ann NY Acad Sci: In press

37. MANITTO P, MONTI D: Acid-catalyzed addition of alcohols and thiols to bilirubin. Experientia 29: 137-139, 1973

38. MANITTO P: Photochemistry of bilirubin. Experientia 27: 1147-1149, 1971

39. MANITTO P, MONTI D: Photoaddition of sulphydryl groups to bilirubin in vitro. Experientia 28: 379-380, 1972.

40. GARBAGNATI E, MANITTO P: A new class of bilirubin photoderivatives obtained in vitro and their possible formation in jaundiced infants. J Pediatr 83: 109-115, 1973

41. MCDONAGH AF, ASSISI F: Direct evidence for the acid-catalyzed isomeric scrambling of bilirubin IX-α. J Chem Soc Chem Commun: 117-119, 1972

42. HUTCHINSON DW, JOHNSON B, KNELL AJ: The reaction between bilirubin and aromatic diazo compounds. Biochem J 127: 907-908, 1972

43. JANSEN PLM: The isomerisation of bilirubin monoglucuronide. Clin Chim Acta 49: 233-240, 1973

44. OSTROW JD: Photocatabolism of labeled bilirubin in the congenitally jaundiced (Gunn) rat. J Clin Invest 50: 707-718, 1971

45. DIAMOND I: Bilirubin binding and kernicterus. Adv Pediatr 16: 99-119, 1969

THE CONJUGATES OF BILIRUBIN

Ellen R. Gordon

Queen Mary Veterans Hospital

Montreal, Quebec, Canada, H3W 1W5

In 1847, over a century ago, Virchow demonstrated that bile pigments arise as a consequence of the metabolism of the porphyrin ring of hemoglobin (1). The end product of this reaction, which occurs in the reticuloendothelial system, and involves the opening of the α methene bridge and release of carbon monoxide, globin and iron, is bilirubin (2). Until 1970, it was generally accepted that bilirubin was secreted in bile conjugated to a glucuronide, even though it had never been isolated as a chemically pure compound (3-5). At that time, this concept was challenged by two groups of investigators (6-12). Their studies indicated that bilirubin was not secreted in bile merely as a simple glucuronide. From dog gallbladder bile Heirwegh and his colleagues isolated and characterized a series of dipyrollic azo-derivatives of bilirubin: an azobilirubin β-D monoxyloside, an azobilirubin β-D monoglucoside, and an azobilirubin β-D monoglucuronide (10-12). However, from human T-tube bile Kuenzle was unable to isolate simple monosaccharide conjugates of bilirubin (7-9). Sophisticated analytical procedures were utilized in both these studies to elucidate the chemical nature of the azoderivatives of bilirubin. Therefore the lack of agreement is rather puzzling.

An examination of the chemical structure of bilirubin reveals the presence of many potential sites for hydrogen binding and the questions can then be raised - why is this compound so insoluble in aqueous media and why is conjugation necessary for bilirubin secretion? It is well known that, in spite of the numerous binding sites, bilirubin is only slightly soluble in an aqueous media. At pH 7.4, ionic strength 0.1M, the solubility is only 0.1μM (0.005 mg/100 ml) (13,14). This is rather remarkable. Recently an explanation for this phenomenon has been obtained from the infra-red and nuclear magnetic sprectra of bilirubin which indicate that internal hydrogen bonding occurs within the molecule (15). Thus the transformation of bilirubin to a more polar compound appears necessary before it can be secreted in bile in any significant amount. This process has been shown to occur in the smooth endoplasmic reticulum of parenchymal cells of the liver (2). Here bilirubin is transformed into a series of polar compounds which are then secreted into bile. Depending on which investigator you believe, the number of conjugated forms of bilirubin which have been isolated from bile varies from two to at least seven (4,6-12,16-18). The multiplicity of the various conjugated forms of bilirubin and the lack of reproducibility have led to a great deal of confusion in this field. However, if an examination is made of the structure of bilirubin it can be seen that there are many potential sites for conjugation in this tetrapyrolle compound. In fact, three different types of linkages are possible: an ester linkage through the propionic acid side chain, an ester linkage in the α position of rings A and D, and a linkage through the N in rings B and C. Thus because of its particular structure many sites are available for conjugation and the forms possible include mono-conjugates, diconjugates, and mixed conjugates.

The fact that bilirubin is so easily degraded in both aqueous and organic solvents has added to the complexity of verifying the number and chemical identity of the conjugates of bilirubin found in bile. Investigators have approached this problem by coupling the bile pigments with diazo reagents, such as sulphanilic acid, para-amino-benzoic acid, ethyl anthranilate, p-iodoaniline or aniline. In these reactions the central methylene carbon of the bilirubin molecule is displaced with the formation of formaldehyde as an end product (19) and the two half molecules (dipyrollic moieties) then react with the coupling reagent (14). The more stable diazo-derivatives of bilirubin are formed which are much easier to handle in analytical procedures (12). However, it should always be kept in mind that only one half of the complete molecule is being analyzed and therefore the actual configuration of the original compound cannot be ascertained unambiguously (20).

Van den Bergh, in 1913, was the first to apply Ehrlich's diazo reaction to quantitate bile pigments in serum. He noted that certain sera containing bile pigments reacted directly with the diazo reagent, while other sera and bilirubin reacted very slowly unless accelerators such as acetone, methanol or alcohol were added to the reaction. This led to the grouping of bile pigments into direct and indirect reacting compounds. However, it was not until 1953 that Barbara Billing actually separated, by reverse phase chromatography (21), the direct and indirect reacting compounds found in serum. The indirect reactant was found to have the same mobility on the column as bilirubin. The direct reacting component could be separated into two fractions, designated as pigments I and II. These pigment bands were eluted, coupled with aniline and rechromatographed. Bilirubin gave rise to azopigment A, pigment I gave rise to two azopigments A and B, and pigment II gave rise to azopigment B. Further studies indicated that azopigment B was alkali-labile and was hydrolyzed by β-glucuronidase (4,5). At this time it was suggested that in the azopigment bilirubin and glucuronic acid were linked by an ester linkage through the propionic acid side chain of the pigment. From the hexuronic acid and azopigment content of these compounds and because pigment I gave rise to two derivatives, while pigment II gave rise to only one, it was postulated that pigment I was a bilirubin monoglucuronide, and pigment II a bilirubin diglucuronide.

However a great deal of controversy has revolved around the reported existence in bile of a bilirubin monoglucuronide. In fact, it has been reported that pigment I is merely a complex of unconjugated bilirubin and bilirubin diglucuronide and appears as the result of inadequate separation procedures (22,23). However, the evidence to support the existence of monoglucuronide appears to over-rule these criticisms. Small quantities of bilirubin monoglucuronide have been isolated from rat and human bile by two different groups of investigators, Jacobson (24), and Ostrow and Murphy (25). The chemical synthesis of bilirubin mono- and diglucuronide has been accomplished by Thompson and Hofmann (26). A monoglucuronide appears to be the pigment formed in the *in vitro* assay for bilirubin UDP glucuronyl transferase (27). Also it has been shown that in the rat the infusion of bilirubin results in the appearance of bilirubin monoglucuronide in the bile, which can account for up to two-thirds of the conjugated bilirubin secreted (28). These data support the hypothesis that bilirubin can be secreted in bile as a bilirubin monoglucuronide. However before such conclusions are accepted, a more critical evaluation of the evidence presented should be made. The conjugates of bilirubin separated by Ostrow and Murphy were characterized as their azo-derivatives and identified by thin-layer chromatography. Unfortunately these procedures are not sophisticated enough to elucidate the chemical nature of these compounds. The compounds synthesized by Hofmann's group could not be hydrolyzed by β-glucuronidase, indicating their structures were not the same as the compounds found in the native bile. The estimation of bilirubin UDP glucuronyl transferase activity is conducted in an artificial system, and therefore the formation of a bilirubin monoglucuronide in this reaction need not reflect the actual reactions occurring *in vivo*. The evidence for the occurrence of a bilirubin monoglucuronide in bile during the infusion of bilirubin relies on the accuracy of the estimation of these compounds as their azo-derivatives. This determination depends on the diazo reaction in which the bilirubin molecule is split in two - each half molecule reacting with the reagent. Unfortunately, the stability of the unconjugated dipyrollic moiety is not known. In fact several investigators have noted that the diazo reaction does not estimate the total bile pigment content of bile accurately. For instance, the total value for direct reacting pigments (conjugates of bilirubin) is often 25% greater than the value obtained for total bile pigments (29). Recently it was claimed by Jansen, that 2 moles of bilirubin monoglucuronide undergo isomerization in aqueous media, producing one mole of bilirubin and one mole of bilirubin diglucuronide (30). However this again is a very artificial system and its biological significance cannot be evaluated. Therefore, the existence, in bile, of a bilirubin monoglucuronide awaits the perfection of more precise analytical methods.

In the 1960's numerous chromatographic studies suggested that conjugates other than bilirubin glucuronide were secreted in bile (16-18). Sulphate, phosphate and taurine conjugates of bilirubin were all claimed to exist. However, little biological significance was attached to these results, and it was generally agreed that bilirubin was secreted in bile as a glucuronide, even though all the evidence was indirect, and bilirubin glucuronide had not been isolated from bile in sufficient quantity or purity to elucidate its chemical structure.

In this decade, the "single conjugate" concept was supported by one group of investigators but challenged by two other groups (24,25,6-12). In 1970 small quantities of both bilirubin mono- and diglucuronide were isolated from human and rat bile by Ostrow and Murphy (25) in the United States. However, their criteria for the purity of these compounds were very weak, as stated before. At the same time, Kuenzle, in an attempt to define the alkali-stable bile pigments, first noted by Billing and Isselbacher in the late 1950's (4-31) isolated a series of biouronic acids as moieties conjugated to bilirubin (7-9). From human T-tube bile he separated three bile pigments utilizing reverse phase chromatography and a solvent system similar to that described by Billing, Cole and Lathe (4). The bands corresponding to pigment I and II were eluted from the column, and when coupled with aniline the azo-pigments formed were separated by reverse-phase chromatography (Fig.1).

Azopigments A_1, A_2, A_3, were shown by spectral analysis to be the azopigments of bilirubin. Azopigment B was separated into 7 components. However, only three azopigments (B_4, B_5, B_6) were obtained in sufficient amounts to be analyzed. Structural elucidation was accomplished after the conjugated portion was

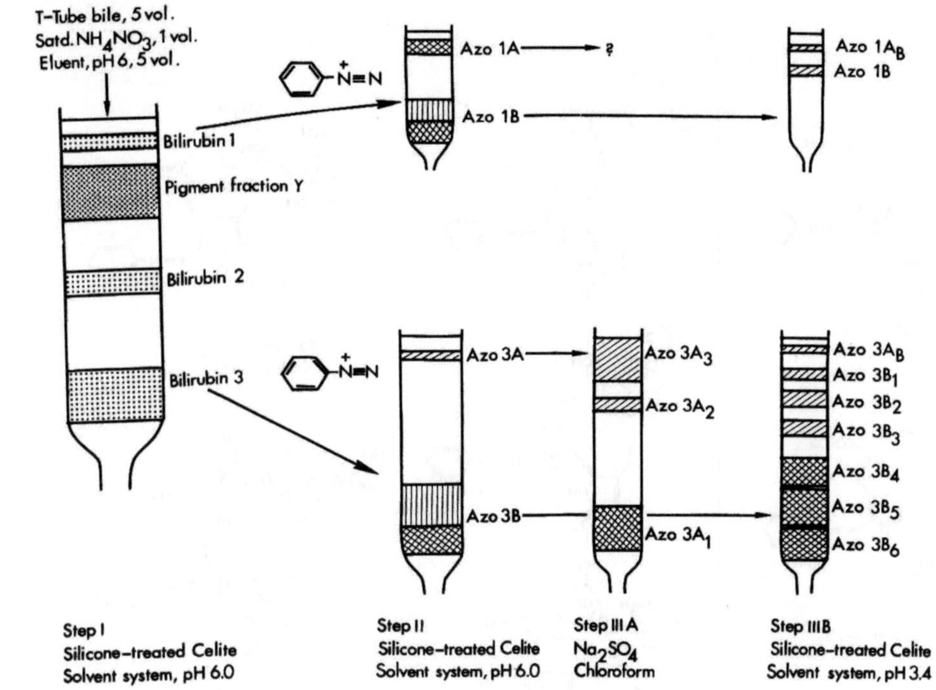

Fig. 1. Separation of bile pigments as outlined by Kuenzle (published with permission of Biochemical Journal).

hydrolyzed from the azopigment by treatment with either mild acid or alkali. The azopigments were then extracted into organic solvents, and the water soluble compounds identified following enzymic and chemical analysis, paper chromatography and finally combined gas liquid chromatography and mass spectrometry. The azopigment B_4 was found to be a mixture, and the moieties conjugated to the azopigment were identified as three aldobiouronic acids, each containing a hexose and a glucuronic acid (Fig.2). The conjugated portion of azopigment B_5 was found to be very complex, consisting of two uronic acids, glucuronic acid, and a hydroxymethylriburonic acid (Fig.2). A pseudobiouronic acid consisting of glucuronic acid and glucose was shown to be the conjugated moiety of azopigment B_6 (Fig.2).

On the other hand, Heirwegh and his colleagues found no evidence for a disaccharide conjugated to bilirubin (6,10-12). This group of investigators separated four major groups of ethyl anthranilate azo-derivatives of bile pigments from dog gall-

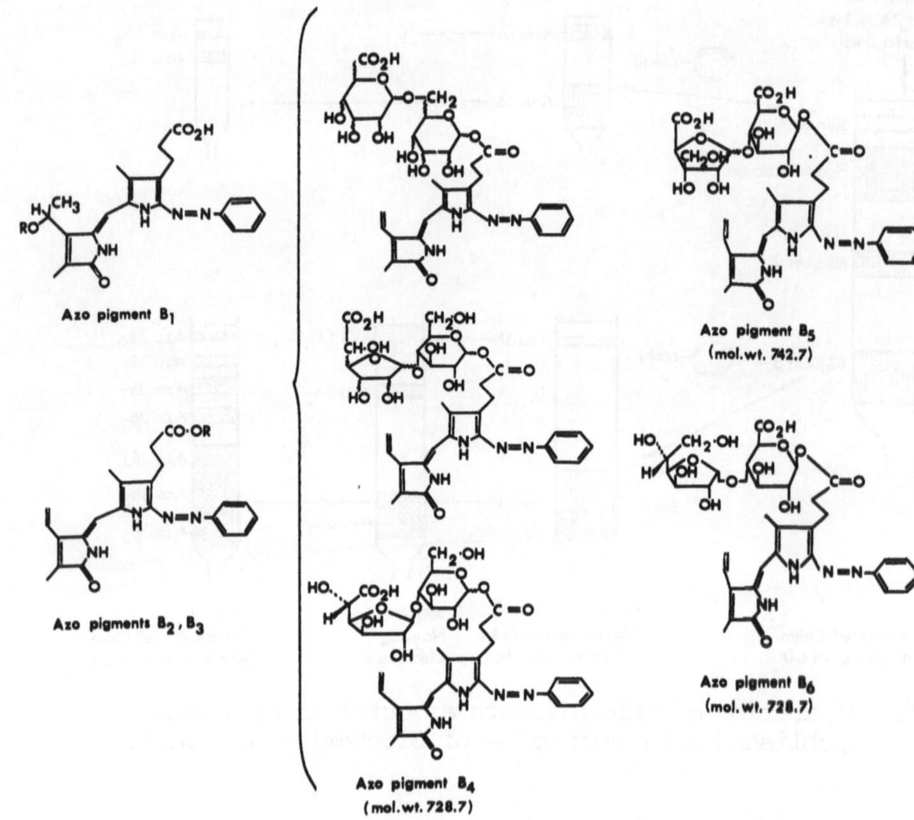

Fig. 2 Structure of biouronic acids as identified by Kuenzle (published with permission of Biochemical Journal).

bladder bile by thin layer chromatography. The azopigments were designated by Greek letters, progressing from alphas to deltas as the compounds became more polar. The non-polar azopigments (α) were separated into at least three components designated as azopigment α_o, α_2 and α_3. The fragmentation pattern of a methylated derivative of the azopigment α_o obtained by mass spectrometry indicated that this compound was derived from the azopigment of bilirubin (32). The azopigments α_2 and α_3 were hydrolyzed by exposure to ammonia vapours. The moieties conjugated to these pigments were then separated and characterized by thin layer chromatography and mass spectrometry and the compounds were identified as β-D monoxyloside and β-D monoglucoside respectively. The azopigments designated as β and γ were shown to contain hexuronic acid but could not be hydrolyzed by β-glucuronidase. The azopigment δ was considered to be a β-D monoglucuronide.

This conclusion was reached by estimating the uronic acid and azopigment content of this component (6-12).

The lack of agreement between these two groups of investigators deserves some comment. One can speculate that the very low yield of the compounds isolated from human bile by Kuenzle might be evidence that in his procedures he lost the simple glucuronide. One might also speculate that in Heirwegh's procedures, even though his azopigment recoveries were high, a portion of the biouronic acid was degraded. Unfortunately Heirwegh's group did not utilize combined gas chromatography and mass spectrometry and some of their identifications are not completely specific.

We also have been investigating the chemical nature of bilirubin as it is secreted in dog bile (33). In order to facilitate this study, these pigments were isolated as the ethyl anthranilate azo-derivatives of bilirubin. The separation of these azopigments by thin layer chromatography is illustrated in Fig. 3. Four major groups were separated in this neutral solvent

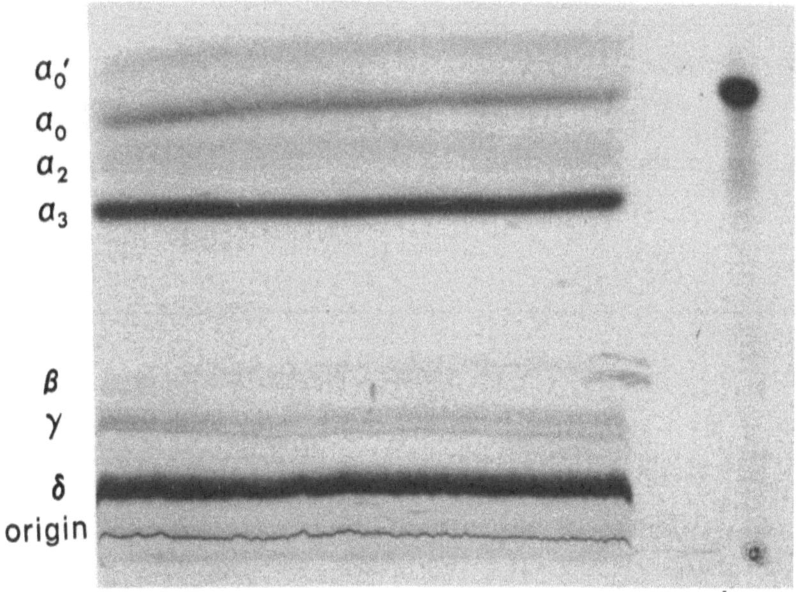

Fig. 3 Separation of the ethyl anthranilate azopigments of bile pigment conjugates isolated from dog gallbladder bile. The azopigments are denoted by Greek letters. Chromatograms were developed in the solvent system chloroform, methanol, water (65:25:3 by vol.).

Table I. Products formed after acid and alkali hydrolysis of azopigment α_3.

Treatment	Chemical Analysis	Distribution of azopigments (%)	
	Glucose	α_o*	α_3
0.15 N HCl 100°C - 1 h	+	85	15
0.10 N HCOOH 100°C - 1 h	+	66	35
0.10 N NH_4OH 100°C - 1 h	-	71	29
0.10 N NaOH 100°C - 1 h	-	100	-
Exposure to NH_3 vapours	+		

* α_o is the azopigment of bilirubin

TABLE II

Effect of enzymes on azopigments α_3

Treatment	No. of experiments	Distribution of Azopigments With enzyme			Without enzyme		
		α_o'	α_o	α_3	α_o'	α_o	α_3
β-Glucosidase	7	13 ± 3	49 ± 7	37 ± 5	11 ± 2	11 ± 1	79 ± 3
β-Glucuronidase	5	7 ± 2	43 ± 6	49 ± 6	11 ± 2	11 ± 1	79 ± 2

The amount of each azopigment detected is presented as a percentage of the total ± SEM. The only water-soluble product formed by the reaction of β-glucosidase and β-glucuronidase on azopigment α_3 was glucose.

system, and since the separation pattern and number of azopigments obtained were similar to those described by Heirwegh his nomenclature was adopted. Our first experiments were carried out on azopigment α_3, because of its apparent simplicity. This azopigment was hydrolyzed by several methods, all of which produced an organic and a water soluble fraction, (Fig.4). The portion of azopigment α_3 not hydrolyzed and the azopigment of bilirubin appear in the organic phase, while the conjugating moieties appear in the water phase. In the initial experiment the azopigment α_3 was found to be both acid and alkali labile (Table I). Glucose was detected by enzymic analysis in the water phase after acid hydrolysis (0.15M HCl and 0.1M formic acid) but was not detected after treatment with alkali (0.1 M NaOH or 0.1M NH_3). This latter observation was expected since monosaccharides are extremely unstable in alkaline media. However exposure of the azopigment α_3 to NH_3 vapours overnight cleaved the compound to its carboxylic acid amide and glucose. These data confirmed the original observations of Fevery (10) i.e. that glucose appeared as the only product after mild alkaline hydrolysis of azopigment α_3. The treatment of azopigment α_3 with β-glucuronidase (bovine liver) and β-glucosidase emulsion produced partial hydrolysis of the pigment under our experimental conditions (Table II). The n-butanol extractable pigments formed during the hydrolysis were shown by thin layer chromatography to be the azopigments of bilirubin. In the water soluble phase glucose was detected by enzymic analysis and thin layer chromatography. Unfortunately this does not prove that other carbohydrates were not present. For this reason the azopigment α_3 was subjected to methanolysis with sodium methoxide at room temperature for two hours and was completely hydrolyzed. The organic soluble products formed were shown by thin layer chromatography and mass spectrometry to be the methyl esters of the azopigments of bilirubin. The water soluble fraction (B) contained the unknown compound conjugated to azopigment α_3. To establish its identity a variety of analytical procedures were conducted as mentioned in Fig. 5. Glucose was detected by enzymic analysis in the water phase. When the amounts of the azopigment hydrolyzed

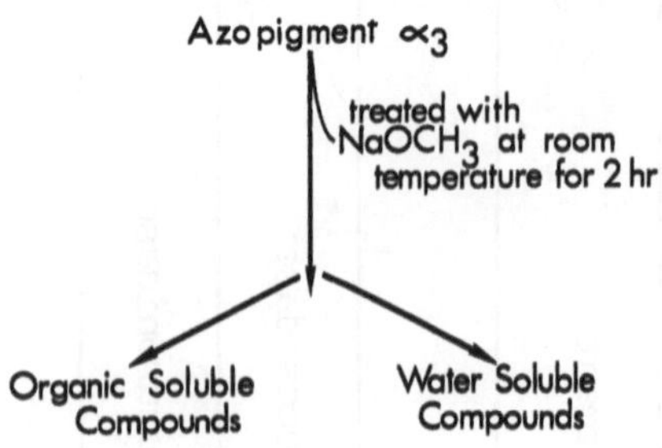

Fig. 4. Phases formed after hydrolysis of azopigment α_3.

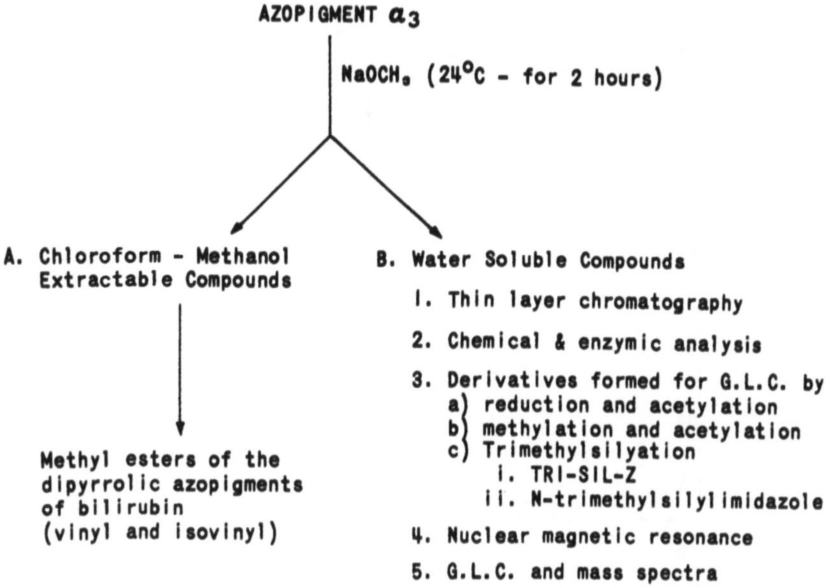

Fig.5. Treatment of azopigment α_3 with sodium methoxide.

and of glucose formed were quantitated, it was found that these compounds existed in a 1:1 molar ratio (Table III). It, therefore, appeared that at least glucose was one constituent of the unknown compound conjugated to bilirubin. Further proof of the chemical nature of the conjugated portion was sought by analyzing the samples of fraction B by gas liquid chromatography. For this analysis samples of fraction B were subjected to a variety of chemical reactions, which resulted in a series of different volatile derivatives. The chromatograms obtained are presented in Fig.6. In each instance, the number of peaks obtained and their observed retention times were identical to those obtained for an authentic sample of α and β-D-glucose. As further proof that fraction B contained only glucose, a dried portion was treated with N-trimethylsilyimidazole and analyzed by combined gas liquid chromatography and mass spectrometry. Two chromatographic peaks were observed. The fragmentation patterns obtained by mass spectrometry of the two chromatographic peaks were identical with those obtained for α and β-D-glucose (Fig.7) and are in agreement with the reported mass spectra of these compounds (34). Furthermore the nuclear magnetic resonance spectrum of fraction B was identical with that obtained for an authentic sample of α and β-D-glucose (Fig.8) and agrees with published data (35). There was no indication that other components were present in this fraction.

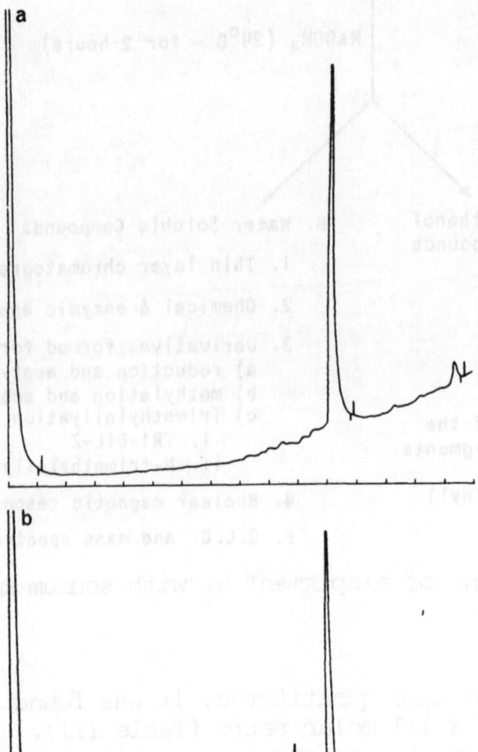
a
b
c
0 2 4 6 8 10 12 14 16 18 20 22 24 26 28 30 32
TIME - minutes

Although the treatment of the azopigment α_3 with sodium methoxide is considered a very mild procedure, there is no proof that this reaction had not destroyed a portion of the moiety conjugated to the azopigment of bilirubin. Therefore the following additional procedure was carried out. The azopigment α_3 was refluxed with super-dry methanol and acetyl chloride for 60 minutes. This reaction should split the ester linkage between the azopigment and the moiety conjugated to it, and simultaneously methylate the unknown conjugating group. Analysis of this sample by gas liquid chromatography indicated that the major component was identical with β-D-glucose treated in a similar manner. No other important products were detected.

These findings support the other evidence presented that the conjugated portion of the azopigment α_3 is β-D-glucopyranose, and confirm the original hypothesis of Fevery et al (10).

Azopigment α_2 was subjected to the same analytical procedures as those described for azopigment α_3. The data obtained from combined gas liquid chromatography and mass spectrometry indicate that β-D-xylose was the moiety conjugated to this azopigment.

Preliminary examination of the major azopigment δ isolated from human, rat, and dog bile indicates that it is composed of at least two major components. Analysis of the polar components formed after hydrolysis of these azopigments with either enzymes or sodium methoxide indicates that both a uronic acid and a hexose are present. Therefore, it would appear that delta may not be a simple azopigment conjugated to a monoglucuronide. Thus, further studies are required to establish the chemical nature of the major bilirubin conjugate that is found secreted in mammalian bile.

Fig. 6 Gas liquid chromatograms of products formed when an aliquot of Fraction B was treated in the following manner.

a) Reduction of aldehyde group with sodium borohydride followed by acetylation.

b) Methylation of acidic or enolic group with diazomethane and acetylation of secondary hydroxyl groups.

c) Formation of the trimethylsilytated derivative of Fraction B.

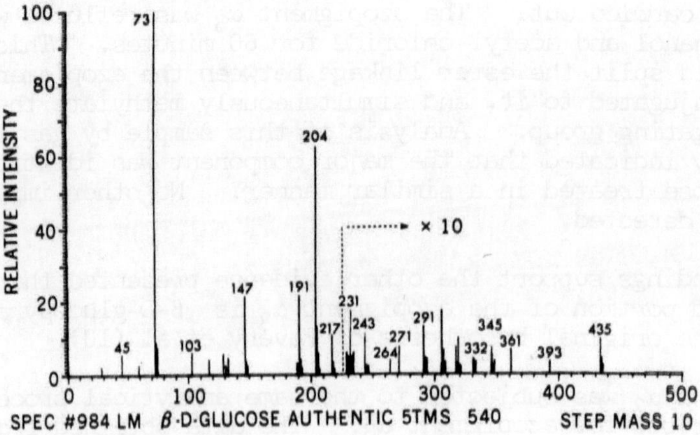

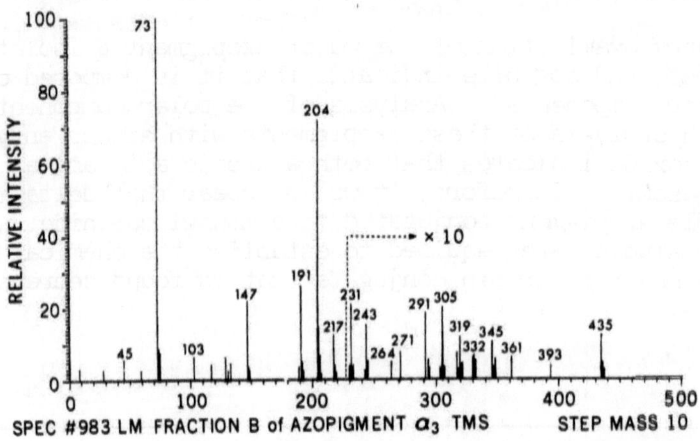

Fig.7. a) The 70 ev mass spectrum of N-trimethylsilyimidazole derivates of an equilibrium mixture of α and β-D-Glucose.

b) The 70 ev mass spectrum of an aliquot of Fraction B treated with N-Trimethylsilyimidazole.

Table III Products formed during hydrolysis of azopigment α_3 with β-glucosidase and sodium methoxide.

Expt. No.	Treatment	Azopigment	Glucose	Ratio (glucose/azopigment)
1	β-Glucosidase	2.38	2.97	1.2
2	β-Glucosidase	1.06	0.99	0.9
3	β-Glucosidase	0.45	0.53	1.2
4	Sodium methoxide	0.20	0.19	1.0
5	Sodium methoxide	0.41	0.45	1.1
6	Sodium methoxide	0.28	0.31	1.1

Details of analysis are outlined in the text. Results are expressed as µmol of azopigment α_3 converted into azopigment α_o after treatment with β-glucosidase, or into azopigment α_o' after treatment with ($NaOCH_3$) and as µmol of glucose cleaved from azopigment α_3.

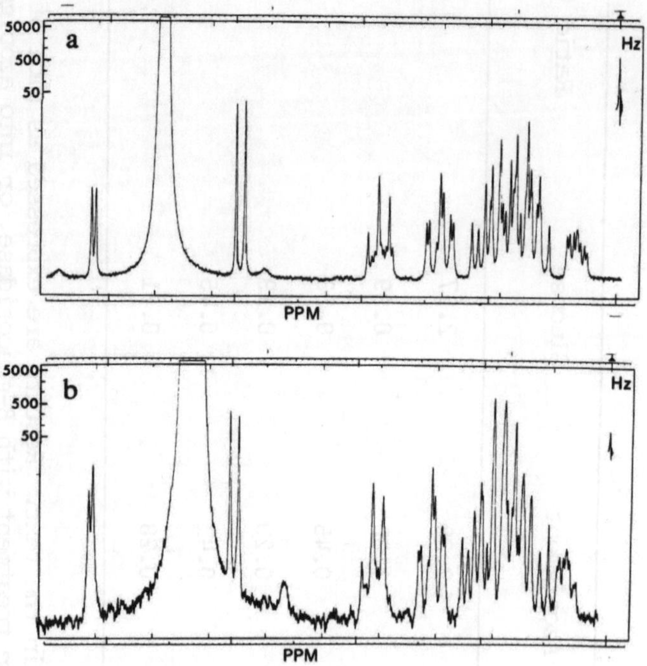

Fig. 8 a) The nuclear magnetic resonance spectrum of a mixture of α and β-D-glucose in pyridine at 210 MHZ.

b) The nuclear magnetic resonance spectrum of an aliquot of Fraction B.

SUMMARY

For many years it has been assumed that bilirubin is secreted in bile as bilirubin glucuronide, even though this compound has never been isolated from bile in a chemically pure form. Recently this basic assumption has been challenged and experiments have been under way in at least three laboratories to identify conclusively the bile pigments secreted in both human and dog bile. Because of bilirubin's instability, it has been necessary to carry out this identification somewhat indirectly using their azoderivatives. Kuenzle separated a series of biouronic acids from human fistula bile in low yields as the conjugates of the azopigment of bilirubin. Three aldohexuronic acids consisting of glucuronic acid, and a hydroxymethylriburonic acid, and a pseudobiouronic acid consisting of glucose and glucuronic acid were characterized utilizing sophisticated analytical techniques. On the other hand, Heirwegh's group, using dog gallbladder bile, isolated a series of simple monosaccharides conjugated to the azopigment of bilirubin - a β-D-monoxyloside, a β-D-monoglucoside, and a β-D-monoglucuronide. We also have characterized, by means of thin layer chromatography enzymic analysis, nuclear magnetic resonance and combined gas liquid chromatography and mass spectrometry, an azobilirubin β-D-monoxyloside and an azobilirubin β-D-monoglucoside which were derived from dog gallbladder bile. However, a simple azobilirubin β-D-monoglucuronide has not yet been isolated.

ACKNOWLEDGEMENT

The author is greatly indebted to the Department of Veterans' Affairs of Canada for its financial support of this project. I also would like to express my appreciation for the cooperation and assistance given by Drs. Carl A. Goresky, Tak-Hang Chan, and A.S. Perlin.

REFERENCES

1. WITH, TK: Formation and Fate of Bile Pigments in the Body, in Bile Pigments. Acad.Press., 1968, pp. 89-162.

2. SCHMID, R: Bilirubin metabolism I. Formation of bilirubin. In Liver and its Diseases. Edited by F. Schaffner, S. Sherlock, C.M. Leevy. Intercontinental Medical Book Corp., N.Y., 1974. pp. 85-96.

3. TALAFANT, E: Properties and composition of the bile pigment giving a direct diazo reaction. Nature 178: 312, 1956.

4. BILLING, BH, COLE, PG and LATHE, GH: The excretion of bilirubin as a diglucuronide giving the direct Van Den Bergh reaction. Biochem J 65: 774-784, 1957.

5. SCHMID, R: The identification of direct reacting bilirubin as a bilirubin glucuronide. J Biol Chem 229:881-888, 1957.

6. HEIRWEGH, KPM, VAN HEES, GP, LEROY, R et al: Heterogeneity of bile pigment conjugates as revealed by chromatography of their ethyl anthranilate azopigments. Biochem J 120: 877-890, 1970.

7. KUENZLE, C: Bilirubin conjugates of human bile. Isolation of phenylazo derivatives of bile bilirubin. Biochem J 119: 387-394, 1970.

8. KUENZLE, C: Bilirubin conjugates of human bile. Nuclear magnetic resonance infrared, and optical spectra of model compounds. Biochem J 119: 395-410, 1970.

9. KUENZLE, C: Bilirubin conjugates of human bile. The excretion of bilirubin as the acyl glycosides of aldobiouronic acid, pseudoaldobiouronic acid and hexuronosylhexuronic acid with branch-chain hexuronic acid as one of the components of the hexuronosylhexuronide. Biochem J 119: 411-435, 1970.

10. FEVERY, J, VAN HEES, GP, LE ROY P et al: Excretion in dog bile of glucose and xylose conjugates of bilirubin. Biochem J 125: 803-810, 1971.

11. COMPERNOLLE, F, JANSEN, FH and HEIRWEGH, KPM: Mass spectrometric study of the azopigments obtained from bile pigments with diazotized ethyl anthranilate. Biochem J 120: 891-894, 1970.

12. HEIRWEGH, KPM, COMPERNOLLE, F, DESMET, V et al: Recent advances in separation and analysis of diazo-positive bile pigments. Methods of Biochem Anal 21, 1973.

13. BRODERSEN, R, and THEILGAARD, J: Bilirubin colloid formation in neutral aqueous solution. Scand J Clin Lab Invest 24: 395-398, 1969.

14. OVERBEEK, J, TH, G, VINK, CLJ et al: The solubility of bilirubin. Recl Trav Chim Pays-Bas Belg 74: 81-84, 1955.

15. HUTCHINSON, DW, JOHNSON, B and KNELL, AJ: Tautomerism and hydrogen bonding in bilirubin. Biochem J 123: 483-484, 1971.

16. WITH, TK: Recent Studies on the Chemistry of Free and Conjugated Bilirubin, in Bile Pigments. Acad Press, pp. 361-386, 1968.

17. ISSELBACHER, KJ and McCARTHY, EA: Identification of a sulfate conjugate of bilirubin in bile. Biochim Biophys Acta 29: 658-659, 1958.

18. NOIR, BA, GROSZMAN, RJ and DE WALZ, AT: Studies on bilirubin sulfate. Biochim Biophys Acta 117: 297-304, 1966.

19. HUTCHINSON, DW, JOHNSON, B and KNELL, AJ: The reaction between bilirubin and aromatic diazo compounds. Biochem J 127: 907-908, 1972.

20. LATHE, GH: Degradation of haem by mammals and its excretion as conjugated bilirubin. Essays in Biochemistry 8: 107-148, 1972.

21. COLE, PG, LATHE, GH and BILLING, BH: Separation of bile pigments of serum, bile and urine. Biochem J 57: 514-518, 1954.

22. GREGORY, CH: Studies of conjugated bilirubin.III. Pigment 1 a complex of conjugated and free bilirubin. J Lab Clin Med 61: 917-925, 1963.

23. WEBER, APH, SCHALM, L and WITMANS, J: Bilirubin monoglucuronide (Pigment 1). A complex. Acad Med Scand 173: 19-24, 1963.

24. JACOBSEN, JA: A chromatographic separation of bilirubin glucuronides from human bile. Acta Chem Scand 23: 3023-3025, 1969.

25. OSTROW, JD and MURPHY, NH: Isolation and properties of conjugated bilirubin in bile. Biochem J 120: 311-327, 1970.

26. THOMPSON, RPH and HOFMANN, AF: Direct chemical synthesis of a bilirubin diglucosiduronic acid. Gastroenterology 60: 202 (abstract), 1971.

27. STREBEL, L and ODELL, GB: UDP glucuronyl transferase in rat liver; genetic variation and maturation. Ped Res 3: 351 (abstract), 1969.

28. BILLING, BH: The formation and excretion of bile pigments. In The Liver. Edited by E.A. Gall, F.K. Mostofi. The Williams and Wilkins Co., 1973. pp. 1-20.

29. FEVERY, J: Recent Developments in Bilirubin Conjugation. Thesis, University of Leuven, Belgium, 1972, p.10.

30. JANSEN, PLM: The isomerisation of bilirubin monoglucuronide. Clinica Chimica Acta 49: 233-240, 1973.

31. ISSELBACHER, KJ and McCARTHY, E: Studies on bilirubin sulfate and other nonglucuronide conjugates of bilirubin. J Clin Invest 38: 645-651, 1959.

32. JANSEN, FH and STOLL, MS: Separation and structural analysis of vinyl and isovinyl-azobilirubin derivatives. Biochem J 125: 585-597, 1971.

33. GORDON, ER, DADOUN, M, GORESKY, CA et al: The isolation of an azobilirubin β-D-monoglucoride from dog gall bladder bile. Biochem J 143: 97-105, 1974.

34. DE JONHG, DC, RADFORD, T, HRIBAR, JD et al: Analysis of trimethylsylil derivatives of carbohydrates by gas chromatography and mass spectrometry. J Amer Chem Soc 91: 1728-1740, 1969.

35. KOCH, HJ and PERLIN, A: Synthesis and carbon 13 NMR spectrum of D-glucose *3-d*. Carbohydrate Res 15: 403-410, 1970.

DISCUSSION OF PAPERS ON BILIRUBIN CHEMISTRY

CHAIRMAN: R. SCHMID

LUCEY: Is there any evidence that photo-isomerization occurs in vivo?

McDONAGH: No. We have tried to find this in Gunn rats, both with and without ligated bile ducts and we have never found any detectable amounts of isomers in the serum following prolonged intensive light treatment. However, this doesn't mean that that type of reaction doesn't occur in vivo. If you irradiate bilirubin in vitro with albumin in solution, you don't get isomerization, but you do get some free radical reaction. So in vivo you could get the initial steps of the reaction, the free radical formation, but these radicals might not recombine to give you the isomers of bilirubin. So the fact that you don't see isomers in vivo doesn't mean necessarily that the free radical reaction doesn't occur. In practice you can't detect the reaction in vivo, and in vitro the reaction is rather slow and requires intense light, and so I don't think that it does occur in vivo to any significant extent.

LAMOLA: It seems to me that the kind of photocleavage mechanism you are invoking to produce the photo-isomerization in vitro means that the reaction ought to be induced by simple thermal mechanisms. Is there any evidence that thermal isomerizations give the same kind of products?

McDONAGH: The reaction in the dark in the presence of oxygen is a thermal reaction. This and the photochemical reaction may proceed in the same way.

LAMOLA: What is the form of bilirubin? Is it a di-keto tautomer, or a di-enol?

McDONAGH: The bulk of the evidence on this point comes from spectroscopic studies. This indicates that bilirubin is a di-keto tautomer.

SASS-KORTSAK: Is it possible that in vivo the photo-cleavage reactions only apply to that very small fraction of bilirubin which is in aqueous solution, not attached to albumin? This could easily account for a slow reaction in vivo. More bilirubin would dissociate, and the reaction would continue.

McDONAGH: The nature of the photo-chemical reactions in vivo is not at all clear. The evidence, such as it is, seems to suggest that most of the degradation occurs in the skin and not in the plasma. However, an alternate mechanism may be occuring. The auto-oxidation of bilirubin which occurs in water at physiological pH, may also occur in vivo, even in the dark, in children with marked unconjugated hyperbilirubinemia or with the Crigler-Najjar syndrome. In these infants the bilirubin level does not continue to rise indefinitely. Bilirubin is broken down by alternate pathways and it also seems likely that there is autooxidation of bilirubin not bound to albumin.

THALER: You have shown that isomerization occurs in aqueous solutions and that albumin inhibits these reactions. Since much of the bilirubin which is accessible to break-down by light in vivo is probably bound to lipid in skin, have you looked at photo-isomerization in chloroform or other non-polar solvents?

McDONAGH: Bilirubin does not photo-isomerize in chloroform to any significant extent. On prolonged irradiation small amounts of isomers are formed, but not in significant amounts.

LESTER: I would like to ask Dr.Gordon whether the only form of bilirubin excreted is the glucuronide, and whether the other conjugates are the result of transesterification reactions? At a recent conference in Israel, Dr. Odell stated that when he administered the methyl ester of bilirubin intravenously to rats, only one form of conjugate appeared to be excreted, the glucuronide.

GORDON: This question will only be answered when the exact chemical forms of the conjugates of bilirubin are known and adequate assay techniques developed.

LESTER: Are other conjugates generated from the azopigments isolated from bile, when they are recycled through your isolation system?

GORDON: We have taken mixtures of the azopigments and rechromatographed them. We recover the original azopigments.

SCHMID: I would like to ask Dr. McDonagh whether he thinks that the exchange isomerization, the 3α,9α,12α interchange, can also occur with conjugates. If this is the case, then all sorts of exchange mechanisms may be present, and will account for the multiplicity of the conjugates identified.

McDONAGH: The reaction does occur in vitro with conjugates and this has recently been shown by Jansen, who took bilirubin monoglucuronide and incubated it for a short period of time in aqueous solution. This produced free bilirubin and bilirubin diglucuronide. These results show that the halves of the molecule can exchange, even when conjugated (Jansen, P.M., Clin Chim Acta 49: 233-240, 1973). Now whether this can occur in the micellar medium of bile is a different question.

I would like to make one other comment about the conjugates. One major problem is that methods for isolation and direct fractionation of the bilirubin conjugates have seldom been used, because of the instability of the compounds. Instead indirect methods, such as the preparation of azo-derivatives, have been used and artefacts may have been produced.

JANSEN: We have incubated monoglucuronide and bilirubin in aqueous media and have found that, in this mixture, there is apparent production of the diglucuronide (Jansen, P.L.M., Clin Chim Acta 49: 233-240, 1973). In this reaction two moles of bilirubin monoglucuronide are converted to one mole of bilirubin and one mole of bilirubin diglucuronide. Mainly the IIIα and IXα isomers of bilirubin were formed. The bilirubin formed was assessed by reaction with ethyl anthranilate, in the presence and absence of organic solvents, and chromatography of the resulting azo pigments. The bilirubin diglucuronide was not isolated, as a separate compound.

GORDON: The methodology which you have used depends on complete conversion of both bilirubin and its conjugates to azo derivatives. Without this, the calculations will not be valid.

SCHMID: There is another aspect of this problem. In those

children in whom there appears to be a defect in glucuronide formation (the Crigler-Najjar syndrome) other conjugating mechanisms are present in a minor form and do not take over quantitatively for the missing glucuronide system. This is very peculiar. Perhaps Dr. Arias would like to comment.

ARIAS: The other sugar conjugates are essentially absent from bile, in the Crigler-Najjar syndrome. The question then becomes what is the relationship between the bilirubin incubation studies which have been done with crude microsomes, and with UDP, and glucose or xylose as substrates, and the absence of these conjugates. It raises the question of whether the bilirubin glucuronyl transferase may not be capable under some circumstances of reacting with different substrates, for example glucose or xylose. I wonder what your response to that would be.

GORDON: It has been shown that the UDP transferase systems interact with a multiplicity of substrates, and that there is probably a multiplicity of corresponding enzyme forms (Vessey, Goldenber and Zakin, Biochim Biophys Acta 309: 75-82, 1973). Pure bilirubin glucuronyl transferase has not yet been characterized, so its reactivities are not known.

JAVITT: I wonder if Dr. Schmid would be kind enough to summarize for us his data on the homozygote Gunn rat, which has an absolute defect in bilirubin glucuronide formation. If one looks at other data it appears that the Gunn rat can form other glucuronides.

SCHMID: Dr. Javitt has alluded to the possibility, mentioned several times in the literature, that the specific Gunn rat defect is not an absence of enzyme. Subsequent information indicates that the enzyme may be present and there may be something which prevents the substrate from getting to the active site of the enzyme. I think that you have said correctly that the defect in glucuronide formation is present for some substrates but not for others in the Gunn rat. In Dutton's group the rate of conjugation of p-nitrophenol with glucuronic acid was found to be about 5% of normal, in the Gunn rat. This could be restored to normal by the addition of diethylnitrosamine, a detergent, to the Gunn rat microsomes. It appears that the enzyme is present, but that a steric mechanism prevents the substrate from reacting with the enzyme (Dutton, GJ, Glucuronic acid, Academic Press, New York, 1966, p. 233). If this is the case, it is easier to understand why these other conjugates are not formed as well in the Crigler-Najjar children and the Gunn rats. This is just a hypothesis but I think it is one possible explanation for the question which Dr. Arias raised.

BILIRUBIN METABOLISM: AN OVERVIEW

Rudi Schmid

University of California, San Francisco

San Francisco, California 94122

1. Chemical and physiological properties of bilirubin

Bilirubin is an open-chain tetrapyrrole with an approximate molecular weight of 585. The four pyrrole rings are linked by three carbon bridges of which two are unsaturated (outside) and one is saturated (central). The nature and order of the eight side chains located on the β-carbons of the pyrrole rings are the same as in protoporphyrin IX. This finding led Fischer and his associates(1) to the conclusion that naturally-occurring bilirubin is derived from ferroprotoporphyrin IX (protoheme) by cleavage of the porphyrin ring at its α-methene carbon bridge; hence the resulting bilirubin is designated as IXα(1). Biliverdin IXα, a green-blue tetrapyrrole formed as an intermediate in the conversion of ferroprotoporphyrin IX to bilirubin IXα, possesses two hydrogen atoms less than bilirubin. It is probable that all bilirubin formed under biologic conditions has the IXα configuration(1), as cleavage of protoheme at carbon bridges other than the α-carbon bridge has not been demonstrated in vivo. The only known exception to this rule is the integumental pigment of a butterfly species (Pieris brassicae) which has been identified as biliverdin IXγ(2). It should be noted, however, that the naturally occurring bilirubin IXα can undergo isomeric scrambling about the central saturated carbon bridge, in that the molecule can split in the middle, permitting two left or two right dipyrrylmethenes to reassemble with themselves(3). This leads to formation of the isomeric forms bilirubin IIIα and XIIIα, both of which are present as minor constituents in commercially produced bilirubin extracted from bile(3). It has not been established, however, whether bilirubin isomers are formed in vivo or are produced only during the process of extraction and purification.

Bilirubin is moderately soluble in many organic solvents, but is only sparingly soluble in aqueous solution at physiological pH. In the plasma, a major fraction of the bilirubin is present in its unionized form which limits its water solubility but renders it soluble in lipid media. Because of these solubility properties the unionized pigment fraction may diffuse freely across lipoid surfaces and cell membranes. For example, unconjugated bilirubin has been shown to be absorbed from the intestine(4) and gallbladder(5), to cross the placenta(6) and to penetrate the blood-brain barrier(7). This physiological behavior of the pigment is drastically altered by the hepatic conversion of the lipid-soluble bilirubin to larger, charged, and hence, water-soluble conjugates. Many lipoid membranes such as the placenta, the blood-brain barrier, and the epithelial lining of the gallbladder and gut are virtually impermeable to organic anions of the size and charge of conjugated bilirubin(8). This fact is of critical importance for the excretion of the pigment in the alimentary canal, because if bilirubin were excreted in its unconjugated lipid-soluble form, back diffusion across the mucosal surface of the biliary tree and the intestinal tract would severely compromise the efficiency of the elimination process. Thus, conjugation confers on the pigment properties that limit its reabsorption and consequently its enterohepatic circulation.

2. Formation of bilirubin

The concept that bile pigment is derived from blood pigment is probably very old, but the first experimental support was provided by Virchow(9), who isolated bilirubin crystals from old blood extravasations. Later, Whipple and Hooper(10), Aschoff(11), and Mann et al.(12) showed beyond all doubt that bilirubin is formed by the breakdown of hemoglobin in the spleen, liver, and a number of other tissues. The nature of this conversion in the intact organism was recently clarified by the identification of a microsomal enzyme system, which converts heme to equimolar amounts of bilirubin and carbon monoxide(13); the latter originates from the α-methene bridge carbon where the porphyrin ring undergoes fissure. This enzyme system, heme oxygenase, consists of at least two components. The first is a microsomal enzyme that requires NADPH and molecular oxygen(13). It resembles the drug-metabolizing enzyme systems of the smooth endoplasmic reticulum of the liver, in that it appears to utilize cytochrome P450 as the terminal oxidase(14). The products of this enzymatic reaction are Fe, CO, and biliverdin: the last is converted to bilirubin by soluble NADPH-dependent biliverdin reductase(15). In this system, the microsomal heme oxygenase usually is rate-limiting, while biliverdin reductase seems to be present in excess.

Microsomal heme oxygenase is an inducible enzyme permitting substrate-mediated regulatory control in spleen, kidney, macrophages, and other tissues(16). For example, after splenectomy the specific activity of the enzyme in the sinusoidal cells of the liver is increased reflecting the role of the liver as an alternate site of red cell breakdown(17). Similarly, in hemoglobinuria, heme oxygenase activity appears in the proximal tubules of the kidney where filtered hemoglobin is reabsorbed and degraded(18). In tissue macrophages, heme oxygenase activity normally is barely detectable, but after these cells have been exposed to extravasated blood, enzyme activity sharply rises in these phagocytic cells(19). The heme oxygenase-catalyzed reaction accounts for the characteristic progressive color change of subcutaneous hematomas from dark purple (heme) to blue-green (biliverdin) and eventually to yellow (bilirubin).

The prosthetic heme group of hemoglobin is the major source of bilirubin in man and accounts for approximately 80 per cent of the 250 to 350 mg of pigment formed in 24 hours. Senescent red blood cells are sequestered in the reticuloendothelial cells of the spleen, bone marrow, and liver, and their hemoglobin-heme is converted in situ to bilirubin. In hemolytic states and in conditions associated with ineffective erythropoiesis, the rate of bilirubin production may be increased several times over that occurring under normal conditions. When hemoglobin is dissolved in the plasma (e.g. in intravascular hemolysis) the epithelial cells of the renal tubules(18) and the hepatic parenchymal cells (17) may assume an important role in the conversion of hemoglobin-heme to bilirubin.

In addition to hemoglobin, bilirubin is formed from catabolism of other hemoproteins, including myoglobin, cytochromes, catalase, and peroxidases. For example, all mammalian cells contain cytochromes essential for oxidative metabolism, which when degraded yield bile pigments. The relative contribution of these hemoproteins to the overall bilirubin production in the body depends primarily on their cellular concentration and rate of turnover. Under physiologic conditions, approximately 20 per cent of all bile pigment formed in man appears to be derived from hemoproteins other than hemoglobin(20).

The liver has a key role in this process, because it represents a relatively large mass of tissue containing an abundance of heme-containing enzymes. The most important among these are the microsomal cytochromes P450 and b_5, which catalyze the biotransformation of many hormones, drugs, and toxins(21). These heme enzymes are present in hepatocytes in high concentration, and their level may be further increased by administration of the very compounds in whose catabolism they are involved(21). Since the biologic half-life of these hepatic cytochromes is only one to two days, their rate of metabolic turnover is much more rapid than that of the hemoglobin of circulating red blood cells(22). Thus, after administration of a radioactive metabolic precursor of heme (e.g., glycine-2-^{14}C or ^{14}C-δ-aminolevulinic acid), isotopically labeled bilirubin produced from heme turnover in the liver appears within one to two days ("early-labeled" bilirubin) (23), whereas formation of labeled bile pigment from hemoglobin of red cells is delayed for approximately 100 to 140 days, which is the time required for the erythrocytes initially labeled with the precursor to reach the end of their physiological life span (24). Since the "early-labeled" bilirubin fraction contains a minor component that is labeled within one to two hours after isotope administration, it is likely that, in addition to various hemoproteins, the liver contains a small pool of free heme that turns over very rapidly(25). Bilirubin that is formed in hepatocytes from intrinsic heme compounds may appear in the plasma, but it is probable that, at least in part, it is excreted directly in the bile(26).

3. Metabolic fate of bilirubin

Because of its poor solubility in water, almost all of the bilirubin in the plasma is bound to albumin, leaving only a minute fraction unbound(27). Since only unbound bilirubin, but not albumin-bound pigment, can diffuse across cell membranes, albumin tends to retain the pigment within the plasma compartment and thereby limits the accumulation of potentially dangerous concentrations of bilirubin in the tissues. Moreover, plasma albumin has a strong affinity for the pigment so that the equilibrium between extravascular and intravascular binding forces is overwhelmingly in favor of the plasma. Consequently, even at elevated bilirubin levels, little pigment may gain access to the cells. It is noteworthy, however, that organic anions in the plasma, for example fatty acids and a variety of drugs(28), may compete with bilirubin for shared binding sites on the albumin molecule; this may result in an increase of the fraction of unbound pigment that is available for diffusion into the cells. Thus, at a given pigment load, treatment with salicylate lowers the total plasma pigment level at the expense of enhanced entry of bilirubin into tissues(29), including the brain(7). In neonatal icterus, displacement of bound bilirubin from albumin by competing organic anions may explain the occurrence of brain damage in association with relatively low plasma bilirubin concentrations(27). Conversely, intravenous administration of albumin may increase the binding capacity of the plasma so that bilirubin is pulled out of the tissues into the circulation, resulting in a temporary rise of the plasma pigment level associated with a reduction of bilirubin concentration of tissues (29). A similar exchange of bilirubin occurs across the placental barrier which functionally represents a lipoid membrane separating two vascular systems with different binding capacities. Since the fetal albumin concentration generally is lower than that of the mother, a diffusion gradient is established which facilitates transfer of bilirubin from the fetal to the maternal blood. Since the latter is continuously cleared of pigment by the maternal liver, this permits the fetal organism to rid itself of endogenously produced bilirubin at a time when its own hepatic conjugating and excretory mechanisms are functioning poorly(6).

The plasma membrane of the hepatocytes resembles other lipoid membranes in that it excludes the large water-soluble pigment-albumin complex, but is readily permeable for unbound lipid-soluble bilirubin. Because the pigment and other organic anions are taken up very rapidly by the liver, it has been suggested that the hepatic plasma membrane may contain specific carrier mechanisms that facilitate bi-directional flux in and out of the liver cell. Most of the bilirubin that has gained access to the liver is bound to cytoplasmic proteins which are believed to function as intracellular acceptors of the pigment. Two such soluble protein fractions of low molecular weight, designated as Y and Z, have tentatively been identified and characterized(30). In addition to bilirubin, they bind other organic anions which are excreted in the bile and may compete with bilirubin for available binding sites in the liver. Thus, in its most simplified static form, the system may be described as an extracellular (plasma) and an intracellular (liver) compartment, separated by a membrane that is permeable to unbound, but not to albumin-bound, bilirubin. In this system, the ultimate equilibration of the pigment between the hepatocellular compartment and the sinusoidal plasma depends primarily on the relative binding forces on either side of the membrane. To this extent, bilirubin uptake in the liver may differ little from that in other organs, except that the liver has a higher intracellular binding capacity for the pigment than most tissues.

What confers on the liver its unique capacity to remove bilirubin from the plasma is its ability to convert intracellular pigment to water-soluble conjugates(8). Their ionic nature and increased molecular weight largely prevent their diffusion across the plasma membrane. Moreover, they readily are excreted into the bile, presumably because their structural configuration provides a better "fit" for the secretory apparatus than does unconjugated bilirubin. By these mechanisms, the hepatocytes continuously reduce their concentration of unconjugated bilirubin, thereby creating a concentration gradient across the plasma membrane resulting in flow of additional pigment from the sinosoids into the cells. It is apparent, therefore, that hepatic uptake of bilirubin is determined by several factors, including the level and binding of unconjugated pigment in the plasma, its binding to intracellular acceptors and the rate of its conjugation in the hepatocyte. In addition, it is possible that the intrahepatic concentration or the rate of biliary excretion of conjugated bilirubin indirectly may influence the uptake of unconjugated pigment by the liver.

The conjugation of bilirubin is catalyzed by enzymes that are located in the smooth endoplasmic reticulum of the liver cell (8). The most important of these is glucuronyl transferase, which transfers glucuronic acid from the nucleotide uridine diphosphate glucuronic acid (UDPGA) to the two propionic acid groups of the pigment, forming an ester glucuronide. A major fraction of the bilirubin excreted in human bile is a diglucuronide, but a monoglucuronide has also been identified(31). Smaller amounts of pigment appear to be conjugated with other sugar moieties(32,33), but the functional importance of these recently discovered conjugating mechanisms is not clear.

Conjugation is virtually essential for the biliary excretion of the pigment since, except during the perinatal period, only minute amounts of unconjugated bilirubin appear in human bile. Details of the secretory mechanism of the hepatocyte for conjugated bilirubin are poorly understood except that the mechanism may involve the Golgi apparatus and is probably shared by a diverse group of endogenous and exogenous organic compounds that are secreted into the bile. Secretion of the pigment proceeds against a large concentration gradient, competitive inhibition by other cholephils has been demonstrated, and the mechanism is saturable(34). This permits the tentative conclusion that secretion of conjugated bilirubin is carrier-mediated and probably is an energy-consuming process. It is noteworthy that bile salts seem to be excreted by a mechanism distinct from that for conjugated bilirubin and other organic anions(35).

Because of its solubility properties and molecular size, conjugated bilirubin that has been excreted with the bile into the intestinal tract is not appreciably reabsorbed(4). The pigment conjugates probably remain intact during their transit through the small bowel, and consequently there is no significant enterohepatic circulation of bilirubin, except perhaps in the neonatal period(36). Bilirubin glucuronide in part is hydrolyzed in the terminal ileum and large bowel by bacterial β-glucuronidase, while at the same time bilirubin may be reduced to a complex series of colorless tetrapyrrolic compounds, collectively termed urobilinogen(37). It is not known whether reduction of bilirubin to urobilinogen precedes or follows hydrolysis of the conjugates and whether, in part, urobilinogen in the colon is still conjugated. A small fraction of the urobilinogen formed is reabsorbed from the large bowel(38), and is transported in the portal blood to the liver, where it is extracted and re-excreted in the bile. Under physiologic conditions, only trace amounts of urobilinogen are excreted in the urine, but in the presence of excessive bilirubin formation (hemolysis), liver disease, or partial obstruction of the bile ducts, urinary urobilinogen may be increased(37). Renal handling of urobilinogen appears to involve glomerular filtration, tubular reabsorption, and tubular secretion(39), so that urinary urobilinogen excretion is affected not only by the amount of urobilinogen produced, the fraction of this amount absorbed, and hepatic function, but also by renal function, urine volume, and urine pH.

4. Pathophysiology of hyperbilirubinemia

Hyperbilirubinemia may be due to increased plasma levels of unconjugated bilirubin, the presence in the plasma of conjugated pigment, or a combination of the two. Overproduction of pigment, impaired hepatic uptake, or failure of the conjugating mechanism may lead to "retention" of unconjugated bilirubin. "Regurgitation" into the plasma of conjugated bilirubin may result from functional cholestasis, disruption of the hepatic architecture, or extrahepatic biliary obstruction.

In patients with hemolysis or with disorders of red cell formation associated with ineffective erythropoiesis(40), the liver is presented with an increased pigment load that has to be transferred to the bile. This appears to be accomplished by raising the bilirubin concentration in the plasma to levels at which pigment flow into the liver is sufficiently increased to balance the elevated rate of bilirubin production. The unconjugated hyperbilirubinemia of hemolysis, therefore, may be regarded as a compensatory mechanism that functions to establish a new steady state of transhepatic pigment transport.

An analogous situation may exist if, at normal rates of bilirubin production, the concentration or the binding forces of intrahepatic acceptor proteins are reduced. Such a hepatic defect has been postulated to explain the mild unconjugated hyperbilirubinemia commonly referred to as Gilbert's syndrome. Although this seems a reasonable hypothesis, convincing experimental evidence in support of this concept is not available, and other pathogenetic mechanisms, including reduced glucuronide formation(42), have been proposed. The only instance in which unconjugated hyperbilirubinemia definitely can be ascribed to interference with hepatic pigment uptake is in patients treated with male-fern extract for tapeworm infestation. This drug contains flavaspidic acid, which competes with bilirubin for intrahepatic binding sites, thereby causing a moderate elevation of plasma unconjugated bilirubin that is readily reversible on drug withdrawal(43).

Defective conjugation as the sole cause of unconjugated hyperbilirubinemia is rare and usually hereditary. In the Crigler-Najjar syndrome, formation of bilirubin glucuronide is completely lacking, leading to severe unconjugated hyperbilirubinemia and virtual absence of bilirubin excretion in the bile(44). The jaundice is lifelong and is commonly associated with bilirubin encephalopathy, which frequently results in death at an early age. In another group of patients, the conjugating ability of the liver seems to be reduced but not completely absent. This is associated with a more moderate degree of unconjugated hyperbilirubinemia and the bile contains conjugated pigments. In these patients, the jaundice responds favourably to treatment with phenobarbital, whereas phenobarbital is ineffective in the syndrome with complete absence of glucuronide formation(45). The biochemical nature of these genetic defects is unknown; the primary lesion may consist of the absence of the enzyme glucuronyl transferase or of structural or conformational modifications of the enzyme protein or its supporting phospholipid membrane, all of which may lead to reduced or absent enzymatic activity with bilirubin as the substrate.

A selective increase in the plasma of conjugated bilirubin, usually with little, if any, increase of unconjugated pigment, is characteristic of the Dubin-Johnson syndrome(46) and of intrahepatic cholestasis, which most frequently results from exposure to a wide variety of drugs or hormones and occasionally occurs in viral hepatitis. The mechanism by which bilirubin that has been conjugated in the liver gains access to the plasma is poorly understood. It has been proposed that conjugated pigment that cannot be excreted in the bile is transferred to the sinusoidal plasma by means of reversed pinocytosis. Alternatively, it has been postulated that the endothelial lining of the bile ductules may be injured, thus permitting leakage of the secreted conjugated bilirubin into the blood. Structural derangements consistent with either of these postulates have been reported, suggesting that intrahepatic cholestasis may be the result of several independent defects.

In most instances of jaundice due to parenchymal liver disease, the plasma exhibits elevated concentrations of both conjugated and unconjugated bilirubin, but the relative proportion of the two pigment types is highly variable and of little diagnostic significance. Elevation of unconjugated bilirubin may be due to shortened erythrocyte life span sometimes occurring in association with liver disease(47), or may be related to reduction of effective hepatic blood flow or of the liver's capacity to take up or to conjugate the pigment. The mechanisms which lead to raised plasma levels of conjugated bilirubin in the absence of overt mechanical obstruction also are unclear. It is possible that the defect involves primarily the secretory apparatus of the hepatic cell in a manner that results in "regurgitation" of conjugated pigment into the circulation. As an alternative, it has been postulated that the injury directly affects the endothelial lining of the bile ductules, or that flow in the fine radicles of the biliary tree may be blocked, thereby producing an obstructive type of jaundice(8).

SUMMARY

Bilirubin is a yellow lipid-soluble pyrrole pigment which is the major catabolite of the heme group of hemoglobin and other hemoproteins. The conversion of the ferroprotoporphyrin IX ring (heme) to equimolar amounts of the linear tetrapyrrole bilirubin IXα and of carbon monoxide is catalyzed by heme oxygenase, which is a microsomal mixed function oxidase requiring NADPH and molecular oxygen; biliverdin is formed as an intermediate. Bilirubin released into the circulation from its sites of formation is bound in the plasma to albumin, which restricts its diffusion into tissues. In the hepatic sinusoids, the pigment detached from its albumin carrier diffuses across the microvillous membrane into the liver cell where it is bound to soluble acceptor proteins. Enzymes located within hepatic smooth endoplasmic reticulum convert the lipid-soluble bilirubin to a series of water-soluble conjugates, among which glucuronides are the most important. These pigment conjugates are then excreted by an energy-requiring secretory mechanism into the bile.

At physiological rates of bilirubin production (about 300 mg per 24 hours), the liver effectively eliminates the pigment from the plasma, and serum bilirubin levels usually do not exceed

1.0 mg per 100 ml. Unconjugated hyperbilirubinemia is the result of increased pigment production (hemolysis), impaired uptake (Gilbert's syndrome?) or defective conjugation (Crigler-Najjar syndrome). In newborn infants transient hyperbilirubinemia frequently is caused by a combination of accelerated erythrocyte breakdown and incomplete development of the hepatic transfer and conjugating apparatus. Inherited or acquired defects in the hepatic secretory mechanism or in the bile ducts lead to conjugated hyperbilirubinemia. Diffuse hepatic injury usually results in retention in the plasma of both conjugated and unconjugated pigment.

REFERENCES

1. FISCHER H, ORTH H: Die Chemie des Pyrrols. Leipzig, Akademische Verlagsgesellschaft m.b.H, 1937.

2. RÜDIGER W, KLOSE W, WUILLAUME M, et al: On the biosynthesis of biliverdin IX-γ in Pieris Brassicae. Experientia 25: 487-488, 1969.

3. McDONAGH AF, ASSISI F: The ready isomerization of bilirubin IX-α in aqueous solution. Biochem J 129: 797-800, 1972.

4. LESTER R, SCHMID R: Intestinal absorption of bile pigments. II. Bilirubin absorption in man. N Engl J Med 269: 178-182, 1963.

5. OSTROW JD: Absorption of bile pigments by the gallbladder. J Clin Invest 46: 2035-2052, 1967.

6. SCHENKER S, DAWBER NH, SCHMID R: Bilirubin metabolism in the fetus. J Clin Invest 43: 32-39, 1964.

7. DIAMOND I, SCHMID R: Experimental bilirubin encephalopathy: the mode of entry of bilirubin-^{14}C into the central nervous system. J Clin Invest 45: 678-689, 1966.

8. SCHMID R: Hyperbilirubinemia. In The Metabolic Basis of Inherited Disease, edited by Stanbury JB, Wyngaarden JB, Fredrickson DS, Boston, McGraw-Hill, 3rd edition, 1972. pp 1141-1178.

9. VIRCHOW R: Die pathologischen Pigmente. Arch für Pathologische Anatomie und Physiologie und Klinische Medizin 1: 379-402, 1847.

10. WHIPPLE GH, HOOPER CW: Bile pigment output influenced by hemoglobin injection, anemia and blood regeneration. Am J Physiol 43: 258-274, 1917.

11. ASCHOFF L: Das reticulo-endotheliale System und seine Beziehungen zur Gallenfarbstoffbildung. Mlichen Med Wochenschr 69: 1352-1356, 1922.

12. MANN FC, SHEARD C, BOLLMAN JL et al: The formation of bile pigment from hemoglobin. Am J Physiol 76: 306-315, 1926.

13. TENHUNEN R, MARVER HS, SCHMID R: Microsomal heme oxygenase: characterization of the enzyme. J Biol Chem 244: 6388-6394, 1969.

14. TENHUNEN R, MARVER HS, PIMSTONE NR et al: Enzymatic degradation of heme. Oxygenative cleavage requiring cytochrome P-450. Biochemistry 11: 1716-1720, 1972.

15. TENHUNEN R, ROSS ME, MARVER HS et al: NADPH-dependent biliverdin reductase: partial purification and characterization. Biochemistry 9: 298-303, 1970.

16. TENHUNEN R, MARVER HS, SCHMID R: The enzymatic catabolism of hemoglobin: stimulation of microsomal heme oxygenase by hemin. J Lab Clin Med 75: 410-421, 1970.

17. BISSELL DM, HAMMAKER L, SCHMID R: Hemoglobin and erythrocyte catabolism in rat liver: the separate roles of parenchymal and sinusoidal cells. Blood 40: 812-822, 1972.

18. PIMSTONE NR, ENGEL P, TENHUNEN R et al: Inducible heme oxygenase in the kidney: a model for the homeostatic control of hemoglobin catabolism. J Clin Invest 50: 2042-2050, 1971.

19. GEMSA D, WOO CH, FUDENBERG HH et al: Erythrocyte catabolism by macrophages in vitro. The effect of hydrocortisone on erythrophagocytosis and on the induction of heme oxygenase. J Clin Invest 52: 812-822, 1973.

20. ROBINSON SH: The origin of bilirubin. N Engl J Med 279: 143-149, 1968.

21. CONNEY AH: Pharmacological implications of microsomal enzyme induction. Pharmacol Rev 19: 317-366, 1967.

22. MARVER HS, SCHMID R: Biotransformation in the liver: implications for human disease. Gastroenterology 55: 282-289, 1968.

23. LEVITT M, SCHACTER BA, ZIPURSKY A et al: The nonerythropoietic component of early bilirubin. J Clin Invest 47: 1281-1294, 1968.

24. LANDAW SA, WINCHELL HS: Endogenous production of ^{14}CO: a method for calculation of RBC life-span in vivo. Blood 36: 642-656, 1970.

25. SCHMID R: Synthesis and degradation of microsomal hemoproteins. Drug Metab Disposition 1: 256-258, 1973.

26. JONES EA, SHRAGER R, BLOOMER JR et al: Quantitative studies of the delivery of hepatic-synthesized bilirubin to plasma utilizing δ-aminolevulinic acid-4-^{14}C and bilirubin-^{3}H in man. J Clin Invest 51: 2450-2458, 1972.

27. ODELL GB: The dissociation of bilirubin from albumin and its clinical implications. J Pediatr 55: 268-279, 1959.

28. STERN L: Drug interactions. II. Drugs, the newborn infant, and the binding of bilirubin to albumin. Pediatrics 49: 916-918, 1972.

29. SCHMID R, DIAMOND I, HAMMAKER L et al: The interaction of bilirubin with albumin. Nature (Lond) 206: 1041-1043, 1965.

30. LEVI AJ, GATMAITAN Z, ARIAS IM: Two hepatic cytoplasmic protein fractions, Y and Z, and their possible role in the hepatic uptake of bilirubin, sulfobromophthalein, and other anions. J Clin Invest 48: 2156-2167, 1968.

31. JANSEN FH, BILLING BH: The identification of monoconjugates of bilirubin in bile as amide derivatives. Biochem J 125: 917-919, 1971.

32. KUENZLE CC: Bilirubin conjugates of human bile. The excretion of bilirubin as the acyl glycosides of aldobiouronic acid, pseudoaldobiouronic acid and hexuronosylhexuronic acid, with a branched-chain hexuronic acid as one of the components of the hexuronosylhexuronide. Biochem J 119: 411-435, 1970.

33. FEVERY J, VAN DAMME B, MICHIELS R et al: Bilirubin conjugates in bile of man and rat in the normal state and in liver disease. J Clin Invest 51: 2482-2492, 1972.

34. GORESKY CA: The hepatic uptake and excretion of sulfobromophthalein and bilirubin. Can Med Assoc J 92: 851-857, 1965.

35. ARIAS I, BERNSTEIN L, TOFFLER R et al: Black liver disease in Corriedale sheep: a new mutation affecting hepatic excretory function. J Clin Invest 43: 1249, 1964 (Abs).

36. POLAND RL, ODELL GB: Physiologic jaundice: the enterohepatic circulation of bilirubin. N Engl J Med 284: 1-6, 1971.

37. GRAY CH: Bile Pigments in Health and Disease. Springfield, Illinois, Charles C. Thomas, 1961.

38. LESTER R, SCHUMER W, SCHMID R: Intestinal absorption of bile pigments. IV. Urobilinogen absorption in man. N Engl J Med 272: 939-948, 1965.

39. LEVY M, LESTER R, LEVINSKY NG: Renal excretion of urobilinogen in the dog. J Clin Invest 47: 2117-2124, 1968.

40. ROBINSON SH, VANIER T, DESFORGES JF et al: Jaundice in thalassemia minor; a consequence of ineffective erythropoiesis. N Engl J Med 267: 523-529, 1962.

41. BERK PD, BLOOMER JR, HOWE RB et al: Constitutional hepatic dysfunction (Gilbert's syndrome). A new definition based on kinetic studies with unconjugated radiobilirubin. Am J Med 49: 296-305, 1970.

42. BLACK M, FEVERY J, PARKER D et al: Effect of phenobarbitone on plasma ^{14}C-bilirubin clearance in patients with unconjugated hyperbilirubinaemia. Clin Sci Mol Med 46: 1-17, 1974.

43. HAMMAKER L, SCHMID R: Interference with bile pigment uptake in the liver by flavaspidic acid. Gastroenterology 53: 31-37, 1967.

44. CRIGLER JF, NAJJAR VA: Congenital familial nonhemolytic jaundice with kernicterus. Pediatrics 10: 169-179, 1952.

45. ARIAS IM, GARTNER LM, COHEN M et al: Chronic nonhemolytic unconjugated hyperbilirubinemia with glucuronyl transferase deficiency. Clinical, biochemical, pharmacologic and genetic evidence for heterogeneity. Am J Med 47: 395-409, 1969.

46. ARIAS IM: Chronic idiopathic jaundice. In Ikterus, edited by Beck K, Stuttgart, FK Schattauer, 1968.

47. JANDL JH: Anemia of liver disease: observations on its mechanism. J Clin Invest 34: 390-404, 1955.

BILIRUBIN PRODUCTION FROM NON-ERYTHROID SOURCES

Stephen H. Robinson

Harvard Medical School

Boston, Mass. 02215

It has become clear over the past several years that a small but significant portion of the total bilirubin production is derived from sources other than the hemoglobin of red blood cells. In retrospect this is not surprising since bilirubin is the product of the degradation of heme, and heme is present in virtually all tissues of the body in the form of a number of enzymes and cytochromes, myoglobin in muscle and hemoglobin in red cells. Quantitatively, most heme is present in red cell hemoglobin. The second richest source of heme synthesis is the liver. Not surprisingly, therefore, most of the bilirubin produced under normal conditions is derived from erythroid and hepatic sources, although there is presumably a small contribution from other tissues as well.

Our present understanding of the sources of bilirubin production is based on the observations of several investigators over the past 25 years. I shall summarize some of the historical landmarks in this work but shall not describe the findings of others in the detail that they deserve. In 1950 two groups of investigators (1,2) used ^{15}N-labeled glycine to study the relationship between hemoglobin and bile pigment production. Glycine is a physiologic precursor of heme and thus is incorporated into the hemoglobin of newly developed red cells. After a brief lag period a cohort of labeled cells entered the circulation and survived for approximately 120 days (Fig. 1). As the labeled cells left the circulation and were destroyed, a large late peak of labeled bile pigment production was observed. Measurements made during the first few days also revealed an "early-labeled peak" of pigment production which preceded the entry of significant numbers of labeled red cells into the peripheral blood. Under normal

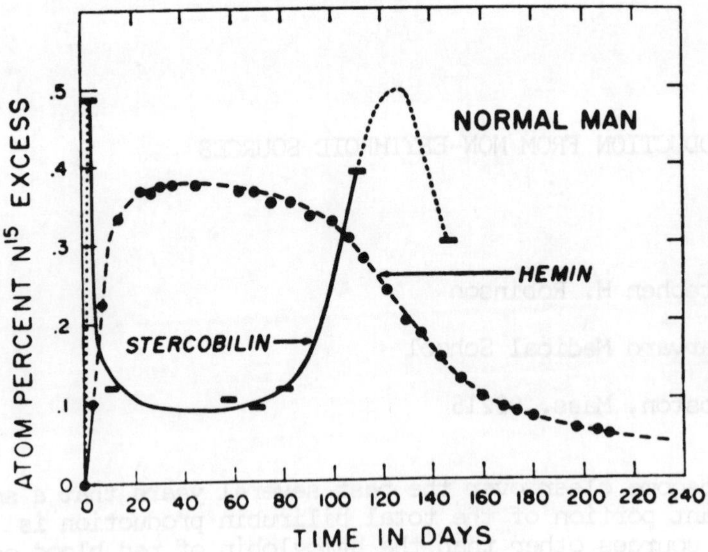

Fig. 1. Labeling of red cell hemoglobin and fecal stercobilin in a normal human subject given glycine-^{15}N orally. (By permission of the publisher (1)).

conditions this early peak accounted for approximately 15% of the total labeled pigment and clearly was derived from sources other than the hemoglobin of senescent red blood cells.

At first, it appeared that the early-labeled fraction was related to hemoglobin metabolism in maturing red cell precursors in the bone marrow, probably as the result of ineffective erythropoiesis. Indeed, there is substantial evidence that erythropoietic mechanisms do play a major role in the production of early-labeled bilirubin, particularly in certain hematologic diseases (2-8). However, more recent studies have shown conclusively that the early-labeled peak is derived to a significant extent from non-erythroid sources, primarily in the liver. Perhaps the first real evidence was the observation of Watson James III that early-labeled bile pigment was produced in substantial quantity in a patient with aplastic anemia, i.e., in the absence of erythropoietic activity and hemoglobin synthesis (9). Later Israels and coworkers performed experiments in which labeled pigment formation was measured as bilirubin in the plasma rather than stercobilin in the stools, as in earlier studies. These workers reported that there were two discrete peaks of early bilirubin production (10,11). The first occurred within the first 24 hours after administration of glycine-^{14}C and appeared to be totally independent of erythroid activity; the second occurred at 3-5 days and varied in relation to the rate of erythropoiesis. Israels et al also made a second major observation, based on an earlier finding by Berlin, Neuberger and Scott (12): that labeled delta-aminolevulinic acid (ALA) is a preferential precursor of non-erythroid sources of bile pigment (10,11).

Our laboratory had also become involved in studies of labeled bilirubin production. Many of our experiments were based on measurements of labeled bilirubin in the plasma of rats (13) and patients (14) who were jaundiced because of impairment of bilirubin excretion but in whom the pattern of bilirubin production was normal. I shall not elaborate on the methodology here, but suffice it to say that it circumvented several problems inherent in other techniques (13,15). Additional studies were performed in normal rats with external drainage of bile and the findings were comparable in both experimental models (13). The results of a representative experiment are shown in Fig. 2. As in human subjects

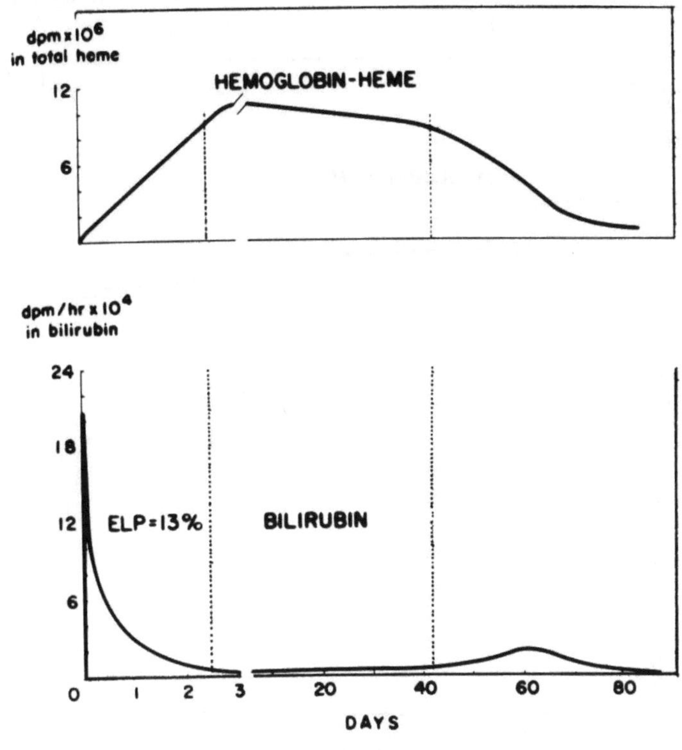

Fig. 2. Labeling of red cell hemoglobin heme and plasma bilirubin in the rat, with glycine-2-^{14}C as precursor. Note that the time scale is condensed after 3 days. (By permission of the publisher (13)).

there was a large late peak of labeled bilirubin production that corresponded to the destruction of circulating red cells at the end of their physiologic life span. Again, an early-labeled peak was observed, accounting for approximately 15% of the total labeled bilirubin. However, in contrast to all earlier findings, the production of early-labeled pigment proceeded at an extraordinarily rapid rate, with peak activity only 1-2 hours after the glycine was given. Thereafter, there was a gradual "plateau" phase which continued over the ensuing 2-3 days.

The rapidity with which the initial sharp component was formed made it seem unlikely that it could be derived from prematurely destroyed red cell precursors. This surmise was further borne out when ALA-^{14}C was used as a precursor rather than glycine-^{14}C (Fig. 3). Although the incorporation of ALA into hemoglobin was smaller than that of glycine, its incorporation into the initial bilirubin component was higher by a factor of 1,000 (13). This confirmed earlier observations (10-12) that ALA labels a bilirubin fraction which is independent of hemoglobin synthesis.

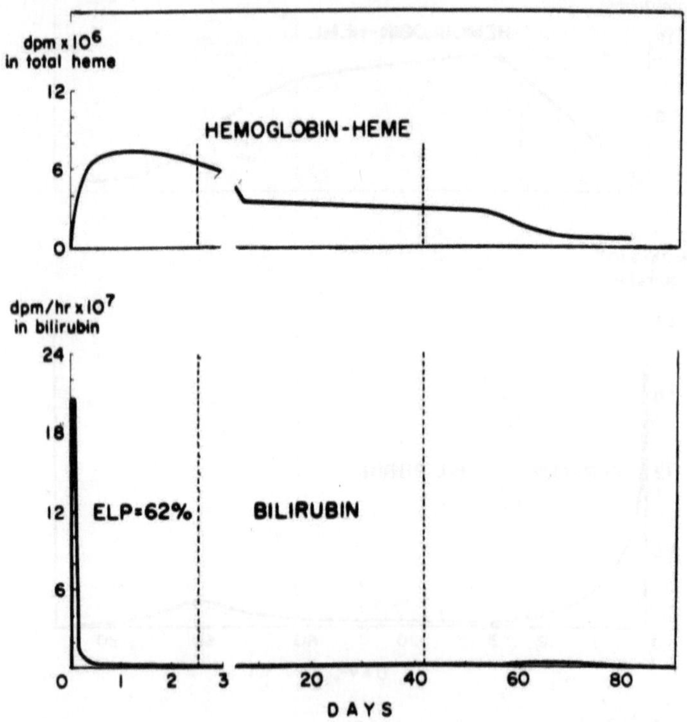

Fig. 3. Labeling of red cell hemoglobin heme and plasma bilirubin in the rat, with ALA-4-^{14}C as precursor. (By permission of the publisher (13)).

The late peak, which is derived from the hemoglobin of circulating red cells, is virtually imperceptible in experiments with ALA, and most of the labeled bile pigment is formed within the first two hours. This is clearly an unphysiologic finding, but serves to underline the existence of non-erythroid sources of bilirubin production. The reason that ALA is incorporated selectively into non-erythroid sources of bilirubin has not yet been ascertained, although several hypotheses have been suggested (13,15).

These findings led to experiments with isolated rat livers. As illustrated in Fig. 4, with ALA as precursor the isolated perfused liver produces labeled bilirubin at both a rate and magnitude comparable to those observed in the intact rat (16). Labeled bilirubin production was also observed with glycine-^{14}C as precursor, but to a much smaller extent than with ALA, as with the findings *in vivo*. At about this time Schwartz reported rapid labeling of hemes in both the liver and kidney of dogs given

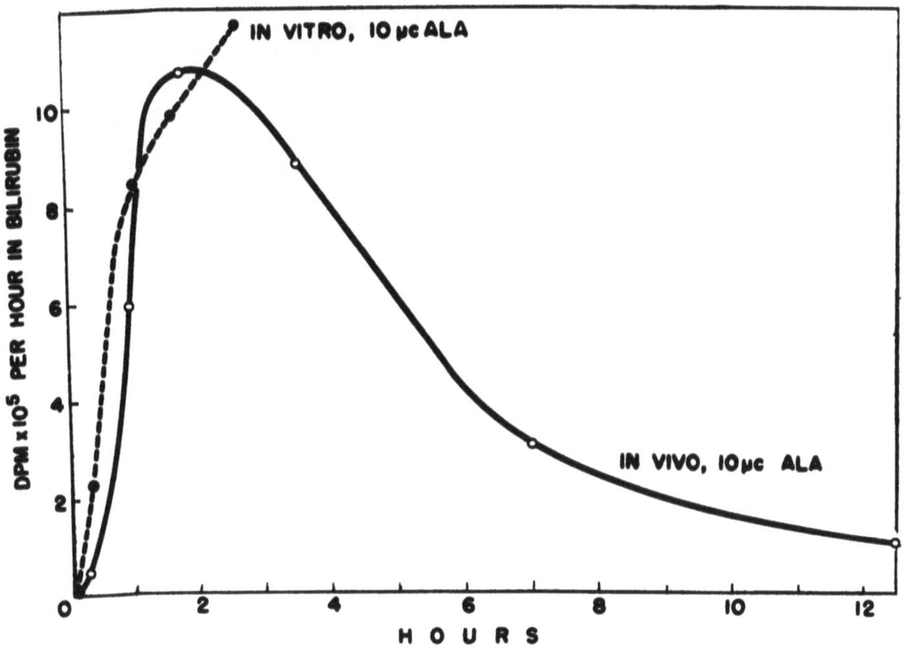

Fig. 4. Excretion of bilirubin-^{14}C in bile from an isolated perfused rat liver after injection of ALA-4-^{14}C. The experiment was terminated at 3 hours. Shown for comparison is the curve of bilirubin-^{14}C excretion in the bile of an intact rat after ALA-^{14}C administration. (By permission of the publisher (16)).

labeled ALA (17). The rise and fall of heme specific activity just preceded the excretion of bilirubin-^{14}C into the bile, suggesting a precursor-product relationship. White et al also demonstrated that liver homogenates incubated in vitro with glycine-^{14}C produce both labeled carbon monoxide and bilirubin (18), indicating that the latter is formed as the result of the degradation of heme, the only metabolic source of carbon monoxide formation. On the basis of these in situ experiments it could be concluded with certainty that some bilirubin is derived from sources unrelated to hemoglobin, chiefly from the turnover of hepatic hemes.

From our studies in rats, the following scheme of bile pigment formation was formulated (Fig.5). Approximately 2/3 of the bilirubin normally produced is derived from red cells at the end of their physiologic life-spans. The early-labeled pigment fraction comprises about 15% of the total and this in turn is divided into at least two phases: an early sharp component, which arises primarily from the turnover of hepatic hemes, and a later slow phase. In rats this later phase is also derived largely from non-erythroid sources under normal conditions but contains a small erythropoietic component which may become markedly enlarged under conditions in which erythropoiesis is either accelerated or abnormal (8,13). Finally, there is a long middle segment of the curve between about 3 and 40 days, bridging the early and late peaks. Its origin is not entirely clear, although it may be derived in part from some random destruction of labeled erythrocytes

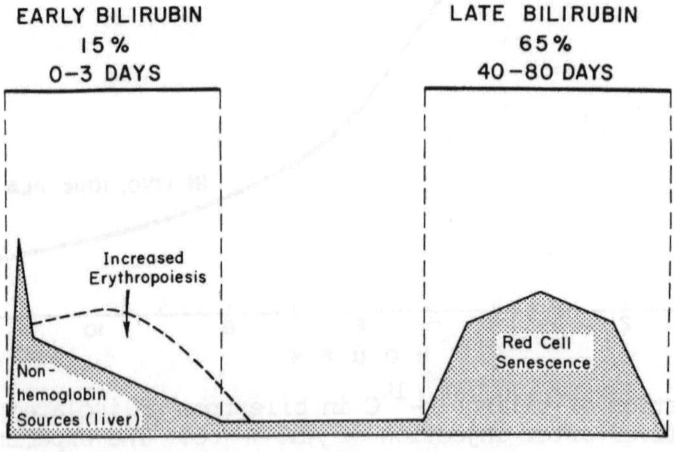

Fig. 5. Sources of bilirubin production in the rat, as adduced from studies of the labeling of plasma bilirubin in Gunn rats and bile bilirubin in normal rats after the injection of glycine-2-^{14}C. (By permission of the publisher (25)).

and in part from the turnover of tissue hemes with rather long half-lives.

It seems probable that much of the bilirubin produced during the early-labeling period is the result of the renewal of a variety of species of heme with different rates of biological turnover. Precisely which heme-containing substances contribute to which phases of non-erythroid bilirubin formation, and to what extent, are largely unresolved questions, and the source of the dramatic early sharp component remains entirely enigmatic. The proposal originally made by Israels et al (19) that the latter is due to the rapid turnover of a free heme pool in the liver becomes more and more attractive as this early component continues to defy our attempts to discern its origin.

It should be added that, although the scheme shown in Fig. 5 is based on findings in rats, observations in a human subject (14) indicate that it is also applicable to man, except for a difference in time course in the two species. Other investigators have reported that erythropoietic mechanisms make a greater contribution to the early bilirubin fraction in man than in the rat (7,10,11,17), although recent studies have suggested that the hepatic fraction may normally contribute as much as 20% of the total bilirubin production in human subjects (20,21).

The next question that we asked was whether the production of bilirubin from hepatic sources has significance with regard to disease states. Bilirubin production from glycine-^{14}C was measured in rats with alterations in liver function produced by a variety of techniques (22). The initial sharp component, i.e. the liver fraction, was found to be increased after administration of phenobarbital or hydrocortisone, after induction of cirrhosis by the chronic administration of carbon tetrachloride, and during the active phase of liver regeneration after partial hepatectomy. Immediately following partial hepatectomy, however, there was a marked reduction in the early bilirubin component, as would be anticipated if this normally originated in the liver. It should be noted that the observation that phenobarbital stimulates early-labeled pigment production was first made by Schmid, Marver and Hammaker who suggested that this might be related to corresponding increases in hepatic cytochromes P-450 and by b_5 (23). In addition, a marked rise in hepatic bilirubin production was observed in iron deficient rats responding acutely to iron therapy (8) and in rats with inflammatory disease provoked by the intramuscular injection of turpentine (22). These observations in rats suggest that enlargement of the hepatic bilirubin component may be a common concomitant of changes in liver metabolism and raise the intriguing possibility that jaundice in liver disease may sometimes be the result not only of impaired bilirubin excretion by the liver but also of increased bilirubin production by this organ.

I will finish by describing some recent experiments in which we have been examining directly the heme sources of the hepatic bilirubin component (24). Glycine-^{14}C was given to rats which were sacrificed at frequent intervals for assay of heme labeling in total liver and in mitochondrial and microsomal fractions. In contrast to some earlier studies, glycine rather than ALA was used as a precursor since it almost certainly yields a more physiologic representation. As shown in Fig.6, there is a rapidly labeled component of hepatic heme synthesis which conforms to the initial sharp component of labeled bilirubin formation. Soon thereafter, between 2 - 8 hours, there is a second, less marked peak followed by a gradual decline in heme labeling over the ensuing 2 - 3 days. Rather similar patterns are observed in both the mitochondrial and microsomal fractions. Thus, a substantial amount of labeled heme is produced in the liver following the formation of the initial component. Indeed, calculations indicate that the changes in hepatic heme labeling are sufficient to account for most of the early-labeled bilirubin fraction observed over 3 days in the intact animal. Significant alterations in these patterns occur in rats with iron deficiency or acutely treated iron deficiency (24).

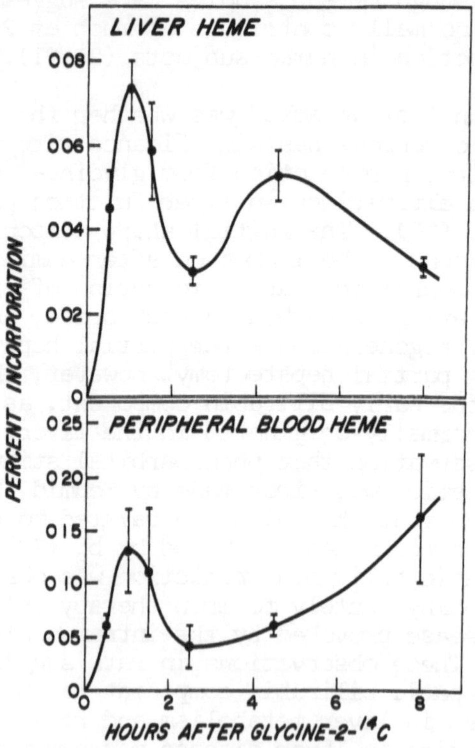

Fig. 6. Labeling of heme in liver and peripheral blood from rats at early intervals after injection of glycine-2-^{14}C.

During the course of these experiments glycine-^{14}C incorporation into peripheral blood heme was measured at very early time points. To our surprise, an initial peak of heme labeling was consistently observed at 1 hour, followed by a brief fall and finally a progressive rise as originally expected. The basis for this "early peak" of erythrocyte heme labeling is not yet known, although it seems possible that this also represents the turnover of a species of non-hemoglobin heme similar to that which accounts for the initial heme component in the liver. This early peak appears to vary in relation to the rate of hemoglobin synthesis, perhaps explaining our recent puzzling observation that the initial "non-erythroid" component of bilirubin is moderately increased with marked stimulation of erythropoiesis (26).

The finding of a labeled heme component of apparently very rapid turnover in both hepatic and erythroid tissue suggests that this is a characteristic of all cells in which heme is made. Perhaps this does represent a pool of free or unassigned heme (19) which could subserve two functions: to serve as the prosthetic group for heme-requiring apoproteins and to stimulate initiation (27,28) of the synthesis of cellular proteins both related and unrelated to heme as a prosthetic group.

SUMMARY

The evidence leading to the demonstration of bilirubin production from nonhemoglobin sources in the liver has been reviewed. In both rats and humans there is a remarkably early sharp peak of labeled bilirubin production occurring only 1 - 2 hours after the administration of glycine-2-^{14}C. This peak is largely independent of erythroid activity and is markedly exaggerated when ALA-^{14}C rather than glycine-^{14}C is used as a precursor; by contrast, ALA is poorly incorporated into hemoglobin heme. Moreover, the initial bilirubin peak formed from ALA-^{14}C can be virtually reproduced in the isolated perfused rat liver. Following the initial sharp peak of bilirubin production from glycine-^{14}C there is a long slow phase which is also derived largely from non-erythroid sources, although it contains a small erythropoietic component.

Enlargement of the non-erythroid bilirubin fraction is readily induced in rats by pathologic or pharmacologic alterations in liver function, and increased hepatic bilirubin synthesis is a possible contributor to jaundice in liver disease.

Recent studies of heme labeling in the livers of rats given glycine-^{14}C demonstrate an initial peak, analogous to the first sharp bilirubin component, followed by a second smaller peak and then a slow decay in radioactivity; hepatic heme turnover is sufficient to account for most of the labeled bilirubin fraction that is formed over 3 days in intact rats. In addition, there is an early peak of heme labeling at 1 - 1.5 hours in the peripheral blood that appears to vary with the rate of erythropoiesis.

ACKNOWLEDGEMENT

Some of the work reported here was supported by USPHS grant AM 09834.

REFERENCES

1. LONDON IM, WEST R, SHEMIN D et al: On origin of bile pigment in normal man. J Biol Chem 184: 351-358, 1950.

2. NEUBERGER A, SNEATH PHA: Studies in congenital porphyria. II. Incorporation of ^{15}N in stercobilin in normal and in porphyric. Biochem J 47: 87-92, 1950.

3. LONDON IM, WEST R: Formation of bile pigment in pernicious anemia. J Biol Chem 184: 359-364, 1950.

4. GRINSTEIN M, BANNERMAN RM, VAVRA JD et al: Hemoglobin metabolism in thalassemia: in vivo studies. Am J Med 29: 18-32, 1960.

5. ROBINSON SH, VANIER T, DESFORGES JF et al: Jaundice in thalassemia minor: consequence of "ineffective erythropoiesis". New Engl J Med 267: 523-529, 1962.

6. ISRAELS LG, ZIPURSKY A: Primary shunt hyperbilirubinaemia. Nature (Lond) 193: 73-74, 1962.

7. BARRETT PVD, CLINE MJ, BERLIN NI: Association of urobilin "early peak" and erythropoiesis in man. J Clin Invest 45: 1657-1667, 1966.

8. ROBINSON SH: Increased formation of early-labeled bilirubin in rats with iron deficiency anemia: evidence for ineffective erythropoiesis. Blood 33: 909-917, 1969.

9. JAMES GW, III, ABBOTT LD, Jr: Stercobilin ^{15}N excretion in refractory anemia. Trans Am Clin Climat Ass 73: 110-120, 1961.

10. ISRAELS LG, YAMAMOTO T, SKANDERBEG J et al: Shunt bilirubin: evidence for two components. Science 139: 1054-1055, 1963.

11. ISRAELS LG, YAMAMOTO T, SKANDERBEG J et al: Early appearing bilirubin: evidence for two components. J Clin Invest 44: 31-44, 1965.

12. BERLIN NI, NEUBERGER A, SCOTT JJ: Metabolism of δ-aminolevulinic acid. II. Normal pathways studied with aid of C^{14}. Biochem J 64: 90-100, 1956.

13. ROBINSON SH, TSONG M, BROWN BW et al: Sources of bile pigment in rat: studies of "early-labeled" fraction. J Clin Invest 45: 1569-1586, 1966.

14. ROBINSON SH, LESTER R, CRIGLER JF Jr, et al: Early-labeled peak of bile pigment in man: studies with glycine-^{14}C and delta-aminolevulinic acid-^{3}H. New Engl J Med 277: 1323-1329, 1967.

15. ROBINSON SH: Formation of bilirubin from erythroid and non-erythroid sources. Semin Hemat 9: 43-53, 1972.

16. ROBINSON SH, OWEN CA Jr, FLOCK EV et al: Bilirubin formation in liver from nonhemoglobin sources. Blood 26: 823-829, 1965.

17. SCHWARTZ S: Quantitation of erythropoietic and non-erythropoietic contribution to early labeling of bile pigments. In Bilirubin Metabolism, edited by Bouchier IAD and Billing BH. Oxford, Blackwell, 1967. p. 15.

18. WHITE P, SILVERS AA, ROSHER ML et al: Hepatic production of bilirubin and carbon monoxide in vitro. J Clin Invest 45: 1085-1086, 1966 (Abs).

19. LEVITT M, SCHACTER BA, ZIPURSKY A et al: The nonerythropoietic component of early bilirubin. J Clin Invest 47: 1281-1294, 1968.

20. JONES EA, BLOOMER JR, BERLIN NI: The measurement of the synthetic rate of bilirubin from hepatic hemes in patients with acute intermittent porphyria. J Clin Invest 50: 2259-2265, 1971.

21. BERK PD, RODKEY FL, BLASCHKE TF et al: Comparison of plasma bilirubin turnover and carbon monoxide production in man. J Lab Clin Med 83: 29-37, 1974.

22. ROBINSON SH: Increased bilirubin formation from nonhemoglobin sources in rats with disorders of the liver. J Lab Clin Med 73: 668-676, 1969.

23. SCHMID R, MARVER JS, HAMMAKER L: Enhanced formation of rapidly labeled bilirubin by phenobarbital: hepatic microsomal cytochromes as possible source. Biochem Biophys Res Commun 24: 319-328, 1966.

24. YANNONI CZ, ROBINSON SH: Manuscript in preparation.

25. ROBINSON SH: Ineffective erythropoiesis and the erythropoietic component of early-labeled bilirubin. In Hemopoietic Cellular Proliferation, edited by Stohlman F Jr, New York, Grune & Stratton, 1970. pp 180-188.

26. ROBINSON SH, TSONG M: Hemolysis of "stress" reticulocytes: a source of erythropoietic bilirubin formation. J Clin Invest 49: 1025-1034, 1970.

27. BEUZARD Y, RODVIEN R, LONDON IM: Effect of hemin on the synthesis of hemoglobin and other proteins in mammalian cells. Proc Nat Acad Sci 70: 1022-1026, 1973.

28, GROSS M, RABINOVITZ M: Control of globin synthesis in cell-free preparations of reticulocytes by formation of a translational repressor that is inactivated by hemin. Proc Nat Acad Sci 69: 1565-1568, 1972.

BILIRUBIN PRODUCTION FROM ERYTHROID SOURCES

Ursula Muller-Eberhard and Eric F. Johnson

Scripps Clinic and Research Foundation

La Jolla, California 92037

A major portion of bilirubin is produced from catabolism of hemoglobin following red cell destruction. Information regarding erythrocyte degradation has been derived primarily from studies of hemolytic states, as the mechanism of red cell aging remains uncertain (1). Deformability of the red cell membrane is prerequisite for their passage through the sinusoids of various organs (2). Increased membrane rigidity or fragmentation (3) leads to red cell sequestration in the reticuloendothelial system (RES) or intravascular lysis. Hemoglobin and heme released into the plasma are carried to liver parenchymal cells by two plasma proteins, haptoglobin and hemopexin respectively. Bilirubin formation from hemoglobin liberated during erythrocyte breakdown occurs in cells of the RES and hepatocytes (4).

The main causes of increased red cell destruction are summarized in the following Table. They are either cellular or extracellular events which result in loss of membrane deformability or fragmentation. Chemical changes affecting the sulfhydryl groups of proteins integral to the membrane or changes in membrane lipid composition result in cellular rigidity. Cellular ATP depletion is also detrimental to membrane deformability. Osmotic swelling of the cells decreases the ratio of surface area to volume and thus limits the cell to a more spherical shape. Osmotic changes are often associated with an imbalance of the Na^+/K^+ ion pump (3,5).

Main Causes For Premature Erythrocyte Destruction

CELLULAR	
Chemical	SH groups, Lipids, ATP depletion
Osmotic	Na^+ Influx, K^+ Efflux
Hemoglobin	Amino acid substitution, oxidation or aggregation
Serum Protein Coating	Immunoglobulins, Complement
EXTRACELLULAR	
Abnormal Turbulence	Valvular disease
Narrowed Passages	Septal defect or capillary obstruction
Trauma	Bruises, burns and frost bites

Various hemoglobin abnormalities are associated with increased red cell destruction (6). Altered hemoglobin can change the intracellular viscosity or can result in hemoglobin chain precipitation. Both occurrences decrease cell pliability. A prominent example of increased viscosity is gelled deoxygenated sickle cell hemoglobin. In the thalassemias, surplus α and β chains precipitate forming the so-called Heinz bodies. Heinz bodies also form when amino acid substitution in the heme pocket region produces an "unstable hemoglobin", or when red cells are exposed to strong oxidants, especially if they are deficient in glucose-6-phosphate dehydrogenase (7). Coating of red cells with immunoglobulins and complement in autoimmune hemolytic diseases enhances red cell aggregation and lysis (8).

Extracellular red cell destruction is usually due to mechanical disruption. Fragmentation and lysis ensue during regurgitation of blood in cardiac valvular disease. Disruption takes place when red cells squeeze through minute septal defects or narrowed arterioles(9). Most commonly, red cells are lysed in tissues damaged by bruising, burning or freezing.

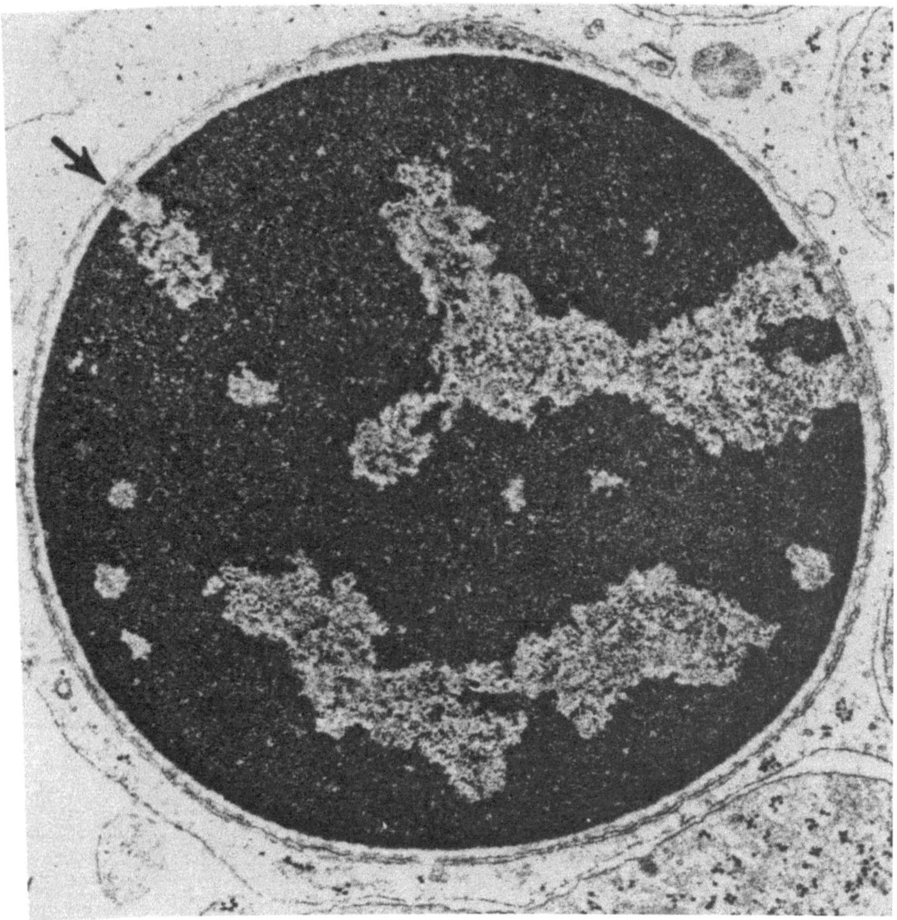

Fig. 1 Extruded nucleus of an erythroblast is seen within the cytoplasm of a bone marrow macrophage. Note the perinuclear rim of hemoglobin which is continuous with intra-nuclear hemoglobin through nuclear pores; one of which is indicated by an arrow. Original magnification is 13,750. Reprinted by permission. From the Journal of the Reticuloendothelial Society 15: 163-169, 1974

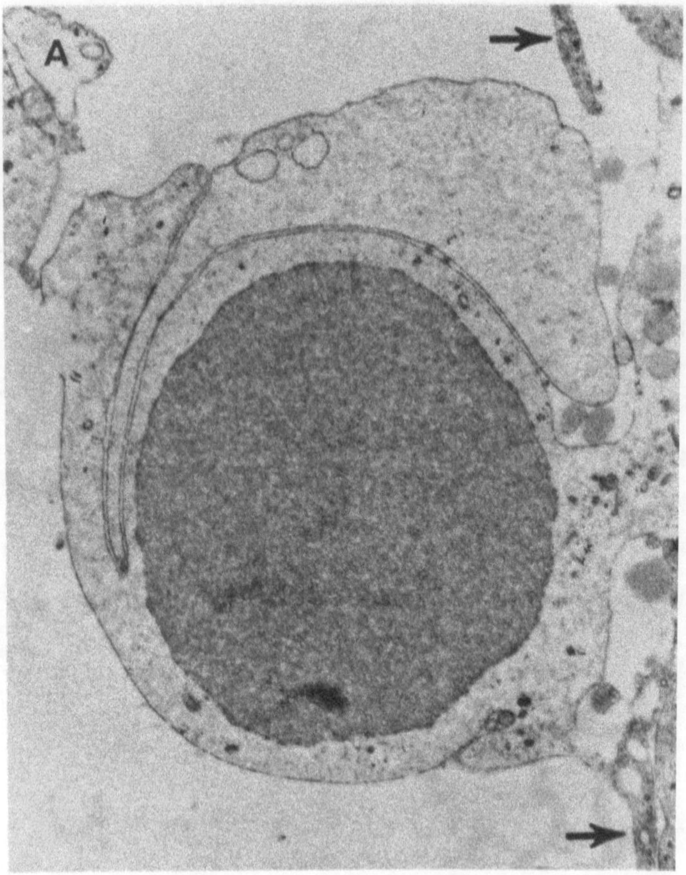

Fig. 2A A mature red cell is seen within the cytoplasm of a bone marrow macrophage which has extended into the lumen of a sinus. The sinus endothelium is identified by arrows. Original magnification is 16,810. reprinted by permission. From the Journal of the Reticuloendothelial Society 15: 163-169, 1974.

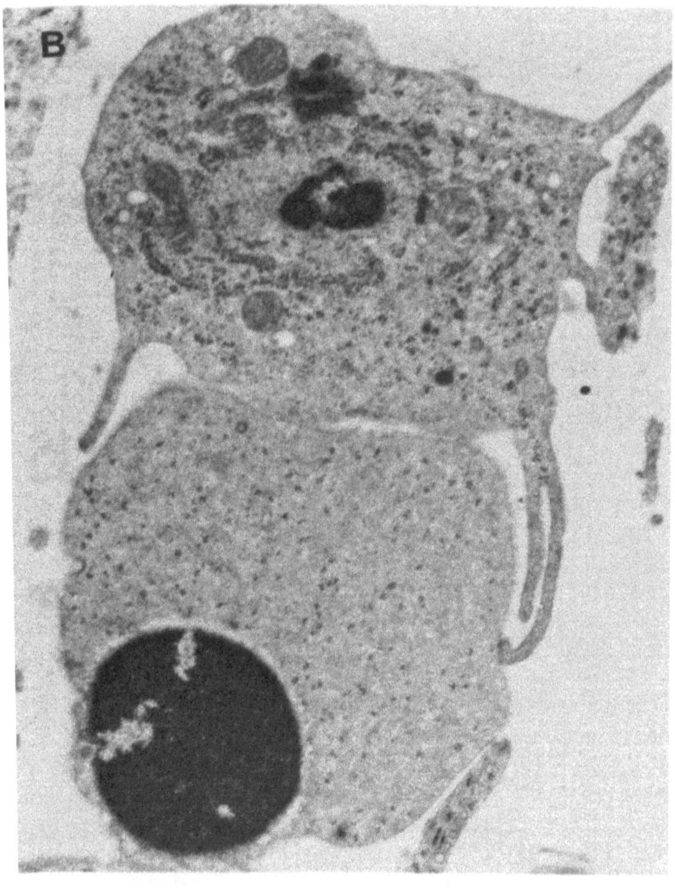

Fig. 2B The pseudopods of a bone macrophage have begun to engulf a normoblast, the nucleus of which is in the process of extrusion. Original magnification is 16,420. Reprinted by permission. From the Journal of the Reticuloendothelial Society 15: 163-169, 1974

The site of erythrocyte sequestration depends upon the extent of membrane damage. Subtly damaged red cells are trapped in the sinusoids of the spleen or die before leaving the bone marrow. Moderately altered erythrocytes are removed by the liver and those grossly deformed are engulfed by all cells of the reticuloendothelial system(3).

Dr. Robinson has already outlined the various sources of bilirubin formation(10). In addition to the large contribution made by erythrocyte degradation at the end of their lifespan, some bilirubin is formed during erythropoiesis(11). This may be produced from hemoglobin extruded with the nucleus during normal erythrocyte maturation as shown in Figure 1. The nucleus with its associated perinuclear rim of hemoglobin is seen within the cytoplasm of a macrophage. Figure 2A depicts phagocytosis of an erythrocyte by a macrophage which extends into the lumen of a bone marrow sinusoid, and Figure 2B shows a nucleated red cell in the process of being engulfed by another macrophage. Both loss of hemoglobin during maturation and erythrophagocytosis may explain increased bilirubin formation concomitant with elevated erythropoiesis(12).

Thus far, we have discussed entrapment of damaged erythrocytes in the RES. Now, we would like to stress intravascular events. Under physiological conditions, 0.8 g of hemoglobin is released into the circulation daily. This represents 10% of the hemoglobin turnover(13). In hemolytic states, hemoglobin levels may be elevated several fold(14).

Our current concept of plasma hemoglobin disposal is summarized schematically in Figure 3. Hemoglobin dissociates into $\alpha\beta$ dimers(15). The dimers are bound by plasma haptoglobin (16,17) and are engulfed by liver parenchymal cells(18,19). Hemoglobin dimers in excess of the haptoglobin binding capacity either enter hepatocytes (18,19,20) or pass the glomeruli and are reabsorbed by the tubular epithelial cells, another site of bilirubin formation(21). In addition, the iron of circulating hemoglobin is oxidized. The methemoglobin formed readily dissociates its heme moiety(15). Dissociated heme is bound by albumin forming methemalbumin(22) and by hemopexin(23,24) forming heme-hemopexin(25). Hemopexin has a greater affinity for heme than albumin(26,27) and is responsible for the transport of heme into hepatocytes(28,19). Albumin is probably not instrumental in this transport(27). We would like to emphasize that hemoglobin as well as hemoglobin-haptoglobin(18,19) and heme-hemopexin(28) are catabolized predominantly by hepatocytes but not by cells of the reticuloendothelial system. Haptoglobin levels are easily depleted with minor hemolytic episodes, whereas hemopexin levels are lowered only with elevated plasma heme levels. Hemopexin

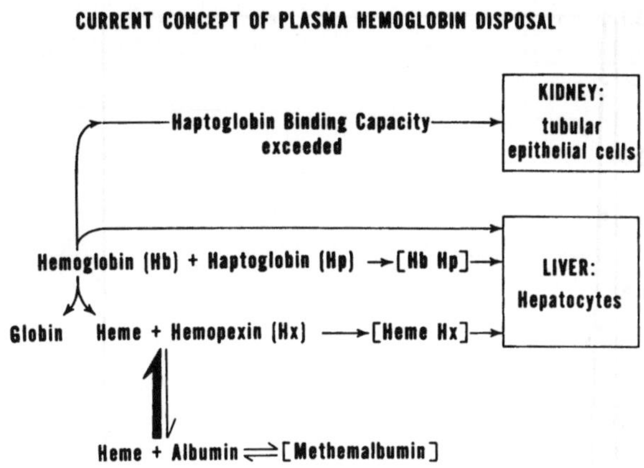

Fig. 3

levels are inversely proportional to those of heme as shown in Figure 4(29). The plasma hemopexin level has been shown to be an excellent guide to assess the severity of cardiac hemolysis(30).

Several experiments suggest a role for hemopexin in plasma heme catabolism. Figure 5 shows the effect of hematin injection on plasma hemopexin turnover in a human subject. Six days after intra- and extra-vascular equilibration of ^{125}I-hemopexin, 250 mg of hematin were given intravenously. The rapid decline of serum ^{125}I-hemopexin is concomitant with that of total hemopexin and heme(31). The serum half-clearance time of the isotope-labeled hemopexin was reduced tenfold. A similar observation was made by Sears by measuring hemopexin levels(32).

Heme was also injected as hematin, hemoglobin or methemoglobin into rabbits which had received both ^{131}I-albumin and ^{125}I-hemopexin. Whereas plasma ^{125}I-hemopexin is rapidly eliminated after injection of heme in either form, the rate of albumin catabolism is not affected(33). These experiments support the hypothesis that albumin is not directly responsible for heme transport(27).

Modification of the heme binding site on hemopexin blocks the effects of heme injection on hemopexin catabolism. Illumination of the hemopexin molecule *in vitro* in the presence of rose bengal, a photo-oxidizing agent, modifies histidine residues. Short-term photo-oxidation partially destroys heme-binding. After heme injection, the catabolism of photo-oxidized hemopexin proceeds at a rate comparable to that of apo-hemopexin once the residual heme-binding capacity is exceeded(34). These experiments suggest that heme-hemopexin complex formation is an important determinant in hemopexin turnover.

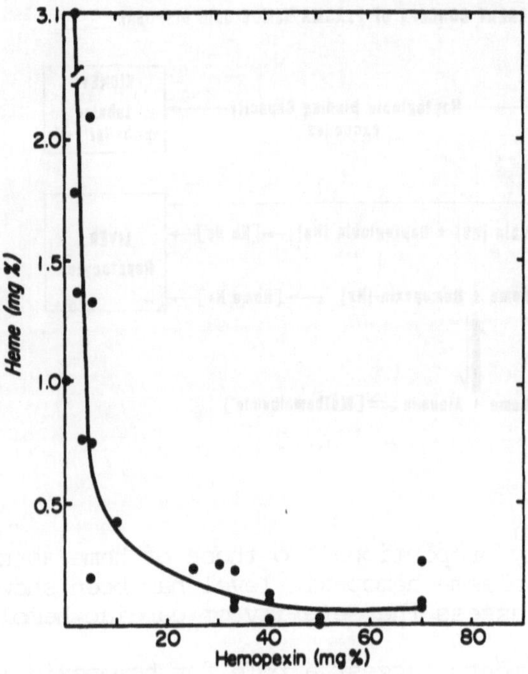

Fig. 4 Plasma concentrations of heme and of hemopexin in patients with hemolytic conditions. Reprinted by permission. From Blood 32: 811-815, 1968

The site of heme-hemopexin uptake was investigated using radioautography. Sixty minutes after intravenous administration of either ^{3}H-heme or ^{125}I-hemopexin, rabbits and rats were sacrificed and various tissues were examined by light and electron microscopy. The distribution of ^{125}I-hemopexin is shown in Figure 6. Silver grains are associated with liver parenchymal cells but not Kupffer cells. Examination of tissues from other organs failed to reveal any associated silver grains(28). Injection of partially aggregated hemopexin results in hemopexin uptake by the macrophages of lung, spleen, kidney and liver. If aggregated instead of monomeric hemopexin is given, one may arrive at an erroneous conclusion with respect to its cellular uptake(35). Data implicating cells of the reticuloendothelial system as the site of uptake for hemoglobin and hemoglobin-haptoglobin may have been influenced by aggregation(36,37). Recent investigations have shown that removal of both entities from the plasma is achieved by the liver parenchymal, but not by the Kupffer cells(18,19).

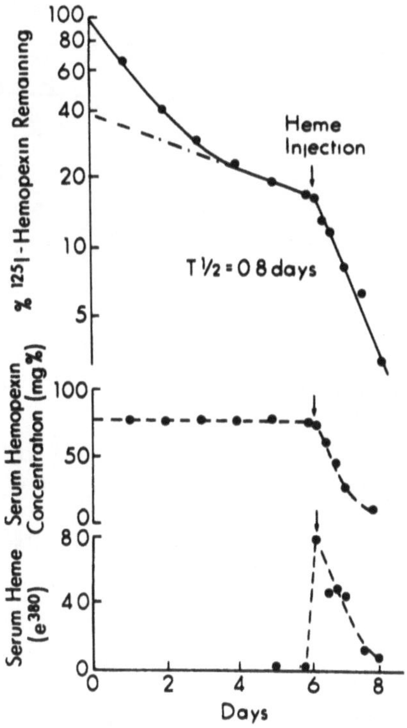

Fig. 5 Effects of hematin injection on ^{125}I-hemopexin metabolism and hemopexin concentration in a human subject, with levels of spectroscopically estimated heme (e^{380}) remaining in the plasma. Reprinted by permission. From the New England Journal of Medicine 290: 822-826, 1974

Figure 7 depicts the intracellular localization of ^{125}I-hemopexin in the liver. The upper portion demonstrates localization of silver grains in the hepatocytes. Kupffer cells, plasma and nuclear membranes show no grains. Similar distribution was observed by Hershko, Cook and Finch(19), when they injected ^{59}Fe-heme and subsequently isolated parenchymal and Kupffer cells. The lower portion of the Figure reveals silver grains associated with the endoplasmic reticulum. Heme oxygenase, the first enzyme implicated in heme degradation, is located in the endoplasmic reticulum(4). It is conceivable that hemopexin delivers heme directly to the site of bilirubin formation. Thus, the liver parenchymal cells appear to play the major role in catabolism of plasma hemoglobin and heme-hemoglobin.

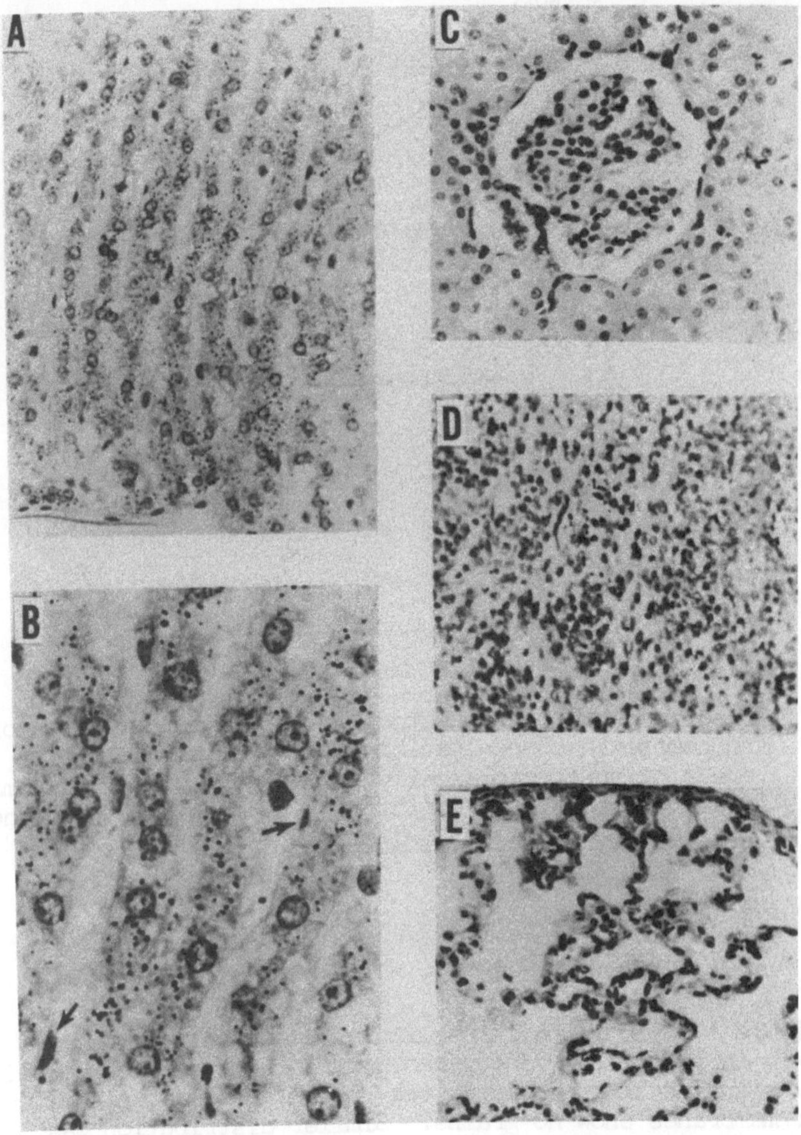

Fig. 6 ^{125}I-rabbit hemopexin found by autoradiography, in the hepatocytes. Arrows in B indicate Kupffer cells which are free of silver grains. Also shown are a glomerulus(C), spleen tissue(D), and alveoli(E). Original magnifications are x 200(A), x 700(B), and x500(C,D, and E). Reprinted by permission. From the Journal of Laboratory and Clinical Medicine 76: 426-431, 1970.

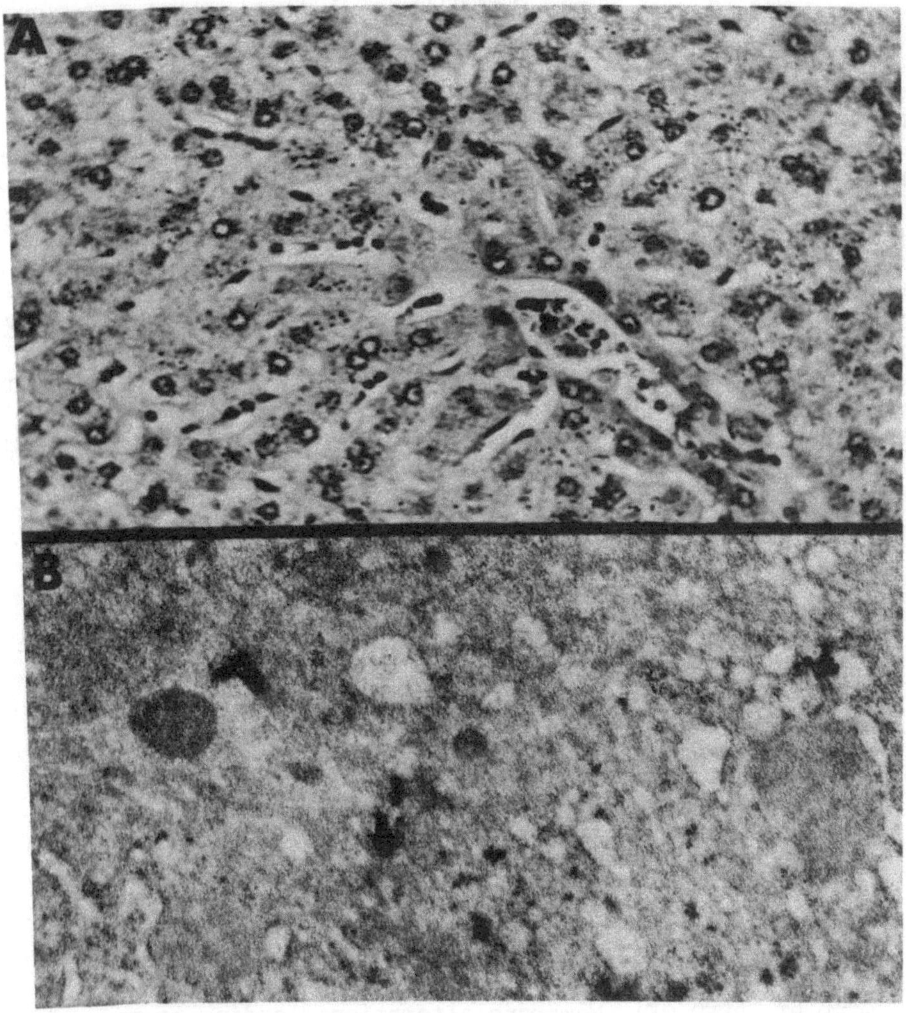

Fig. 7A ^{3}H-heme shown by autoradiography to be confined to the liver parenchyma(A). This rabbit was sacrificed 60 minutes after intravenous injection of ^{3}H-cyanmethemoglobin. Original magnification is x 300. Reprinted by permission. From the Journal of Laboratory and Clinical Medicine 76: 426-431, 1970.

Fig. 7B Subcellular localization of ^{3}H-heme in hepatocyte of the rabbit. Radioautographic grains are associated with endoplasmic reticulum and microbodies. Magnification x 17,5000. Performed by Dr. M. Tavassoli.

SUMMARY

Catabolism of hemoglobin is a major source of bilirubin formation. Destruction of some nucleated and mature red blood cells occurring in the bone marrow contributes to bilirubin formation. The deformability of red cells ensures their survival in the circulation. Alteration of the erythrocyte membrane or fragmentation results in filtration from the circulation by the reticuloendothelial system. The site of sequestration depends on the degree of red cell damage. Alternatively red cells lyse intravascularly and release hemoglobin. Plasma hemoglobin is bound by haptoglobin. Unbound plasma hemoglobin oxidizes readily and loses its heme moiety which is complexed with albumin and hemopexin. Whereas heme associated with albumin merely circulates, hemoglobin, hemoglobin-haptoglobin, and heme-hemopexin are taken up by the liver parenchymal cells, a major site of bilirubin production.

REFERENCES

1. BUNN HF: Erythrocyte destruction and hemoglobin catabolism. Seminars Hemat 9: 3-17, 1972

2. LA CELLE, PL: Alteration of membrane deformability in hemolytic anemias. Seminars Hemat 7: 355-371, 1970.

3. COOPER RA, JANDL JH: Destruction of erythrocytes. In Hematology, edited by WILLIAMS WJ, BEUTLER E, ERSLEV AJ, et al, New York, McGraw-Hill, Inc., 1972, p 178-190.

4. TENHUNEN R: The enzymatic degradation of heme. Seminars Hemat 9: 19-29, 1972

5. WEED RI, REED CF: Membrane alterations leading to red cell destruction. Amer J Med 41: 681-698, 1966

6. JENSEN WN, LESSIN LS: Membrane alterations associated with hemoglobinopathies. Seminars Hemat 7: 409-426, 1970

7. JACOB HS: Mechanisms of Heinz body formation and attachment to red cell membrane. Seminars Hemat 7: 341-354, 1970

8. SPIEGELBERG HL, MIESCHER PA, BENACERRAF B: Studies on the role of complement in the immune clearance of *Escherichia coli* and rat erythrocytes by the reticuloendothelial system in mice. J Immunol 90: 751-759, 1963

9. MARSH GW, LEWIS SM: Cardiac haemolytic anaemia. Seminars Hemat 6: 133-149, 1969

10. ROBINSON SH: Bilirubin production from non-erythroid sources. In Jaundice, edited by C.A. GORESKY and M.M. FISHER, Plenum Press, New York 1975.

11. ROBINSON SH: Formation of bilirubin from erythroid and nonerythroid sources. Seminars Hemat 9: 43-53, 1972

12. TAVASSOLI M: Bone marrow erythroclasia: The function of perisinal macrophages relative to the uptake of erythroid cells. J Reticuloendothel Soc 15: 163-169, 1974

13. GARBY L, NOYES WD: Studies on hemoglobin metabolism. II. Pathways of hemoglobin iron metabolism in normal man. J Clin Invest 38: 1484-1486, 1959

14. CROSBY WH, DAMESHEK W: The significance of hemoglobinemia and associated hemosiderinuria, with particular reference to various types of hemolytic anemia. J Lab Clin Med 38: 829-841, 1951

15. BUNN HF, JANDL JH: Exchange of heme among hemoglobins and between hemoglobin and albumin. J Biol Chem 243: 465-475, 1968

16. NAGEL RL, GIBSON QH: Kinetics and mechanism of complex formation between hemoglobin and haptoglobin. J Biol Chem 242: 3428-3434, 1967

17. PEACOCK AC, PASTEWKA JV, REED RA, et al: Haptoglobin-hemoglobin interaction. Stoichiometry. Biochemistry 9: 2275 - 2279, 1970

18. BISSELL DM, HAMMAKER L, SCHMID R: Hemoglobin and erythrocyte catabolism in rat liver: The separate roles of parenchymal and sinusoidal cells. Blood 40: 812-822, 1972

19. HERSHKO C, COOK JD, FINCH CA: Storage iron kinetics. II. The uptake of hemoglobin iron by hepatic parenchymal cells. J Lab Clin Med 80: 624-634, 1972

20. GOLDFISCHER S, NOVIKOFF AB, ALBALA A, et al: Hemoglobin uptake by rat hepatocytes and its breakdown within lysosomes. J Cell Biol 44: 513-529, 1970

21. PIMSTONE NR: Renal degradation of hemoglobin. Seminars Hemat 9: 31-42, 1972

22. FAIRLEY NH: Methaemalbumin. Part I, Clinical Aspects. Quart J Med 10: 95-114, 1941

23. BRAUN HJ: Übersichten. Eigenschaften, funktion und serumkonzentration des menschlichen hämopexins. Klin Wschr 49: 445-451, 1971

24. MULLER-EBERHARD U, LIEM HH: Hemopexin, the heme-binding serum β-glycoprotein. Structure and Function of Plasma Proteins (in press), Plenum Press, London.

25. HRKAL Z, VODRAZKA Z, KALOUSEK I: Transfer of heme from ferrihemoglobin and ferrihemoglobin isolated chains to hemopexin. Europ J Biochem 43: 73-78, 1974

26. SEERY VL, MULLER-EBERHARD U: Binding of porphyrins to rabbit hemopexin and albumin. J Biol Chem 248: 3796-3800, 1973

27. LIEM HH: Hepatic uptake of heme and hemopexin but not albumin. Biochim Biophys Acta 343: 546-550, 1974

28. MULLER-EBERHARD U, BOSMAN C, LIEM HH: Tissue localization of the heme-hemopexin complex in the rabbit and the rat as studied by light microscopy with the use of radioisotopes. J Lab Clin Med 76: 426-431, 1970

29. MULLER-EBERHARD U, JAVID J, LIEM HH, et al: Plasma concentrations of hemopexin, haptoglobin and heme in patients with various hemolytic diseases. Blood 32: 811-815, 1968

30. EYSTER ME, EDGINGTON TS, LIEM HH, et al: Plasma hemopexin levels following aortic valve replacement: A valuable screening test for assessing the severity of cardiac hemolysis. J Lab Clin Med 80: 112-116, 1972

31. WOCHNER RD, SPILBERG I, IIO A, et al: Hemopexin metabolism in sickle-cell disease, porphyrias and control subjects - Effects of heme injection. New Engl J Med 290: 822-826, 1974

32. SEARS DA: Disposal of plasma heme in normal man and patients with intravascular hemolysis. J Clin Invest 49: 5-14, 1970.

33. Manuscript in preparation

34. Manuscript in preparation

35. Manuscript in preparation

36. WADA T, OHARA H, WATANABE K, et al: Autoradiographic study on the site of uptake of the haptoglobin-hemoglobin complex. J Reticuloendothel Soc 8: 185-193, 1970

37. OKUYAMA S, ITO Y: Reticuloendothelial uptake of hemoglobin assessed with radiocolloid: An experimental approach to intravascular hemolytic sequelae. J Reticuloendothel Soc 14: 68-78, 1973

INDUCTION MECHANISMS FOR BILE PIGMENT FORMATION

Brent A. Schacter

University of Manitoba and The Manitoba Institute of

Cell Biology, Winnipeg, Manitoba, R3E 0V9

Detailed knowledge of the mechanisms by which bile pigment production may be stimulated has been accelerated by the recent delineation of the enzymatic mechanism for heme catabolism, microsomal heme oxygenase, and the regulatory processes which control this step in bile pigment production. Microsomal heme oxygenase catalyzes the conversion of heme to biliverdin by oxidative fission of the α-methene bridge of heme (1,2). This enzyme system is related to and dependent on the activity of the microsomal electron transport system (1-4) which comprises cytochrome P-450 and NADPH-cytochrome c reductase. Biliverdin formed is then converted to bilirubin by the soluble NADPH-dependent enzyme, biliverdin reductase (5). Although in rats hemoglobin administration enhances hepatic biliverdin reductase activity (6) this induction mechanism is probably of little importance in view of the fact that biliverdin reductase is present in excess and is not rate-limiting in the over-all conversion of heme to bilirubin.

Substrate-mediated induction of rat liver microsomal heme oxygenase by hematin was first demonstrated by Tenhunen, Marver and Schmid (7). A six-fold induction of hepatic heme oxygenase activity was produced by hematin given as methemalbumin (MHA) over a 48 hour period. Less marked induction of the hepatic enzyme was produced by injections of hemoglobin, or by the production of a hemolytic anemia in rats with phenylhydrazine or red cell antibodies. In contrast splenic heme oxygenase activity was not much affected by these manipulations, although the total activity of splenic heme oxygenase increased two to three-fold as the result of splenic hypertrophy (7). Fig. 1 demonstrates that the induction of hepatic heme oxygenase begins within two hours of intravenous injection of

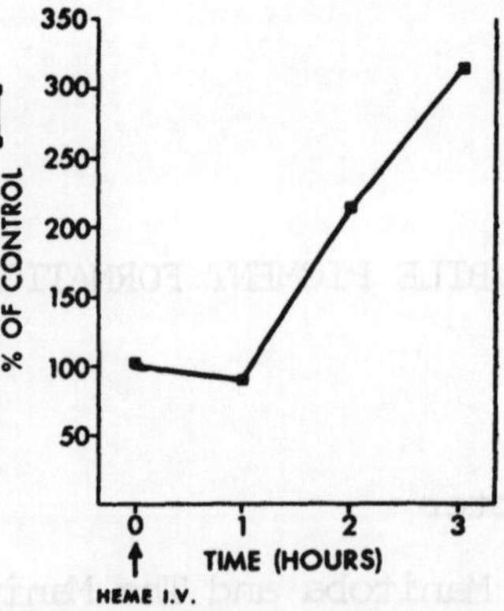

Fig. 1. Early changes in rat hepatic heme oxygenase activity after intravenous injection of methemalbumin (2.55 μmoles heme/100 gm body weight).

methemalbumin (2.55 μmoles heme/100 gm). A similar time of onset of induction of heme oxygenase has also been demonstrated in rat kidney (8) and liver parenchymal cells (9) following intravenous injection of hemoglobin and in rat peritoneal macrophages incubated <u>in vitro</u> with antibody-coated erythrocytes (10). The time course of hepatic heme oxygenase induction following a single intraperitoneal injection of methemalbumin (4 μmoles/100 gm) is shown in Fig. 2 where maximal induction of hepatic heme oxygenase is seen 24 hours following heme injection, with return to pre-

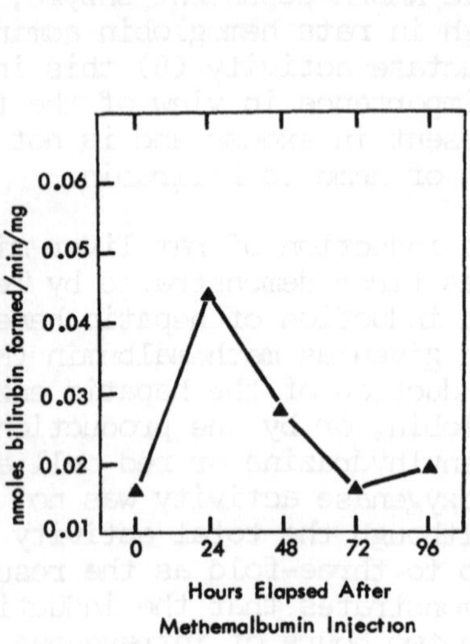

Fig. 2. Time course of induction of rat hepatic heme oxygenase after intraperitoneal injection of methemalbumin (4 μmoles heme/100 gm body weight).

injection levels within 72 hours. If heme is given intravenously as hemoglobin, heme oxygenase activity returns to basal levels within 24-48 hours in rat kidney (8) and hepatic parenchymal cells (9). This difference in the time course of induction may be related to the nature of the substrate (MHA or hemoglobin) and to the mode of administration (IV or IP).

Table I demonstrates that administration of MHA to rats in vivo causes no change in NADPH-cytochrome c reductase (3,19) and a decrease in cytochrome P-450 levels (3,19) despite four-fold induction of hepatic heme oxygenase (3). This interesting dissociation between induction of hepatic heme oxygenase and the lack of any inductive response in the components of the microsomal electron transport system, which are known to support heme oxygenase activity (2-4), suggests that other as yet undefined factors may influence the activity and induction of heme oxygenase.

A number of classes of drugs known to induce the various elements of the microsomal electron transport system (11,12) and drug metabolism (13) have no inductive effect on the activity of heme oxygenase in liver and spleen (14-16) (Table II).

Several possibilities may be entertained to explain these peculiar dichotomies in induction of heme oxygenase by various classes of compounds:
(1) A specific cytochrome P-450 species may exist to facilitate

TABLE I

Effect of Methemalbumin Administration to Rats in vivo on the Activities of Heme Oxygenase, NADPH-Cytochrome c Reductase, and on Microsomal Cytochrome P-450 Levels in Rat Liver[a]

	Cytochrome P-450 (nmoles/mg)	NADPH-Cytochrome c Reductase (nmoles/mg/min)	Heme Oxygenase (nmoles/mg/min)
Control	1.19 ± 0.10	86.8 ± 20.9	0.015 ± 0.004
MHA	0.87 ± 0.33	89.7 ± 11.4	0.055 ± 0.017
% of control	73	103	367

a Total dose of methemalbumin given intraperitoneally to each group of rats varied from 4 - 12 μmoles/100 gm body weight given in from 1 to 4 injections. Results are expressed as means ± standard deviation. Reproduced by permission of the Journal of Biological Chemistry (3).

TABLE II

The Effect of Various Microsomal Inducers on Hepatic and Splenic Heme Oxygenase[a]

Treatment	Heme Oxygenase (nmoles/mg/min)	
	Spleen	Liver
Untreated	0.230 ± 0.032 (6)	0.025 ± 0.002 (14)
Phenobarbital (40 mg/kg IP x 4 days)	0.221 ± 0.014 (7)	0.022 ± 0.002 (7)
3-Methylcholanthrene (13 mg/kg IP x 4 days)	0.114 ± 0.013 (5)[b]	0.016 ± 0.001 (5)[b]
3,4 Benzpyrene (20 mg/kg IP x 4 days)	0.146 ± 0.020 (3)	0.025 ± 0.001 (3)
PCN[c] (50 mg/kg PO x 3 days)	0.228 ± 0.017 (3)	0.017 ± 0.001 (3)

[a] Figures in brackets represent the number of groups of animals tested. Each group comprised 6-10 rats, and the values are expressed as mean ± S.E.M. Reproduced by permission of Archives of Biochemistry and Biophysics (14).

[b] $\underline{P} < 0.02$ [c] PCN= Pregnenolone-16α-carbonitrile

heme catabolism; (2) a specific binding protein which facilitates heme catabolism may be found at the microsomal level; or (3) an undefined enzyme moiety related to the microsomal electron transport system but responsible specifically for heme catabolism may be present (14).

The presence of any of these factors might modify the induction of heme oxygenase as compared with the induction of elements of the microsomal electron transport system. At the present time, no qualitatively distinct cytochrome P-450 species or specific binding protein has been identified, although the control of induction of splenic cytochrome P-450 appears to be different from that of hepatic cytochrome P-450 (14). An in vivo model for heme catabolism proposed by Kondo, Nicholson, Jackson and Kenner (17) postulates intermediates in heme catabolism that might require an additional enzyme moiety, but there is as yet no direct evidence. What is of interest is the fact that although phenobarbital is known to induce delta-aminolevulinic acid (ALA) synthetase, stimulate hepatic heme synthesis (19) and synthesis of microsomal hemoproteins (20), increase the activity of hepatic UDP-glucuronyl transferase (21-24) and levels of Y protein

(25), and stimulate hepatic bilirubin uptake (26), it has no effect on hepatic or splenic heme oxygenase activity (14-16). It would therefore appear that the well defined phenobarbital-induced decrease in unconjugated bilirubin in normals (27-29) and patients with Gilbert's syndrome (30) cannot be attributed to any change in capacity for enzymatic heme catabolism. The fact that increased hepatic hemoprotein turnover produced in animals by phenobarbital pre-treatment is not associated with increased activity of hepatic heme oxygenase may help provide an explanation for the observation that phenobarbital treatment does not significantly increase bile bilirubin excretion in rats (31).

A single pulse dose of intravenous heme has been shown by Tschudy et al (32) to cause a series of cyclic oscillations in hepatic ALA-synthetase activity after the initial decrease caused by end-product repression (18,32,33) and possibly inhibition (34) of hepatic ALA synthetase by heme. We have recently demonstrated that a single intravenous pulse dose of heme in rats also produces cyclic oscillations in hepatic heme oxygenase that appear to be reciprocally related to the oscillations in hepatic ALA-synthetase (fig.3). 150 gm female Sprague-Dawley rats that had been fasted for 48 hours were given 2.55 µmoles heme/100 gm as MHA intravenously by tail vein injection, and groups of rats were killed at various time intervals and assays of hepatic heme oxygenase and ALA synthetase were done. ALA-synthetase activity drops to 45% of control activity 4 hours after heme administration, and then rises to levels 250% above control at 8 to 12 hours. Progressively damped cyclic oscillations in ALA synthetase activity are seen at

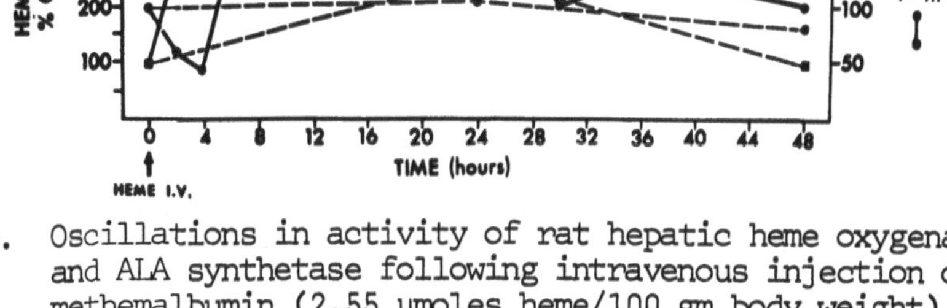

Fig. 3. Oscillations in activity of rat hepatic heme oxygenase and ALA synthetase following intravenous injection of methemalbumin (2.55 µmoles heme/100 gm body weight). The dotted lines represent values in control groups given 2.5% (W/V) human serum albumin instead of methemalbumin.

24 and 36 hours after injection before declining to control levels again at 48 hours. Heme oxygenase activity however, demonstrates a rapid initial increase to 350% of control levels at 4 hours, followed by a series of oscillations at 20, 30 and 48 hours following heme administration. Control rats given albumin demonstrated levels of activity of heme oxygenase and ALA-synthetase at 24 and 48 hours that did not differ significantly from the control values. These complimentary oscillations in ALA-synthetase and heme oxygenase suggest that the perturbation in hepatic heme metabolism evoked by a pulse dose of heme results in rapid changes in both heme synthesis and catabolism designed to restore metabolic homeostasis. The resultant overshoots in, first, heme catabolism, and then in heme synthesis result in a series of progressively damped secondary inductive effects on both enzyme systems until homeostasis in hepatic heme metabolism is again attained.

These adaptive changes in hepatic heme oxygenase in response to varying substrate load may be of importance in regulating intracellular hepatic heme levels and their disposition in response to hepatic heme synthesis, hepatic heme and hemoprotein turnover (19, 20,31), and also in the catabolism of hemoglobin presented to hepatic parenchymal cells (9).

Bissell, Hammaker and Schmid have recently shown that the manner of presentation of hemoglobin to the liver greatly influences the mechanism of its catabolism to bile pigment at that site (9). Working with pure isolates of hepatic parenchymal and sinusoidal cells, they were able to demonstrate that the intravenous infusion of free hemoglobin caused a four-fold increase in hepatic parenchymal cell heme oxygenase activity with quantitatively insignificant induction of hepatic sinusoidal cell heme oxygenase activity (9). In contrast, infusion of spherocytic red cells containing a comparable total amount of hemoglobin produced a doubling of sinusoidal cell heme oxygenase activity with no detectable change in parenchymal cell activity. Studies with isotopically-labelled hemoglobin demonstrated that at least 85% of the labelled hemoglobin was taken up and degraded by hepatic parenchymal cells, while almost all of the Fe^{59}-labelled heat-damaged spherocytic red cells were phagocytosed by hepatic sinusoidal cells. These experiments demonstrate that both hepatic parenchymal and sinusoidal cells can participate in hemoglobin catabolism, but their roles are quite different; parenchymal cells have the capacity to catabolize plasma hemoglobin and parenchymal cell heme oxygenase can be stimulated by free hemoglobin, while sinusoidal cell capacity for heme catabolism is responsive primarily to requirements for destruction of phagocytosed red cells.

The important role of the reticuloendothelial cell in hemoglobin catabolism is therefore evident on the basis of the high specific and total activity of splenic heme oxygenase (1,7,14,15) the great capacity for induction of rabbit alveolar macrophage and rat peritoneal macrophage heme oxygenase activity by exposure to hemoglobin (10) or MHA (35) and the capacity of hepatic sinusoidal cells for erythrophagocytosis and heme catabolism (9).

These observations suggest that the primary function of the adaptive response of heme oxygenase in reticuloendothelial cells is directed towards changes in requirements for catabolism of hemoglobin from breakdown of senescent red cells, while the function of the adaptive response of hepatic parenchymal cell heme oxygenase may be confined to variations in the fractional catabolic rate of hepatic heme and hemoproteins and to catabolism of plasma hemoglobin derived from intravascular hemolysis.

Although rat kidney contains negligible basal levels of heme oxygenase activity, a 30 to 100-fold increase in activity follows the production of hemoglobinuria by injection of hemoglobin in amounts in excess of the plasma haptoglobin-binding capacity (8). This activity is confined mainly to renal cortex, and was identified in dissected proximal tubular cells (8). Hemoglobin filtered by the renal glomerulus appears to regulate this process, and the suggestion has been made that induction of heme oxygenase occurs in response to the presentation of hemoglobin to the renal tubular epithelial cells in a process designed to maintain renal functional homeostasis and minimize renal iron loss by reabsorption and catabolism of part of the filtered hemoglobin load in situations where the plasma binding capacity for hemoglobin is depleted by chronic intravascular hemolysis (8).

At the present time, there is limited evidence available as to whether the mechanism of induction of heme oxygenase involves the synthesis of some new enzyme moiety or binding protein, enzyme stabilization, or to an increase in some active cell type. It is known that the induction of heme oxygenase in rat kidney can be inhibited by cycloheximide, puromycin, and actinomycin D (8), and puromycin and actinomycin D also inhibit heme oxygenase induction in peritoneal macrophages (10). Hepatic heme oxygenase induction by methemalbumin _in vivo_ is also inhibited by cycloheximide, but not to a significant degree by pre-treatment with actinomycin D (fig.4). These data suggest that the functional adaptation to allow heme catabolism via heme oxygenase is dependent on protein synthesis, but the requirement for transcriptional processes in the induction process is not yet clearly defined in some organs. The addition of heme to hepatic microsomes in concentrations known to be reached by _in vivo_ administration of heme (1 nmole heme/mg microsomal protein) (19) and pre-incubation of the treated microsomes for two hours at 10°C does not result in any induction of hepatic heme oxygenase (36). This implies a role for an active process involved in heme

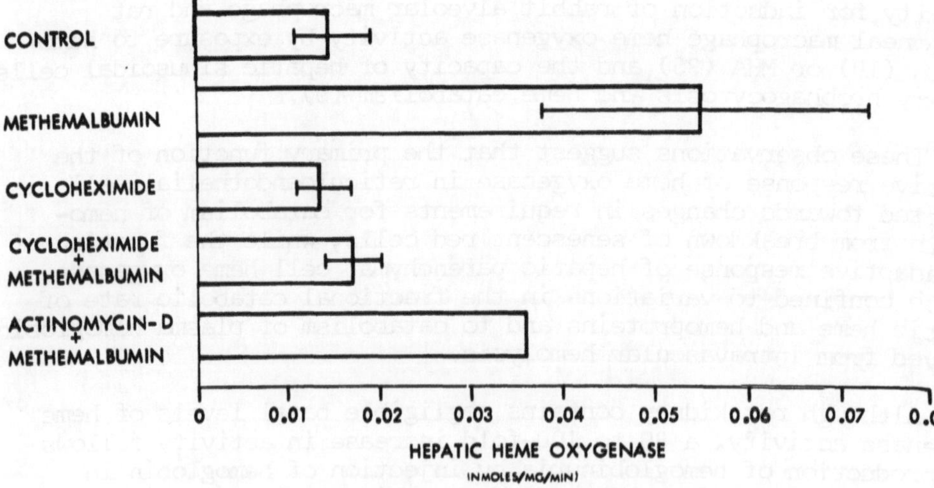

Fig. 4. The effect of cycloheximide and actinomycin D on the induction of hepatic heme oxygenase in vivo. At 0 time groups of rats, fasted for 24 hours, were given either cycloheximide (1.8 mg/kg) or actinomycin D (1.5 mg/kg) or 0.9% NaCl subcutaneously. At 1 hour certain groups received methemalbumin IP (4 µmoles/100 gm body weight) and at 15 hours all groups were killed. Hepatic heme oxygenase activity was measured as previously described (3).

oxygenase induction which does not involve activation of pre-formed enzyme by substrate.

Several other metabolic parameters which modify heme oxygenase activity and the rate of heme catabolism have recently been defined. Bakken, Thaler, and Schmid have demonstrated that fasting rats for up to 72 hours produces a three-fold induction of hepatic heme oxygenase (37) and these results have been confirmed, although the time course of induction was shorter and less pronounced (15). Refeeding rats within this time period caused a rapid return of hepatic heme oxygenase to basal levels. Insulin or mannose-induced hypoglycemia also produced marked induction of hepatic heme oxygenase which was reduced or abolished by concomitant administration of glucose (37). Glucagon and epinephrine also caused induction of hepatic heme oxygenase, and their effects were additive (37). Cyclic AMP and di-butyryl cyclic AMP, which are known to mediate the action of epinephrine and glucagon, also induced hepatic heme oxygenase. Thyroxin and hydrocortisone had no effect on hepatic heme oxygenase activity. Neither fasting nor any of these agents has any effect on splenic heme oxygenase. Fasting of pregnant rats for 3 days produced a 20% increase in heme oxygenase activity of fetuses and newborns (38).

A sudden increase in hepatic heme oxygenase activity has been observed in newborn rats within 10 hours of birth, and this high activity reaches a peak at seven days, followed by a slow decline to adult levels at weaning (38). In contrast, newborn splenic heme oxygenase did not demonstrate this response. There is speculation that this increase in hepatic heme oxygenase activity occurs as the result of the relative hypoglycemia resulting from interruption of maternal glucose supplies and low newborn hepatic glycogen levels. This hypoglycemia may lead to induction of hepatic heme oxygenase through increased release of glucagon and epinephrine (37,38). Taking into consideration the low levels of UDP-glucuronyl transferase in the newborn, it has been postulated that the disparity between the increased potential to produce bilirubin and the relative inability to conjugate it may be responsible for the severe unconjugated hyperbilirubinemia seen in premature infants and infants of diabetic mothers, who are prone to hypoglycemia in the perinatal period (38). It has also been shown that epinephrine and glucagon cause a 3 - 5 fold increase in CO production from non-erythrocytic heme sources and a significant expansion of the total bilirubin pool without any evident hemolysis (39). Fasting also augments CO production in man (40).

These results suggest that the origin of the fasting hyperbilirubinemia which has been described in both normal man (41-43) and patients with Gilbert's syndrome (44) may in part be related to the marked induction of hepatic heme oxygenase and the consequent increased capacity for bilirubin production demonstrated experimentally in rats fasted or treated with hormones such as glucagon and epinephrine which are released during the fasting hypoglycemic state (45). However, it should be mentioned that although prolonged fasting does not appear to affect plasma bilirubin turnover in man nor whole body bilirubin turnover in Gunn rats it does significantly decrease plasma bilirubin clearance (43), so that this might be an additional factor of importance in the etiology of fasting hyperbilirubinemia. Another factor whose importance has not been quantitated is the "glucose effect" on ALA synthetase, the rate controlling enzyme in heme biosynthesis. Since the induction of hepatic ALA synthetase can be blocked by carbohydrate intake (46,47), it is possible that induction of ALA synthetase and heme synthesis might take place in the absence of sufficient carbohydrate intake (i.e. fasting) (48,49) producing a significant increase in the substrate load presented to heme oxygenase.

While the fasting state appears to promote induction of hepatic heme oxygenase, the availability of glucose seems to have a much different effect on heme catabolism in peritoneal macrophages. Gemsa et al (10) have shown that adding hydrocortisone in concentrations of 0.1 mg/ml of medium to an in vitro system containing rat peritoneal macrophages and antibody-coated erythrocytes completely inhibited heme oxygenase induction without any

TABLE III

Sites and Mechanisms of Induction of Bile Pigment Formation

Site	Effect on Heme Oxygenase	Effector	References
Liver Parenchymal Cells	Increased activity	Heme	3, 6, 7
		Hemoglobin	9
		Hypoglycemia	37
		Glucagon	37
		Epinephrine	37
		Cyclic AMP	37
		Endotoxin	55
Liver Sinusoidal Cells	Increased activity	Phagocytosed Erythrocytes	9
		Endotoxin	37
Liver	No effect	Phenobarbital	14, 15, 16
		3,4-Benzpyrene	14
		Pregnenolone-16α-carbonitrile	14
		Hydrocortisone	37
		Thyroxin	37
		Adrenalectomy	7, 37
		Oophorectomy	37
		Dicarbethoxydihydrocollidine	15
	Decreased activity	3-Methylcholanthrene	14
		Allylisopropylacetamide	15
Spleen	Increased activity	Zymosan	7
		Hemolytic anemia	7

(TABLE III cont'd)

Spleen	No effect	Phenobarbital	14, 15
		3,4 Benzpyrene	14
		Pregnenolene-16α-carbonitrile	14
		Hypoglycemia	37
		Glucagon	37
		Epinephrine	37
		Adrenalectomy	37
	Decreased activity	3-Methylcholanthrene	14
Macrophages	Increased activity	Heme	35
		Phagocytosed erythrocytes	10
		Glucose ± insulin	10
		Endotoxin	55
	Inhibits induction	Hydrocortisone	10
	No effect	Zymosan	35
		BCG	35
Kidney	Increased activity	Hemoglobin	8

suppression of erythrophagocytosis. The suppressive effect of hydrocortisone on heme oxygenase induction was reversible by the addition of glucose or glucose and insulin to the incubation medium, if added within three hours of the start of incubation. Hydrocortisone decreased glucose removal from the macrophage incubation medium and decreased CO_2 production from glucose via the hexose monophosphate shunt. Both these effects were reversed by glucose and insulin. These findings suggest that heme catabolism in reticuloendothelial cells is dependent on adequate glucose transport or metabolism, and that hydrocortisone interferes with this process. The exact nature of this steroid effect and of the requirement of macrophage heme oxygenase induction for glucose remains to be explained, but it does highlight several interesting points: It appears from these data (10) that glucose is required for induction of reticuloendothelial cell heme oxygenase, but glucose deprivation leads to induction of hepatic parenchymal cell heme oxygenase (15, 37,38). Thus the control of induction by glucose in these two cell types is quite different as may be the nature of the regulatory processes. Also, since erythrophagocytosis may proceed without hindrance at pharmacological levels of hydrocortisone, the disposition of macrophage-ingested hemoglobin heme in these situations is not clear at the present time, although it has been suggested that heme may simply accumulate in the macrophages or may be degraded by alternate pathways to catabolic products other than bilirubin (10). There is no direct evidence as yet for either of these possibilities, although alternate degradative pathways may in fact exist (50-52). On the basis of these studies, it has been hypothesized that the amelioration of hyperbilirubinemia by steroids observed in patients with parenchymal or obstructive liver disease (53,54) may result from decreased bile pigment formation from phagocytosed erythrocytes during steroid therapy (10).

Bacterial endotoxin has recently been shown to enhance induction of heme oxygenase activity in rat peritoneal macrophages active in erythrophagocytosis (55). Endotoxin produced this change without evidence of injury to the incubated erythrocytes, without enhancement of erythrophagocytosis itself, and without evidence of stimulation of carbohydrate, protein or RNA metabolism in the incubated macrophages (55). Endotoxin given in vivo also stimulated induction of hepatic parenchymal and sinusoidal cell heme oxygenase activity two or three-fold. On the basis of these findings, it has been postulated that endotoxin directly stimulates heme oxygenase by an as yet undefined mechanism (55). This experimental observation offers a possible explanation for the hyperbilirubinemia sometimes observed in gram-negative bacteremia in man (56).

Table III summarizes the effects of various agents and manoeuvres on heme oxygenase activity in various tissues that have been studied. The conclusion to be drawn from all the information that has recently accrued is that mechanisms do exist to facilitate and enhance the formation of bile pigments as the substrate load varies, whether the substrate is heme, hemoglobin, or other hemoproteins. These mechanisms would appear to be regulated to a degree by some hormones, by the nutritional status of the animal, and by some exogenous influences (e.g. endotoxin), but the over-all activity of this system is clearly designed to allow efficient catabolism of whatever substrate load is presented at various sites and in various forms.

SUMMARY

Bile pigment formation is regulated primarily by heme oxygenase, a microsomal enzyme which promotes the oxidative catabolism of heme. Substrate-mediated induction of heme oxygenase has been demonstrated in liver, kidney, and macrophages, and this is the most important mode of regulation of enzyme activity and of the rate of bile pigment formation. Induction of heme oxygenase is dependent on protein synthesis, may be influenced by the rate of endogenous heme synthesis, and is regulated by heme in different forms in different tissues (e.g. hemoglobin in hepatic parenchymal cells; phagocytosed erythrocytes in hepatic sinusoidal cells). The fasting state, some hormones, the availability of glucose to macrophages, and bacterial endotoxin also promote induction of heme oxygenase and increased formation of bile pigment, but the regulation of bilirubin formation is most closely related to accommodating the changing requirements for heme and hemoglobin catabolism in reticuloendothelial and other tissues.

ACKNOWLEDGEMENT

Supported by a grant from the Medical Research Council of Canada.

REFERENCES

1. TENHUNEN R, MARVER HS, SCHMID R: The enzymatic conversion of heme to bilirubin by microsomal heme oxygenase. Proc Nat Acad Sci USA 61: 748-754, 1968.

2. TENHUNEN R, MARVER HS, SCHMID R: Microsomal heme oxygenase, characterization of the enzyme. J Biol Chem 244: 6388-6394, 1969.

3. SCHACTER BA, NELSON EB, MARVER HS et al: Immunochemical evidence for an association of heme oxygenase with the microsomal electron transport system. J Biol Chem 247: 3601-3607, 1972.

4. TENHUNEN R, MARVER H, PIMSTONE NR et al: Enzymatic degradation of heme. Oxygenative cleavage requiring cytochrome P-450. Biochem 11: 1716-1720, 1972.

5. TENHUNEN R, ROSS ME, MARVER HS et al: Reduced nicotinamide-adenine dinucleotide phosphate dependent biliverdin reductase: Partial purification and characterization. Biochem 9: 298-303, 1970.

6. TENHUNEN R: The enzymatic degradation of heme. Sem Hemat 9: 19-29, 1972.

7. TENHUNEN R, MARVER HS, SCHMID R: The enzymatic catabolism of hemoglobin: Stimulation of microsomal heme oxygenase by hemin. J Lab Clin Med 75: 410-421, 1970.

8. PIMSTONE NR, ENGEL P, TENHUNEN R et al: Inducible heme oxygenase in the kidney: A model for the homeostatic control of hemoglobin catabolism. J Clin Invest 50: 2042-2050, 1971.

9. BISSELL DM, HAMMAKER L, SCHMID R: Hemoglobin and erythrocyte catabolism in rat liver: The separate roles of parenchymal and sinusoidal cells. Blood 40: 812-822, 1972.

10. GEMSA D, WOO CH, FUDENBERG HH et al: Erythrocyte catabolism by macrophages in vitro. The effect of hydrocortisone on erythrophagocytosis and on the induction of heme oxygenase. J Clin Invest 52: 812-822, 1973.

11. GILLETTE JR: Biochemistry of drug oxidation and reduction by enzymes in hepatic endoplasmic reticulum. Advan Pharmacol 4: 219-261, 1966.

12. SLADEK NE, MANNERING GJ: Evidence for a new P-450 hemoprotein in hepatic microsomes from methylcholanthrene treated rats. Biochem Biophys Res Commun 24: 668-674, 1966.

13. CONNEY AH: Pharmacological implications of microsomal enzyme induction. Pharmacol Rev 19: 317-366, 1967.

14. SCHACTER BA, MASON JI: The effect of phenobarbital, 3-methylcholanthrene, 3,4-benzpyrene, and pregnenolone-16α-carbonitrile on microsomal heme oxygenase and splenic cytochrome P-450. Arch Biochem Biophys 160: 274-278, 1974.

15. ROTHWELL JD, LACROIX S, SWEENEY GD: Evidence against a regulatory role for heme oxygenase in hepatic heme synthesis. Biochim Biophys Acta 304: 871-874, 1973.

16. HUPKA AL, KARLER R: Biotransformation of ethylmorphine and heme by isolated parenchymal and reticuloendothelial cells of rat liver. J Reticuloendothel Soc 14: 225-241, 1973.

17. KONDO T, NICHOLSON DC, JACKSON AH et al: Isotopic studies of the conversion of oxophlorins and their ferrihaems into bile pigments in the rat. Biochem J 121: 601-607, 1971.

18. GRANICK S: The induction in vitro of the synthesis of delta-aminolevulinic acid synthetase in chemical porphyria: A response to certain drugs, sex hormones, and foreign chemicals. J Biol Chem 241: 1359-1375, 1966.

19. MARVER HS: The role of heme in the synthesis and repression of microsomal protein, in Microsomes and Drug Oxidations, edited by GILLETTE JR, CONNEY AH, COSMIDES GJ, ESTABROOK RW, FOUTS JR, MANNERING GJ, New York, Academic Press, 1969. p. 495.

20. REMMER H, MERKER HJ: Effect of drugs on the formation of smooth endoplasmic reticulum and drug-metabolizing enzymes. Ann NY Acad Sci 123: 79-97, 1965.

21. DE LEON A, GARTNER LM, ARIAS IM: The effect of phenobarbital on hyperbilirubinemia in glucuronyl transferase deficient rats. J Lab Clin Med 70: 273-278, 1967.

22. CATZ C, YAFFE SJ: Barbiturate enhancement of bilirubin conjugation and excretion in young and adult animals. Pediat Res 2: 361-370, 1968.

23. WINSNES A: Studies on the activation in vitro of glucuronyl transferase. Biochim Biophys Acta 91: 279-291, 1969.

24. POTREPKA RF, SPRATT JL: Effect of phenobarbital and 3-methylcholanthrene pretreatment on guinea pig hepatic microsomal bilirubin glucoronyltransferase activity. Biochem Pharm 20: 861-867, 1971.

25. REYES H, LEVI AJ, GATMAITAN Z et al: Studies of Y and Z, two hepatic cytoplasmic organic anion-binding proteins: Effect of drugs, chemicals, hormones, and cholestasis. J Clin Invest 50: 2242-2252, 1971.

26. ROBERTS RJ, PLAA GL: Effect of phenobarbital on the excretion of an exogenous bilirubin load. Biochem Pharm 16: 827-835, 1967.

27. TROLLE D: Decrease of total serum bilirubin concentration in newborn infants after phenobarbitone treatment. Lancet 2: 705-708, 1968.

28. THOMPSON RPH, EDDLESTON ALWF, WILLIAMS R: Low plasma bilirubin in epileptics on phenobarbitone. Lancet 1: 21-22, 1969.

29. YEUNG CY, FIELD CE: Phenobarbitone therapy in neonatal hyperbilirubinemia. Lancet 2: 135-140, 1969.

30. BLACK M, SHERLOCK S: Treatment of Gilbert's Syndrome with phenobarbitone. Lancet 1: 1359-1362, 1970.

31. LEVITT M, SCHACTER BA, ZIPURSKY A et al: The nonerythropoietic component of early bilirubin. J Clin Invest 47: 1281-1294, 1968.

32. WAXMAN AD, COLLINS A, TSCHUDY DP: Oscillations of hepatic delta-aminolevulinic acid synthetase produced in vivo by heme. Biochem Biophys Res Commun 24: 675-683, 1966.

33. MARVER HS, TSCHUDY DP, PERLROTH MG et al: Coordinate synthesis of heme and apoenzyme in the formation of tryptophane pyrrolase. Science 154: 501-503, 1966.

34. SCHOLNICK PL, HAMMAKER LE, MARVER HS: Soluble hepatic ALA synthetase: End-product inhibition of the partially purified enzyme. Proc Nat Acad Sci (USA) 63: 65-70, 1969.

35. PIMSTONE NR, TENHUNEN R, SEITZ PT et al: The enzymatic degradation of hemoglobin to bile pigments by macrophages. J Exp Med 133: 1264-1281, 1971.

36. SCHACTER BA: Unpublished observations.

37. BAKKEN AF, THALER MM, SCHMID R: Metabolic regulation of heme catabolism and bilirubin production. I Hormonal control of hepatic heme oxygenase activity. J Clin Invest 51: 530-536, 1972.

38. THALER MM, GEMES DL, BAKKEN AF: Enzymatic conversion of heme to bilirubin in normal and starved fetuses and newborn rats. Pediat Res 6: 197-201, 1972.

39. DAWBER NH, BAKKEN A, SCHMID R et al: Stimulation of bilirubin production by epinephrin and glucagon. (Abstract). Gastroenterology 66: 881, 1974.

40. LUNDH B, JOHANSSON B, MERCKE C et al: Enhancement of heme catabolism by caloric restriction in man. Scand J Lab Clin Invest 30: 421-427, 1972.

41. GILBERT A, HERSCHER M: Sur les variations de la cholemie physiologique. Presse Med 14: 209-211, 1906.

42. BARRETT PVD: Hyperbilirubinemia of fasting. J A M A 217: 1349-1353, 1971.

43. BLOOMER JR, BARRET PV, RODKEY FL et al: Studies on the mechanism of fasting hyperbilirubinemia. Gastroenterol 61: 479-487, 1971.

44. FELSHER BF, RICKARD D, REDEKER AG: The reciprocal relation between caloric intake and the degree of hyperbilirubinemia in Gilbert's syndrome. New Engl J Med 283: 170-172, 1970.

45. SOKAL, JE: Glucagon, an essential hormone. Amer J Med 41: 331-341, 1966.

46. TSCHUDY DP, WELLAND FH, COLLINS A et al: The effect of carbohydrate feeding on the induction of delta-aminolevulinic acid synthetase. Metabolism 13: 396-406, 1964.

47. MARVER HS, COLLINS A, TSCHUDY DP et al: Delta-aminolevulinic acid synthetase. II Induction in rat liver. J Biol Chem 241: 1359-1375, 1966.

48. WELLAND FH, HELLMAN ES, GADDIS EM et al: Factors affecting the excretion of porphyrin precursors by patients with acute intermittent porphyria. I The effect of diet. Metabolism 13: 232-250, 1964.

49. FELSHER BF, REDEKER AG: Acute intermittent porphyria: Effect of diet and griseofulvin. Medicine (Baltimore) 46: 217-223, 1967.

50. GOLDSTEIN GW, HAMMAKER L, SCHMID R: The catabolism of Heinz bodies; An experimental model demonstrating conversion to non-bilirubin catabolites. Blood 31: 388-395, 1968.

51. LANDAW SA, CALLAHAN EW, SCHMID R: Catabolism of heme in vivo: Comparison of the simultaneous production of bilirubin and carbon monoxide. J Clin Invest 49: 914-925, 1970.

52. SCHACTER BA, MARVER HS, MEYER UA: Hemoprotein catabolism during stimulation of microsomal lipid peroxidation. Biochim Biophys Acta 279: 221-227, 1972.

53. KATZ RM, DUCCI H, ALESSANDRI H: Influence of cortisone and prednisolone on hyperbilirubinemia. J Clin Invest 36: 1370-1374, 1957.

54. SCHIFF L: The use of steroids in liver disease. Medicine (Baltimore) 45: 565-573, 1966.

55. GEMSA D, WOO CH, FUDENBERG HH et al: Stimulation of heme oxygenase in macrophages and liver by endotoxin. J Clin Invest 53: 647-651, 1974.

56. VERMILLION SE, GREGG JA, BAGGENSTOSS AH et al: Jaundice associated with bacteremia. Arch Intern Med 124: 611-618, 1969.

CARBON MONOXIDE PRODUCTION AS A MEASUREMENT OF HEME CATABOLISM

Stephen A. Landaw

Veterans Administration Hospital

Syracuse, New York 13210

INTRODUCTION

During the Second World War, Sweden was obliged to use producer gas in place of gasoline for automobile propulsion, and many cases of carbon monoxide (CO) poisoning resulted. While studying CO levels in blood and expired air in affected and control patients, Sjöstrand noted that CO was produced endogenously in normal subjects, and that subjects with increased heme turnover showed increased CO production. These early studies, which have been summarized elsewhere (1) suggested that 1 mole of CO was produced for each mole of heme degraded in vitro and in vivo. Twenty years later, investigators at the University of Pennsylvania were able to confirm and amplify Sjöstrand's original observations in a large series of publications. Over the past 10 years, additional laboratories have become interested in the measurement of endogenous CO production. While, in general, measurement of endogenous CO production is still a research procedure not available outside large teaching institutions, it has become recognized as perhaps the most accurate measure of heme catabolism now available. Coburn has recently reviewed the progress and significance of research in endogenous CO production (2).

TOTAL ENDOGENOUS CO PRODUCTION: MAN

As noted previously, Sjöstrand was responsible for the first observations concerning endogenous CO production in both experimental animals and man. He was able, as had Grehant (3), Nicloux (4), and others, to confirm the presence of a combustible gas in blood, and to show that the concentration of CO was higher in expired air than inspired air. Further, in certain hospitalized patients, blood CO was found to be markedly increased. These patients had in common an increased turnover of hemoglobin, either due to trauma, mismatched blood transfusions, or hematologic disease (5). Sjöstrand's later experiments with myoglobin and hemoglobin solutions indicated that CO could be produced in vitro in an amount equal to the heme content of the solutions (6). Further, he showed that injection of hemolyzed blood and hemoglobin solutions increased endogenous CO production in experimental animals and man in vivo (7). The increased CO production was noted to be approximately one mole of CO for every mole of heme injected.

From these studies, he concluded that the alpha-methene bridge carbon atom of heme, which is lost upon transformation of heme to bile pigment, is excreted intact in the breath as CO. In 1957, Engstedt extended these observations, and noted that there was a strong correlation between blood CO content (COHgb), corrected for estimated circulating hemoglobin mass, and such well-accepted parameters of RBC turnover as reticulocyte percentage, stercobilin excretion, and ^{51}Cr RBC survival (8). Following these publications, a large number of articles appeared, primarily in the Scandinavian literature, indicating the usefulness of these measurements in clinical situations (9-17).

In 1963, Coburn, Blakemore, and Forster published a method for determination of endogenous CO production using a rebreathing apparatus (18). Their study indicated that blood CO content rose linearly with time after placing the patient in a closed rebreathing system with constant pO_2, after a short equilibration time. Total heme mass was determined by the dilution method: i.e. by the observed increment in blood CO content following addition of a known volume of pure CO to the rebreathing system. Endogenous CO production was then calculated as the product of the total heme mass (as defined above) and the rate of increase of COHgb (%/hour). If total body heme mass is stated in micromoles, the result becomes micromoles of CO produced per hour, although the authors originally chose to state their results in terms of ml/hr (STPD). In 10 normal subjects, they found endogenous CO production (V_{CO}) to be 0.42 ± 0.07 (SD) ml/hr.

In a subsequent publication appearing in 1964, Coburn, Williams, and Forster investigated the effect of hemoglobin destruction on endogenous CO production by injecting RBC damaged with N-ethylmaleimide (19), and measuring the effect on CO production in the closed rebreathing system. In 5 subjects, the rate of CO production was found to increase after injection of damaged RBC. The amount of this increase corresponded to a molar yield of CO equalling 97 ± 6 (SE)% of the heme content of the injected RBC. This study provided further confirmation of Sjöstrand's original findings, and helped set up the quantitative basis for the Vco measurement as an accurate estimation of in vivo heme catabolism.

These authors calculated the endogenous CO production to be expected from RBC catabolism, assuming a RBC lifespan of 120 days, and obtained a value of 0.32 ml/hr from this source. They noted that the previously-obtained value of 0.42 ml/hr was greater than this value, and speculated that the additional CO arose from the same sources responsible for "early peak" production of bile pigments. Their value of 23% of total CO production for these sources was in fair agreement with the estimates of 10-15% of total bile pigment production, as obtained by London et al (20).

In 1966, Coburn, Williams and Kahn reported the use of the rebreathing apparatus in 7 subjects with hemolytic anemia (21). In all subjects Vco was increased, although venous COHgb was normal in one subject. Erythrocyte survival was determined in all subjects, using ^{51}Cr, and heme turnover was compared using the ^{51}Cr and Vco data. A strong linear correlation was found ($r = 0.94$) between these independent measures of heme turnover. While the slope of the regression was nearly unity (1.04), Vco exceeded the calculated turnover of circulating RBC by 40%, as compared to their previously published value of 23% in normal controls. The authors concluded that this additional CO production was not artifactual, and may have arisen from co-existing ineffective erythropoiesis. As noted in a previous paper (22), they further concluded that venous COHgb is a relatively imprecise index of RBC survival.

In 1969, Coltman and Dudley reported results in 11 normal subjects, and in 7 subjects with suspected increased heme turnover (23), utilizing the rebreathing method of Coburn and co-workers. Their data supported the original work by Coburn et al (18) in that a linear increase in venous COHgb was found during 2½ hours of rebreathing. Further, their value for Vco in normal subjects (20.2 ± 3.7 (SD) μm/hr) was in excellent agreement with that of Coburn et al (18) (18.8 ± 3.2μm/hr). The authors noted that additional information could be gained by plotting fractional heme turnover (DRf, or the ratio of Vco to total heme mass) versus total heme mass. They suggested that this plot is of value in understanding the hematologic status of the patient (marrow failure, ineffective erythropoiesis, compensated hemolysis, etc.).

An additional method for determination of Vco was presented by Logue et al (24) in 1971. These authors used the rebreathing method of Coburn et al, but measured the increment in CO in the gas phase, rather than in the blood. As with the blood phase method, the authors found a linear increase in gas phase CO with time. Further, they found a strong linear correlation between RBC lifespan (^{32}DFP) and fractional heme turnover (total body heme/Vco) ($r = 0.91$) in 8 patients with hemolytic anemia. However, in 8 studies in normal subjects, Vco averaged 28 μm/hr. This value is approximately 50% larger than that obtained by Coburn et al (18) and by Coltman and Dudley (23). Their conclusion that 42% of endogenous CO production arises from sources other than circulating RBC destruction does not appear to be supported by results using other techniques, such as "early peak" ^{14}CO studies and bilirubin turnover studies (vide infra), all of which suggest that such sources account for not more than about 20% of total CO production.

In 1974, Berk et al (25) reported the comparison of simultaneous measurements of Vco and bilirubin turnover. CO production was measured using the Coburn rebreathing method, and bilirubin turnover was determined from the disappearance of labeled bilirubin (26). The average value for Vco in normals was 22.7 μm/hr, in agreement with values obtained by others using this method (18,23). There was a strong linear correlation between Vco and bilirubin turnover (r = 0.99), with Vco exceeding bilirubin turnover by approximately 14%. Bilirubin turnover, as measured, does not include a portion of hepatic heme turnover, since some of the bilirubin thus derived is excreted directly into the bile without passage through plasma. Since this fraction amounts to 13-21% of bilirubin production (27), it is likely that this fraction accounts for the above discrepancy. The authors concluded, therefore, that bilirubin and CO production are quantitatively equivalent.

It should be pointed out in this regard, that the tests used for comparing Vco to heme turnover do not measure the same phenomena, and that direct comparison of Vco with a fully equivalent test has yet to be performed. Table I indicates a number of these tests and the phenomena which are measured. It is obvious that only Vco measures all phenomena.

TABLE I

PHENOMENA MEASURED BY 3 TESTS EMPLOYED FOR DETERMINING HEME TURNOVER

Study	RBC Destruction	Erythropoiesis-associated heme turnover*	Hepatic heme turnover
RBC survival	Yes	No	No
Bilirubin turnover	Yes	Yes	No
CO production	Yes	Yes	Yes

* Includes "ineffective erythropoiesis"

KINETICS OF ENDOGENOUS CO PRODUCTION

1. In Man:

In 1967, White et al (28) reported on the production of carbon-14 labeled CO in normal subjects, and in several patients with ineffective erythropoiesis. These authors built the study around the observations that the methylene (#2) carbon atom of glycine is the source of the alpha-methene bridge carbon atom of heme (29), which, in turn, is the sole source of endogenously-produced CO in mammals. Earlier studies by Ludwig, Blakemore, and Drabkin in 1957 (30) had shown that the oxidation of ^{14}C-hemin in vitro produced ^{14}CO from one of the 4 methene bridge carbon atoms. The resulting bile pigment was of the alpha-urobilin type, indicating that the ^{14}CO arose from the alpha-methene bridge carbon atom.

In their patients, White et al noted that ^{14}CO was produced in both an "early peak" and a "late peak", as had been noted for the bile pigments (31,32). The "late peak" was maximal at approximately 120 days after glycine-2-^{14}C injection, corresponding to the accepted value for RBC lifespan in man. In one normal subject, the "early peak" appeared within minutes of glycine injection, became maximal in 1-2 days, falling to 20% of peak values at 6 days. The magnitude of this "early labeled peak" (ELP) was estimated at 6.5 to 10% of total potential ^{14}CO production in 2 normal subjects.

Five patients with ineffective erythropoiesis were studied. In 4 of the patients, Vco was increased. In these 4 patients, Vco ranged from 150-410% above that expected from simultaneously-performed ^{51}Cr studies, indicating that the major source for the CO was not derived from circulating RBC. Labeled CO studies were performed in 3 of these subjects, and the ELP represented 49-76% of total potential ^{14}CO production. Together with the increased Vco, increased plasma iron turnover, stercobilin excretion, simultaneous RBC survival, and marrow erythroid hyperplasia, it seems reasonable to conclude that these results are indicative of markedly increased destruction of RBC precursors within the bone marrow (ineffective erythropoiesis).

The shape of the ELP in the normal and abnormal subjects is of some interest. Animal experiments (vide infra), and bilirubin studies (33,34) have suggested that the ELP is made up of at least 2 major components -- an initial peak portion representing hepatic heme turnover, and a slower, later portion representing erythropoiesis-associated heme turnover. In the 2 normal subjects, the ELP was maximal or near-maximal on the 2nd day, with the value on the 1st day being 75-117% of the maximal value. In the 3 abnormal patients, the ELP was maximal at 3-4 days. While the shape of the curves differed in all 3 patients, they suggested an accentuation

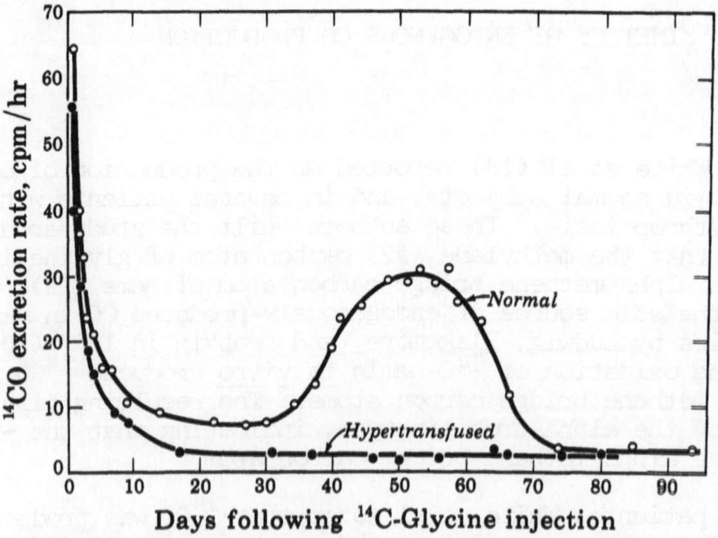

Fig. 1. ^{14}CO production in normal and hypertransfused mice. ^{14}CO production (cpm/hr) is shown in normal (open circles) and plethoric (solid circles) LAF_1 mice following injection of glycine-2-^{14}C. Note that the "late peak" is absent in the plethoric mice, identifying this component with destruction of labeled, senescent RBC. The "early peak" (downslope only shown) is still present, although reduced in magnitude. Reprinted by permission of Science (JR GOLDSMITH & SA LANDAW, Science 162: 1352-1359, 1968). Copyright 1968 by the American Association for the Advancement of Science.

of the later portion of the ELP, with one ELP being clearly biphasic. In a subsequent publication, the ELP for a patient with porphyria cutanea tarda is shown (35), and suggests an increase in the initial (or hepatic heme) portion of the ELP. While the studies in both normal and abnormal patients must be considered preliminary, these studies suggest that the separation of the ELP into its component parts is possible in man.

2. In experimental animals:

In 1966, Landow and Winchell (36) reported obtaining an "early peak" and "late peak" for ^{14}CO in the rat (Fig. 1). The "late peak" was maximal at 63-68 days, in agreement with prior studies for RBC-lifespan in this species. The ELP magnitude was originally estimated at from 15-30% of total circulating hemoglobin heme activity, in the range reported previously for bile pigment studies in man (31). A more detailed analysis of the ELP was presented in 1970 (37), in which an attempt was made to separate erythropoietic and non-erythropoietic components of the ELP. This separation was attempted by the following procedures:

1. Comparison of the ELP in normal mice with the ELP in plethoric mice. The latter have erythropoiesis virtually completely suppressed, and their ELP thus contains only non-erythropoietic components.

2. Selective increase in hepatic heme turnover using such agents as allylisopropylacetamide (AIA) and phenobarbital.

3. Selective increase in the erythropoietic component of the ELP by experimentally-produced (iron deficiency) or genetically-determined ineffective erythropoiesis.

In all these studies, as in pioneer and parallel studies performed by Robinson (38) using ^{14}C-bilirubin excretion, a clear pattern has emerged. The initial portion of the ELP (maximum at 1-3 hours after isotope injection) represents mainly non-hemoglobin heme turnover, whereas the latter portion of the ELP (maximum 8-14 hours after isotope injection) represents erythropoiesis-associated heme turnover. Clearly biphasic curves have been found in iron deficiency (ineffective erythropoiesis, 37,39) and in the intramedullary destruction of RBC precursors found after intravenous injection of lead (40,41).

In further studies (42), a model based upon these assumptions has been able to show that the "erythropoietic portion" of the ELP thus defined bore a linear relationship with the late peak in a series of rats with compensated hemolysis secondary to methylcellulose-induced splenomegaly (43)-- with a doubling of the size of the late peak causing a doubling in the size of this ELP component. This portion of the ELP represented 10% of total erythropoiesis-associated heme turnover. While the exact mechanism for this heme "wastage" in normal animals is not yet known, this value is in the range cited by Bessis as representing the fraction of total hemoglobin in the normoblast attached to the extruded nucleus (3-10%, 44). That this cannot be the complete answer for the genesis of this phase is attested to by the increase in all portions of the ELP in the erythropoietically-stimulated quail, which does not extrude the nucleus from its circulating mature erythrocyte (37,45, 46). As discussed by Levitt et al (47), it is possible that this phase represents the presence of an unassigned heme pool in the developing erythroid precursor, with a rapid turnover. Additionally, since the nucleus in the bird appears to be non-functional, the presence of this phase in birds may represent loss of heme-containing organelles during erythroid maturation.

An additional phase of ^{14}CO production was noted in mice with congenital microcytosis (mk/mk)(48), hemolytic anemia (ha/ha) (37), and in a sibling pair of NZB mice (42). In all 3 cases, an additional distinct "peak" was noted beginning at 18-24 hours after labeled glycine injection, terminating at approximately 72 hours. This time span corresponds to the maximum rate of entry of labeled RBC into the circulation (18-24 hrs) and to the time when all cells in the cohort have entered the circulation (72 hrs). All 3 groups of mice are known to have splenomegaly and hemolysis, suggesting that this phase represents splenic sequestration and destruction of reticulocytes. This was confirmed in mk/mk mice by showing that this additional phase was abolished by prior splenectomy (48).

Quantitative details concerning the "late peak" were outlined in a subsequent publication in 1970 (49). Red cell labeling following glycine injection was assumed to take the form originally proposed by Eadie and Brown (50).

$$\text{Heme}(t) = \frac{Ce^{-kt}}{(1 + e^{a(t-T)})}$$

where Heme(t) is the total activity of ^{14}C in circulating RBC hemoglobin heme (t) days after isotope injection. (C) is the size of the cohort (maximal dpm in RBC Hgb heme), (k) is the rate of random hemolysis (day^{-1}), and (a) is a measure of the spread of lifespans about the mean potential lifespan (time of senescent death, (T)). It was further assumed that death of labeled RBC represented a direct loss from this compartment, and that ^{14}CO production (the rate of labeled RBC destruction) could be represented as the first derivative with respect to time of the heme activity curve (dH/dt). Since glycine labeled 8 carbon atoms in heme, but only one in CO, the rate of ^{14}CO production should be only 1/8th of this first derivative. In rats injected with glycine-labeled, viable RBC, total ^{14}CO recovery in the "late peak" averaged 102 ± 2(SE)% of theoretical (51), confirming the quantitative nature of this ^{14}CO production. By means of a computer program, it was possible to show that ^{14}CO production following injection of labeled RBC did fit the expected function with great accuracy (49)(Fig.2), with the best-fit parameters of such curves approximating those values obtained using more conventional lifespan techniques. When the "late peak" in animals injected with glycine-2-^{14}C was obtained, it was found necessary to account for 2 more phases of ^{14}CO production, namely the long-term continuation of processes associated with non-hemoglobin heme turnover (continuation of the "early peak"), and the recycling of labeled glycine in the body's glycine pool(s) (52). This and subsequent publications have shown the ability of this model to derive useful information concerning RBC lifespan in a number of clinically-relevant experimental conditions (37,41,48,49,53,54). The "late peaks" obtained by White, Coburn, Williams and Coburn et al (28,35,55) in normal man appear to be interpretable using these same techniques.

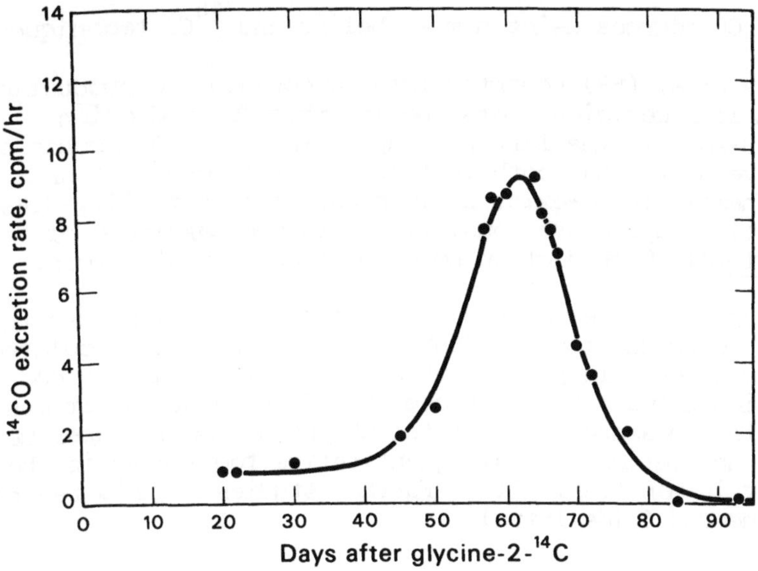

Fig. 2. ^{14}CO production in a normal rat given viable heme-labeled compatible RBC. Glycine-2-^{14}C was given to the donor at day 0, and RBC harvested and injected into host rat at day 14. Subsequent ^{14}CO production by host is shown as solid circles. Least-squares best fit of data points to function described in text is shown as the solid line. Reprinted by permission of Blood (SA LANDAW and HS WINCHELL, Blood 36: 642, 1970).

QUANTITATIVE ASPECTS OF ENDOGENOUS CO PRODUCTION

1. Experimental animals:

Initial studies by Metz and Sjöstrand indicated that several animal species produced CO in excess of that expected from normal heme turnover (56). Since these initial studies were performed with a Hopcalite meter which is not specific for CO, it was not possible to determine whether this was due to a combustible gas other than CO. Our initial studies with guinea pigs (42), however, indicated that a large amount of a gas with the infrared absorption pattern of CO was evolved from guinea pig feces, suggesting that this material was CO. Rodkey, Collison and O'Neal studied CO production in normal germ-free rats and guinea pigs (57), and were able to show that CO production (gas chromatographic method) was 2-4 times that expected from total heme turnover. They concluded that the additional CO arose from sources other than the breakdown of endogenous heme compounds, a conclusion consistent with the inability to show such additional CO sources using heme-labeling and ^{14}CO techniques.

Toskes et al (58) reported total endogenous CO production in normal and iron deficient rats, noting that CO production increased 3-fold in the latter group of animals. Bilirubin and CO studies have shown that both ineffective erythropoiesis and excessive hemolysis co-exist in iron deficient rats (37,39,49); these kinetic studies are consistent with the magnitude of increased total CO production noted by these investigators.

In dogs, Coburn et al (19) and Luomanmaki (59) showed that endogenous CO production was 250% greater than that calculated from RBC heme turnover. In view of these incompletely-understood discrepancies between heme turnover and CO production, it must be concluded that measurement of total CO production in experimental animals is not yet on the same quantitative footing as is the measurement in man (Table II). Further studies in this regard are obviously needed (vide infra).

2. In Man:

In preceding sections, it has been discussed that endogenous CO production in man is approximately 20-30% greater than that expected from turnover of circulating RBC hemoglobin heme, and that estimated non-hemoglobin heme turnover is of approximately the same magnitude as this "excess" CO production. Further, recovery of CO from damaged RBC is quantitatively complete in both animals and man. Based upon these results several authors have shown strong correlation between endogenous CO production and mean RBC lifespan (Fig. 3). It

TABLE II

MEASUREMENT OF TOTAL CO PRODUCTION (Vco)
IN SEVERAL ANIMAL SPECIES

Authors	Animal Species	Total CO Production (µl/kg/hour)
Toskes et al (1973)	Rat	24.6 ± 2.2
Rodkey et al (1972)	Guinea pig	12.9 ± 3.5
"	Rat, male	29.8 ± 22.7
"	Rat, female	15.7 ± 3.7
"	Rat, female, germfree	15.5 ± 7.3
Coburn et al (1967)	Dog	13.5 ± 3.2

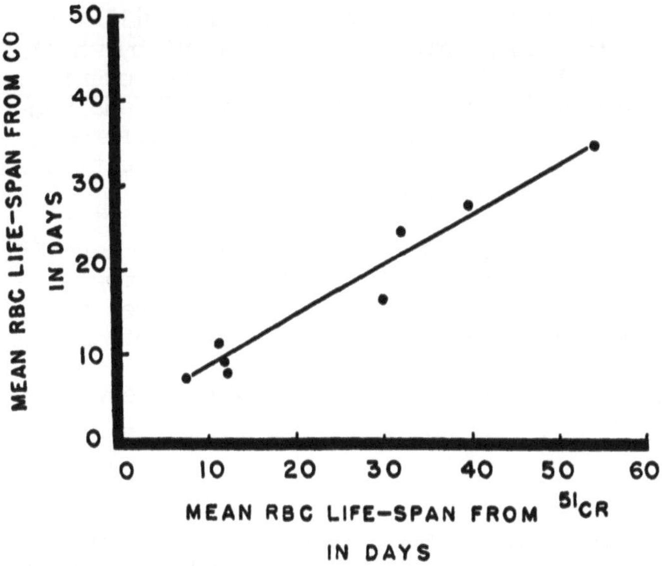

Fig. 3. Comparison of mean RBC lifespans (^{51}Cr and Vco techniques) Mean RBC lifespan derived from ^{51}Cr data (corrected for elution) is plotted on the abscissa and mean RBC lifespan derived from the rate of CO production on the ordinate. (r = 0.94). Reprinted with permission of author and J Clin Invest (RF COBURN, WJ WILLIAMS and SB KAHN, J Clin Invest 45: 460, 1966).

is therefore tempting to determine RBC lifespan from Vco measurements by subtracting a fixed amount of CO as due to non-hemoglobin heme turnover, and assuming that the remainder is due to destruction of circulating RBC. However, as pointed out by Coburn, Williams and Kahn (21), in a study of 8 subjects with hemolysis of varying proportions, Vco averaged 41 ± 28% greater than ^{51}Cr-derived measurements of RBC heme turnover, in excess of that noted for normal subjects (27 ± 8%). Unlabeled CO methods, therefore, cannot distinguish between non-hemoglobin heme turnover, ineffective erythropoiesis, and increased RBC turnover, but the following approaches might be used in conjunction with estimation of Vco to elucidate their relative contributions:

1. Isotopic studies of ^{14}CO production together with determination of total circulating hemoglobin heme activity can estimate the fraction of total heme turnover associated with hepatic heme turnover and ineffective erythropoiesis combined. If the "early peak" can be dissected into its component parts, the desired information can be estimated correctly.

2. Combined RBC survival and Vco determination will yield 2 different values for heme turnover. The amount by which CO production exceeds RBC hemoglobin heme turnover represents the combined processes of ineffective erythropoiesis and non-hemoglobin heme turnover. If bilirubin turnover is also performed, the difference between bilirubin turnover and CO production will be an estimate of non-hemoglobin heme turnover.

3. Iron kinetics models, containing provision for a rapidly-turning over tissue heme compartment, can estimate non-hemoglobin heme turnover (60). Red blood cell survival and ineffective erythropoiesis can be determined from existing iron kinetics models.

A summary of values for Vco from various investigators is shown in Table III.

3. The Newborn:

Maisels, Pathak, and Nelson, utilizing the rebreathing technique, found Vco to average 13.7 ± 3.6 µl/kg/hr in normal newborn infants (61,62), a value which is twice that noted in the adult. In children with Rh disease, values were 3-11 times increased, consistent with increased hemolysis. Vco returned towards normal with treatment and time after birth, indicating that this test is of value in determining both the presence and the extent of neonatal hemolysis, and its response to treatment. Utilizing the direct breathing technique, Fallstrom (13) obtained an average value of 11.4 µl/hr/kg using a Hopcalite meter device, and Landaw, Winchell, and Boone (63) obtained a value of 14.2 ± 6.7 µl/kg/hr using an infra-red device.

Qualitative information has been afforded by estimation of blood levels of CO (as COHgb). In their initial studies, Scandinavian workers found that COHgb levels correlated well with Vco measurements (13-17). Coburn has discussed the relationship between COHgb and Vco in quantitative terms (22), and noted that such variables as CO body burden, and parameters of respiratory function are important in determining the accuracy by which Vco can be estimated from COHgb values. However, in general, a number of authors have been able to show a significant correlation between CO concentration in inspired air and venous blood COHgb, in the form of:

$$\text{COHgb (corrected)} = \text{COHgb (measured)} - k\ \text{CO(air)}$$

The value for (k) in 3 different studies, is shown in Table IV.

TABLE III

AVERAGE VALUES OBTAINED FOR ENDOGENOUS CO PRODUCTION IN ADULTS FROM SEVERAL INVESTIGATORS, USING THE REBREATHING TECHNIQUE (BLOOD OR GAS PHASE METHOD)

Authors	CO Method	CO Production (Vco) um/hr	CO Production (Vco) um/kg/d	Vco/TBH (%/day)*	"Excess CO" (%)#
Coburn et al (18)	Rebreathing Blood phase	18.8	6.5**	1.06	21.4
Coltman, Dudley (23)	"	20.2	6.6	1.12	25.6
Lynch, Moede (72)	" (males)	24.7	7.9	1.17	28.8
	(females)	14.9	6.3	1.24	32.8
Logue et al (24)	Rebreathing Gas phase	28.0	-	1.57	46.9
Berk et al (25)	Rebreathing Blood phase	22.7	7.9	-	-

* Ratio of total CO production to total heme mass (CO dilution space)

CO production in excess of that calculated from RBC Hgb heme turnover (% of Vco)

** Also given as 6.1 μl/kg/hr

TABLE IV

ESTIMATES FOR THE RELATIONSHIP BETWEEN CO(air) AND COHGB IN STUDY SUBJECTS

Author	Subjects Studied	(k) (%COHgb/ppmCO)
Longo (64)	Pregnant female	0.131
Landaw et al (65)	Newborn	0.097
Engel et al (66)	Newborn	0.160

Such corrections were not generally needed in the Scandinavian studies, since CO (air) usually averaged less than 2 ppm (67). However, in the San Francisco Bay Area, values of CO (air) in excess of 10 ppm were often found in the air of newborn nurseries; a value of COHgb of 0.97% would be expected from this source alone. In contrast, in all our normal subjects (65), corrected values for COHgb were less than 1.0%, whereas in all subjects with Rh disease, corrected COHgb values exceeded 1.0%. Preliminary observations by Engel et al (66) indicate that these corrected values correlate well with simultaneously-obtained Vco measurements using the rebreathing technique, and are of value in assessing results of treatment for Coombs positive hemolytic anemia, for judging the severity of Rh hemolytic disease, and for judging the presence of increased hemolysis in infants with prematurity and sepsis (65,66). It has further been possible, as discussed by Longo (64), to detect increased COHgb levels in blood of non-smoking pregnant women in the last trimester before the birth of newborn with Rh disease (68). These preliminary studies, if confirmed, should be of some value in detecting fetal hemolysis and/or distress, and perhaps also in judging the severity of such processes and the results of treatment (fetal exchange transfusions, etc.).

4. Variations in Endogenous CO Production: Additional Considerations

Table V indicates a partial list of conditions which have been considered in the evaluation of alterations in endogenous CO production, and which must be taken into account when assessing the significance of such changes.

Exogenous CO. This source, coming from such diverse processes as cigarette smoking, automobile exhausts, industrial effluents, wood fires, home heaters, etc. (69) is a major source of increased COHgb in the general population. Cigarette smoke contains approximately

TABLE V

FACTORS WHICH MAY ALTER APPARENT ENDOGENOUS CARBON MONOXIDE PRODUCTION

Exogenous sources (tobacco smoke, auto exhaust, etc.)
Alterations in pulmonary function
Physiologic variability (menses, circadian rhythm, fasting (86)
Pharmacologic agents (phenobarbital, steroids, nicotinic acid)
Other heme sources (myopathies?, heme in GI tract, bacterial action)
Non-heme sources (plastics, catechols, etc.)
Oxidation of CO to CO_2 (59,87)
Artifacts, methodology (24,55,84,85)

2% CO, and the average concentration of CO in such smoke as taken into the lungs is approximately 400 ppm. It has been further estimated that smoking of a single cigarette increases venous COHgb by about 1% (70), and that inhalers of smoke tend to have greater COHgb levels than non-inhalers with the same cigarette consumption (69). Such external sources will complicate interpretations based upon COHgb levels, and are usually avoided when determining Vco. Engel, Rodkey, and Krill obtained a qualitative evaluation of COHgb in children suspected of having increased hemolysis by comparison with normal siblings or controls exposed to the same exogenous CO sources (71), and more recently devised a diffusion chamber with uptake and washout parameters similar to that of the newborn (66). By placing this diffusion chamber near the bedside, a time-averaged CO burden from such exogenous sources could be estimated.

Alteration in Pulmonary Function Parameters: Coburn, Forster, and Kane (22) investigated the effect of alterations in pulmonary function on Vco and COHgb levels, and concluded that the principal physiologic parameters of importance were rate of CO production, alveolar ventilation, lung diffusing capacity, mean pulmonary capillary oxygen tension, and concentration of CO in inspired air. Since these factors can be deranged in seriously ill subjects, especially in newborn subjects with assisted respiration, enriched O_2, etc., alterations in Vco and COHgb in such subjects must be interpreted with caution.

Physiologic and Pharmacologic Alterations: Lynch and Moede (72) repeated Vco measurements in 16 normal subjects, and noted significant variations in both men and women. Measurements were significantly higher in women during the premenstrual half of the menstrual cycle, presumably due to an effect of progesterones on hepatic heme turnover (73). They also found a significant correlation between Vco, serum iron, and serum bilirubin (unconjugated) levels, suggesting significant variations in the overall rate of heme catabolism in normal subjects. Similar alterations were found in pregnant women, with progesterone effect, placental transfer of CO and binding by fetal Hgb, increased RBC mass, and fetal CO production as important factors (64).

Gydell (9) studied the effect of nicotinic acid on endogenous CO production and bilirubin values, and concluded that this was due to accelerated hemoglobin catabolism. This was especially pronounced in patients with hemolysis, and was noted to decrease after splenectomy. Coburn noted increased Vco in subjects taking phenobarbital, presumably due to increases in non-hemoglobin heme turnover. The magnitude of this effect was such to increase Vco 50-200% (74,75).

The possibility that a circadian rhythm exists for heme catabolism has been explored in experimental animals. The result of a study of ^{14}CO production in 2 groups of normal mice is shown in Fig. 4. A definite peak in ^{14}CO excretion rate is seen in the early evening in these animals, suggesting a biologic rhythm in either heme catabolism or in certain parameters of pulmonary excretion.

Sources Other than "Endogenous" Heme Turnover: It was originally postulated that CO could be formed "anabolically" from porphyrin precursors, without an intervening heme molecule. All studies to date indicate that heme is an obligatory intermediate for CO production from the porphyrin ring. The present concept regarding "shunt" hyperbilirubinemia and CO production is that this represents heme "shunted" away from hemoproteins (and hemoglobin) rather than bile pigment and/or CO formed without an intervening heme molecule (76,77). However, in rats made porphyric with allylisopropylacetamide (AIA), a discrepancy between ^{14}CO and ^{14}C-bilirubin production was seen. In these animals, more CO was produced than bilirubin, in contrast to the situation in normals, in which the production of these 2 catabolites was equimolar (77). While it was the conclusion from these experiments that the CO production represented true heme turnover and the decreased bilirubin recovery represented alterations in the final pathway to biliary bilirubin excretion (metabolites other than bilirubin, accumulation of "green hemes", etc.)(78), the possibility exists that small amounts of CO arise from non-heme sources. However, ^{14}CO has not been found following

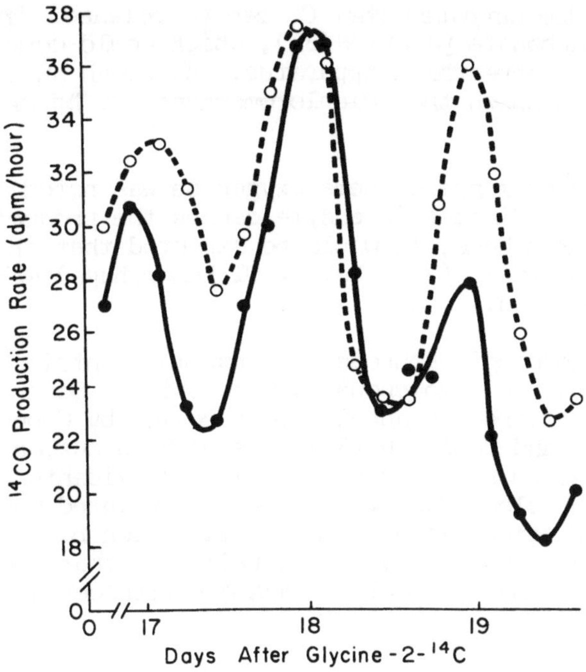

Fig. 4. Variation in ^{14}CO excretion in normal mice. Two groups of normal LAF_1/J mice (5 mice/group) were studied continuously for ^{14}CO excretion 17-20 days after glycine-2-^{14}C injection. Each data point represents a 5-hour collection, located on the graph at the mid-point of the collection period. The time marked on the abscissa (short vertical line) represents 5 PM. Note that ^{14}CO excretion is maximal for both groups in the early evening.

injection of glycine-1-^{14}C, which is not a precursor for any of the carbon atoms of heme (77), ^{14}C-bilirubin (77), or ^{14}C-formate (55). Further, the agreement between total CO production and total bilirubin production in man is such that these sources, if they exist, must be extremely small in magnitude in normal man (25).

As noted previously, CO production is unusually high in the normal male rat, suggesting that non-heme sources contribute CO in these and in other animal species (57). Engel has shown that CO can be evolved by certain bacteria from heme sources (79), and bacterial strains are known which produce CO from non-heme sources (80). Thus, it is possible that some CO may arise from the GI tract, diffuse into the blood stream, and contribute to total "endogenous" CO production.

It has been demonstrated that CO can be released from various acrylic and polycarbonate plastics(81), which could conceivably be incorporated in rebreathing apparatus. Although an unlikely source, it has been shown that dichloromethane may be metabolized to CO in man (82).

Recently, the presence of heme oxygenase was noted in cells of the GI mucosa (83). Since this enzyme causes the production of CO and bile pigment from heme, it would be expected that the absorption of heme from the GI tract (food hemes, GI hemorrhage) would lead to increased CO production.

Finally, methodologic sources of error may contribute to apparent alterations in endogenous CO production. Some of these sources have been covered in an excellent review by Coburn et al (84), while Rodkey and Collison (85) have pointed out an additional source of increased CO recovery resulting from oxidants utilized in *in vitro* assays for blood COHgb. It has been pointed out that the time constants for return to baseline CO excretion rates following exposure to exogenous CO are very long (22), and that true steady-state conditions may be difficult to achieve with certain methods for estimating Vco.

SUMMARY

It has been shown, in both experimental animals and man, that one mole of CO and one mole of bilirubin are produced for each mole of heme degraded *in vivo*. The measurement of CO production has been shown to be a reliable and quantitative measure of *in vivo* heme catabolism. Methods employed consist of the determination of blood CO content (as COHgb), with or without correction for exogenous CO sources, measurement of CO in expired air, and determination of the linear increase in CO content of blood or gas in a closed rebreathing system. These techniques have been valuable in understanding the physiology of heme degradation in normal subjects, and in quantitating heme turnover in clinical situations, such as in hemolytic anemia and neonatal jaundice.

CO kinetics can be studied through the use of glycine-2-^{14}C and delta-aminolevulinic acid-5-^{14}C, isotopic precursors of the alpha methene bridge carbon atom of heme, the sole source of endogenously produced CO in mammals. Endogenous ^{14}CO production can be divided into early and late phases, as for the bile pigments. Study of these separate phases has led to a more complete understanding of the genesis of the early and late "peaks", as well as their relative contribution to total CO production. The ^{14}CO technique has been successfully applied to the study of ineffective erythropoiesis in man, and of various disorders of RBC production and destruction in experimental animals.

REFERENCES

1. SJOSTRAND T: Early studies of CO production. Ann NY Acad Sci 174: 5-10, 1970.

2. COBURN RF: Endogenous carbon monoxide metabolism. Ann Rev Med 24: 241-250, 1973.

3. GREHANT N: Les gas du sang. G. Masson (Paris) 1894.

4. NICLOUX M: Sur l'oxyde de carbone contenu normalement dans le sang. C R Acad Sci (Paris) 126: 1526- 1528, 1898.

5. SJOSTRAND T: Endogenous formation of carbon monoxide in man under normal and pathological conditions. Scand J Clin Lab Invest 1: 201-214, 1949.

6. SJOSTRAND T: The in vitro formation of carbon monoxide in blood. Acta Physiol Scand 24: 314-332, 1951.

7. SJOSTRAND T: The formation of carbon monoxide by the decomposition of haemoglobin in vivo. Acta Physiol Scand 26: 338-344, 1952.

8. ENGSTEDT L: Endogenous formation of carbon monoxide in haemolytic disease. Acta Med Scand (Suppl 332): 1-63, 1957.

9. GYDELL K: Transient effect of nicotinic acid on bilirubin metabolism and formation of carbon monoxide. Acta Med Scand 167: 431-441, 1960.

10. KUSTOV VV, GOFMAN IA and IVANOVA FA: On the endogenous formation of carbon monoxide. Radiobiology (USSR) 2: 187-192, 1961.

11. PALMA CARLOS AG, PALMA CARLOS M-L and DULCA SOARES A: Formation endogene d'oxyde de carbone et catabolisme hemoglobinique. Nouv Rev Francaise d'Hematologie 6: 225-238, 1966.

12. OSKI FA and ALTMAN AA: Carboxyhemoglobin levels in hemolytic disease of the newborn. J. Pediat. 61: 709-719, 1962.

13. FALLSTROM SP: Endogenous formation of carbon monoxide in newborn infants. Acta Paediat Scand 57: 321-329, 1968.

14. FALLSTROM SP: Endogenous formation of carbon monoxide in newborn infants. Acta Paediat Scand 57: 487-494, 1968.

15. FALLSTROM SP: On the endogenous formation of carbon monoxide in full-term newborn infants. Acta Paediat Scand (Suppl 189) 57: 137-144, 1969.

16. WRANNE L: Studies on erythro-kinetics in infancy. Acta Paediat Scand 58: 49-53, 1969.

17. BJURE J and FALLSTROM SP: Endogenous formation of carbon monoxide in newborn infants. Acta Paediat (Stockholm) 52: 361-366, 1963.

18. COBURN RF, BLAKEMORE WS and FORSTER RE: Endogenous carbon monoxide production in man. J Clin Invest 42: 1172, 1963.

19. COBURN RF, WILLIAMS WJ and FORSTER RE: Effect of erythrocyte destruction on carbon monoxide production in man. J Clin Invest 43: 1098-1103, 1964.

20. LONDON IM, WEST R, SHEMIN D and RITTENBERG D: On the origin of bile pigment in normal man. J Biol Chem 184: 351-358, 1950.

21. COBURN RF, WILLIAMS WJ and KAHN SB: Endogenous carbon monoxide production in patients with hemolytic anemia. J Clin Invest 45: 460-468, 1966.

22. COBURN RF, FORSTER RE and KANE PB: Consideration of the physiological variables that determine the blood carboxyhemoglobin concentration in man. J Clin Invest 44: 1899-1910, 1965.

23. COLTMAN CA and DUDLEY GM: The relationship between endogenous carbon monoxide production and total heme mass in normal and abnormal subjects. Am J Med Sci 258: 374-385, 1969.

24. LOGUE GL, ROSSE WF, SMITH WT et al: Endogenous carbon monoxide production measured by gas-phase analysis: an estimation of heme catabolic rate. J Lab Clin Med 77: 867-876, 1971.

25. BERK PD, RODKEY FL, BLASCHKE TF et al: Comparison of plasma bilirubin turnover and carbon monoxide production in man. J Lab Clin Med 83: 29-37, 1974.

26. BERK PD: In Jaundice, edited by CA GORESKY and MM FISHER. Plenum Press, New York, 1975.

27. JONES EA, BLOOMER JR and BERLIN NI: The measurement of the synthetic rate of bilirubin from hepatic hemes in patients with acute intermittent porphyria. J Clin Invest 50: 2259-2265, 1971.

28. WHITE P, COBURN RF, WILLIAMS WJ et al: Carbon monoxide production associated with ineffective erythropoiesis. J Clin Invest 46: 1986-1998, 1967.

29. WITTENBERG J and SHEMIN D: The location in protoporphyrin of the carbon atoms derived from the alpha-carbon atom of glycine. J Biol Chem 185: 103-116, 1950.

30. LUDWIG GD, BLAKEMORE WS and DRABKIN DL: Production of carbon monoxide and bile pigment by haemin oxidation. Biochem J 66: 38p, 1957.

31. GRAY CH, NEUBERGER A and SNEATH PHA: Studies in congenital porphyria. 2. Incorporation of ^{15}N in the stercobilin in the normal and in the porphyric. Biochem J 47: 87-92, 1950.

32. JAMES GW and ABBOTT LD: Stercobilin N^{15} excretion in refractory anemia. Trans Amer Clin Climat Assoc 73: 110-120, 1961.

33. ROBINSON SH: Bilirubin production from non-erythroid sources. In: Jaundice, edited by CA GORESKY and MM FISHER, Plenum Press, New York, 1975.

34. ISRAELS LG, YAMAMOTO T, SKANDERBEG J et al: Shunt bilirubin: evidence for 2 components. Science 139: 1054-1055, 1963.

35. WHITE P: Carbon monoxide production and heme catabolism. Ann NY Acad Sci 174: 23-31, 1970.

36. LANDAW SA and WINCHELL HS: Endogenous production of carbon-14 labeled carbon monoxide; an in vivo technique for the study of heme catabolism. J Nuclear Med 7: 696-707, 1966.

37. LANDAW SA: Kinetic aspects of endogenous carbon monoxide production in experimental animals. Ann NY Acad Sci 174: 32-48, 1970.

38. ROBINSON SH, TSONG M, BROWN B et al: The sources of bile pigment in the rat: studies of the "early labeled" fraction. J Clin Invest 45: 1569-1588, 1966.

39. ROBINSON SH: Increased formation of early-labeled bilirubin in rats with iron deficiency anemia: evidence for ineffective erythropoiesis. Blood 33: 909-917, 1969.

40. MORSE BS, GERMANO GJ and GIULIANI DG: Abnormal erythroid maturation following acute lead toxicity in mice. Blood 39: 713-720, 1972.

41. LANDAW SA and SCHOOLEY JC: Decreased erythropoietin synthesis and ineffective erythropoiesis in acutely lead-poisoned rats. Blood 42: 996, 1973 (abstract).

42. LANDAW SA: Unpublished results.

43. PALMER JG, EICHWALD EJ, CARTWRIGHT GE et al: Experimental production of splenomegaly, anemia, and leukopenia in albino rats. Blood 8: 72-80, 1953.

44. BESSIS M: Quelques donnees cytologiques sur le role du systeme reticulo-endothelial dans l'erythropoiese et l'erythroclasie. In: Role du systeme reticulo-endothelial dans l'immunite antibacterienne et antitumorale. President: MBN HALPERN. Editions du Centre National de la Recherche Scientifique, Paris, 1963, p 447.

45. SCHMID R: Discussion In: Erythropoiesis. Edited by : LO JACOBSON and M DOYLE, Grune & Stratton, New York, 1962, p 242.

46. ISRAELS LG, NOVAK W, FOERSTER J et al: The early-appearing bilirubin in ducks. Canad J Physiol Pharmacol 44: 864-866, 1966.

47. LEVITT M, SCHACTER BA, ZIPURSKY A et al: The non-erythropoietic component of early bilirubin. J Clin Invest 47: 1281, 1968.

48. LANDOW SA, RUSSELL ES and BERNSTEIN SE: Splenic destruction of newly-formed red blood cells and shortened erythrocyte survival in mice with congenital microcytosis. Scand J Haematol 7: 516-524, 1970.

49. LANDAW SA and WINCHELL HS: Endogenous production of ^{14}CO: a method for calculation of RBC lifespan in vivo. Blood 36: 642-656, 1970.

50. EADIE GS and BROWN IW: Red blood cell survival studies. Blood 8: 1110-1136, 1953.

51. LANDAW SA: Quantitative recovery of ^{14}C-labeled carbon monoxide (^{14}CO) from viable heme-labeled red blood cells in the rat. Blood 40: 257-260, 1972.

52. BERLIN NI, HEWITT C and LOTZ C: Hippuric acid synthesis in man after the administration of (alpha-^{14}C) glycine. Biochem J 58: 498-503, 1954.

53. LANDAW SA and BRISTOL SK: Prolongation of RBC survival in the hypophysectomized rat. Proc Soc Exptl Biol Med 138:152-156, 1971.

54. LANDAW SA: Studies of heme metabolism using the endogenous production of carbon-14 labeled carbon monoxide. PhD Thesis. University of California, Berkeley, 1969.

55. COBURN RF: Endogenous carbon monoxide production and body CO stores. Acta Med Scand (Suppl 472): 269-282, 1968.

56. METZ G and SJOSTRAND T: Formation and elimination of CO in mammals. Acta Physiol Scand 31: 384-392, 1954.

57. RODKEY FL, COLLISON HA and O'NEAL JD: Carbon monoxide and methane production in rats, guinea pigs, and germ-free rats. J Applied Physiol 33: 256-260, 1972.

58. TOSKES P, BENSINGER T, GIANELLA R et al: Folic acid abnormalities in iron deficiency. Clin Res 21: 55, 1973 (abstract).

59. LUOMANMAKI K: Studies on the metabolism of carbon monoxide. Ann Med Exp Biol Fenniae 44: (Suppl 2), 1-55, 1966.

60. WINCHELL HS: Quantitation of red cell and heme production and destruction using radioisotope kinetics. In: Progress in Atomic Medicine, edited by JH LAWRENCE, New York, Grune & Stratton, 1968, volume 2, p 85.

61. MAISELS MJ, PATHAK A, NELSON NM et al: Endogenous production of carbon monoxide in normal and erythroblastotic newborn infants. J Clin Invest 50: 1-8, 1971.

62. MAISELS MJ, PATHAK A and NELSON NM: The effect of exchange transfusion of endogenous carbon monoxide production in erythroblastotic infants. J Pediatrics 81: 705-709, 1972.

63. LANDAW SA, WINCHELL HS and BOONE RF: Measurement of endogenous carbon monoxide production in hemolytic disease of the newborn. Clin Res 19: 208, 1971 (abstract).

64. LONGO LD: Carbon monoxide in the pregnant mother and fetus and its exchange across the placenta. Ann NY Acad Sci 174: 312-341, 1970.

65. LANDAW SA, KANDALL SR and THALER MM: Corrected carboxyhemoglobin as an index of hemolysis in "non-hemolytic" neonatal hyperbilirubinemia. Clin Res 21: 321, 1973 (abstract).

66. ENGEL RR, MODLER S, NORBERG W et al: Enhancing the diagnostic value of carboxyhemoglobin (%COHb) determination. Ped Res: 8: 467, 1974 (abstract).

67. ALDEN ER, LYNCH SR and WENNBERG RP: Carboxyhemoglobin determination in evaluating neonatal jaundice. Am J Dis Child 127: 214-217, 1974.

68. CREASEY R, THALER MM, KANDALL SR et al: Unpublished results.

69. GOLDSMITH JR and LANDAW SA: Carbon monoxide and human health. Science 162: 1352-1359, 1968.

70. LANDAW SA: The effects of cigarette smoking on total body burden and excretion rates of carbon monoxide. J Occup Med 15: 231-235, 1973.

71. ENGEL RR, RODKEY FL and KRILL CE: Carboxyhemoglobin levels as an index of hemolysis. Pediatrics 47: 723-730, 1971.

72. LYNCH SR and MOEDE AL: Variation in the rate of endogenous carbon monoxide production in normal human beings. J Lab Clin Med 79: 85- 95, 1972.

73. DELIVORIA-PAPADOPOULOS M, COBURN RF and FORSTER RE: Cyclical variation of rate of heme destruction and carbon monoxide production (V_{CO}) in normal women. Physiologist 13: 178, 1970. (Abstract)

74. COBURN RF: Effect of phenobarbital on endogenous carbon monoxide production in normal man. J Clin Invest 46: 1046, 1967 (abstract).

75. COBURN RF: Endogenous carbon monoxide production. New Engl J Med 282: 207-209, 1970.

76. COBURN RF, WILLIAMS WJ, WHITE P et al: The production of carbon monoxide from hemoglobin in vivo. J Clin Invest 46: 346-356, 1967.

77. LANDAW SA, CALLAHAN EW and SCHMID R: Catabolism of heme in vivo: comparison of the simultaneous production of bilirubin and carbon monoxide. J Clin Invest 49: 914-925, 1970.

78. SCHWARTZ S and IKEDA K: Studies of porphyrin synthesis and inter-conversion, with special reference to certain green porphyrins in animals with experimental hepatic porphyria. In: Ciba Foundation Symposium on Porphyrin Biosynthesis and Metabolism. Edited by GEW WOLSTENHOLME and ECP MILLAR, J & A Churchill, London, 1955, p 209.

79. ENGEL RR, MATSEN JM, CHAPMAN SS et al: Carbon monoxide production from heme compounds by bacteria. J Bacteriol 112: 1310-1315, 1972.

80. WESTLAKE DWS, ROXBURGH JM and TALBOT G: Microbial production of carbon monoxide from flavonoids. Nature 189: 510, 1961.

81. RODKEY FL, COLLISON HA and ENGEL RR: Release of carbon monoxide from acrylic and polycarbonate plastics. J Applied Physiol 27: 554-555, 1969.

82. STEWART RD, FISHER TN, HOSKO MJ et al: Carboxyhemoglobin elevation after exposure to dichloromethane. Science 176: 295-296, 1972.

83. RAFFIN SB, WOO CH and SCHMID R: Role of heme oxygenase in intestinal absorption of hemoglobin iron. J Clin Invest 53: 62a, 1974 (abstract).

84. COBURN RF, DANIELSON GK, BLAKEMORE WS et al: Carbon monoxide in blood: analytical method and sources of error. J Applied Physiol 19: 510-515, 1964.

85. RODKEY FL and COLLISON HA: An artifact in the analysis of oxygenated blood for its low carbon monoxide content. Clin Chem 16: 896-899, 1970.

86. LUNDH B, JOHANNSON M-B, MERCKE C et al: Enhancement of carbon monoxide production by caloric restriction in man. Scand J Lab Clin Invest 30: 421-427, 1972.

87. FENN WO: The burning of CO in tissues. Ann NY Acad Sci 174: 64-71, 1970.

DISCUSSION OF PAPERS ON BILIRUBIN PRODUCTION

CHAIRMAN: R. LESTER

SASS-KORTSAK: I would like to ask Dr. Schmid a question concerning his scheme for the handling of bilirubin by the liver cell. He shows two little arrows through the cell membrane and then the whole explanation seems to be that what goes through, how fast, and so on really just depends on the acceptor proteins which we know about, inside the cell. I would like to submit that perhaps the acceptor proteins would very strongly influence the transport through the cell membrane from the exterior to the interior of the cell because they provide an essential acceptor on the other side. Yet it is quite conceivable that there is some sort of a specific mechanism that provides for entry through the cell membrane. It could be said that since bilirubin is lipid soluble and since the membrane is lipid, the mechanism is dissolution and passive diffusion but I really don't believe that this could be the case. The membrane is covered by glycoprotein and it is now a general hypothesis that most substances entering the cell pass through areas or pores in perforating proteins, so that they indeed do not pass through the lipid phase of the membrane. I think that we should take the viewpoint that there are unknown areas and big questions. I think that this is one of them. Would Dr. Schmid comment?

SCHMID: I think you are entirely right. I did not want to imply that there is not a carrier mechanism in the membrane of the liver cell. There are several suggestions in the literature that carrier transport processes are involved in cell entry. Much of this work has been done with the model compound sulfobromophthalein. The process of entry for this material is reversible, and this reversibility underlies the storage phenomenon (Wheeler, Meltzer, Bradley; J Clin Invest 39: 1131-1144, 1960). Bilirubin can also be shown to enter the cells by a reversible process (Hammaker, Schmid; Gastroenterology, 53: 31-37, 1967). Sulfobromophthalein binding to plasma proteins has been explored and it has been shown by Baker and Bradley that, on the basis of the amount of unbound material in equilibrium with that bound to albumin, it would be appropriate to hypothesize that there is a membrane protein functioning as a carrier, in order to account for the rate of transfer of sulfobromophthalein across the membrane (Baker, Bradley; J Clin Invest 45: 281-287, 1966). And finally Goresky showed that the uptake process for sulfobromophthalein exhibits saturation kinetics (Goresky; Am J Physiol 207: 13-26, 1964). Would Dr. Goresky comment?

GORESKY: I think the problem of defining the membrane carrier transport process for bilirubin is a major one. From the kinetic point of view the presence of saturation must be sought. If the entry process is a non-mediated passive diffusion process, then the proportion of tracer bilirubin taken up by the liver cells will be the same when the plasma bilirubin is low as when it is high. No evidence of saturation will be found. However, if, at the higher level, the proportion of tracer bilirubin removed is less, the data may be construed to show the presence of a carrier-mediated transport system or of some kind of a transport system with capacity limitations. The problem with this approach is that it will not give you the specificities of the process. If there is a protein in the membrane that underlies the shuttle, then the only way one could finally describe this would be to isolate the protein and finally to reconstruct the system. Thus much remains to be done, in the definition of the transport process for bilirubin. I will outline the results from some preliminary experiments with labeled bilirubin later in the Conference.

DORE: In the newborn babies of diabetic mothers, we always have the problem of icterus and I would like to ask Dr. Schacter whether it is produced by the relative hypoglycemia in the fasting newborn.

SCHACTER: Dr. Thaler has in fact investigated this point in newborn rats. His experiments did show an induction of hepatic heme-oxygenase, which began very soon after the rats were born and continued, to reach a peak about 10 days after birth. He hypothesized that the relative hypoglycemia which these animals experience may be responsible for the induction. A similar phenomenon may account for the hyperbilirubinemia seen in babies. There is also obviously a deficiency of glucuronyl transferase at this time.

SASS-KORTSAK: Could I ask whether you really believe that simply an increase in the activity of heme-oxygenase is enough to produce an increased amount of bilirubin? Isn't the amount of bilirubin formed primarily dependent on the amount of substrate given to this enzyme?

SCHACTER: Most studies show that heme-oxygenase appears to function at a maximal rate. Dr. Schmid and his co-workers have shown, in rats, that one can make very good kinetic correlations between the activity of heme-oxygenase and the daily turnover of hemoglobin heme. More recently we have found a similar quantitative correlation with the activity in the human spleen.

GORESKY: In view of the data presented by Dr. Muller-Eberhard, what is the effect of heme-hemopexin on heme-oxygenase?

SCHACTER: I myself have no direct experience with hemopexin as related to heme-oxygenase. A fundamental question arises in this area. Does hemopexin actually enter the liver cell or does it just adhere to the cell membrane?

MULLER-EBERHARD: The data which I have shown indicate that the combined heme-hemopexin molecule actually enters the cell. However, whether this is the only mechanism of entrance of heme into the hepatocyte remains to be seen. I find it very interesting that the induction of microsomal heme-oxygenase peaks at 24 hours, which is exactly the same time it takes for hemopexin levels to rise maximally when you give amounts of heme intravenously to rabbits. A doubling of the hemopexin concentration occurs at that particular time. The same effect, namely hemopexin induction, is seen if a rabbit is bled many times a day. This releases minute amounts of heme into the circulation which are, in themselves, enough of a stimulus for the increased synthesis of hemopexin.

I myself know of no data with regard to the activity of heme-hemopexin on the heme-oxygenase system.

SCHMID: In vitro hemopexin bound heme does serve as a substrate for microsomal heme-oxygenase, so there is no reason a priori why induction should not occur. We have studied isolated cultured liver cells, maintained in a culture medium, free of proteins. If one puts in hemopexin bound heme, a large amount of that heme gets into the liver cell and is copiously converted to bilirubin. In the whole animal, the effects are a little more difficult to ascertain. We have looked at the disappearance of heme from the circulation, presumably as a complex with hemopexin. If, however, we give first a large dose of unlabeled heme, to deplete the hemopexin, and then inject labeled heme the disappearance of this appears very similar to that observed in the undepleted state. This brings up the question of whether the hemopexin represents the only transfer mechanism by which the heme can get into the liver cell or whether there are alternative mechanisms.

MULLER-EBERHARD: In cultured liver cell systems, hemopexin is produced very rapidly and if the same phenomenon occurs in vitro you may not have depleted the circulation of hemopexin.

THALER: The question previously asked is a very crucial question. That is, what is the rate limiting role of heme itself versus that of heme-oxygenase activity. At least in the newborn we have been able to show very clearly, by using labeled precursors of heme, that the specific activity of newly formed bilirubin parallels the activity of heme-oxygenase.

MUSTRIGAN: Might the jaundice in septicemia occur secondary to an excess of heme-oxygenase activity, due to its induction by pyrogen? In most of these patients there is, on biopsy, evidence of cholestasis and there is a conjugated hyperbilirubinemia. Is there clinical evidence of overproduction?

LESTER: In young babies with E. coli sepsis there is first a very definite drop in hemoglobin, with an accompanying indirect reacting hyperbilirubinemia. Later this hemolytic component then switches over into an obstructive "direct reacting" hyperbilirubinemia.

SCHMID: The clinical observations do indicate the presence of a conjugated hyperbilirubinemia in sepsis. It was shown, however, a few years ago, that under the influence of endotoxin, total bilirubin production could be just about doubled and this is really what gave us the idea to look at endotoxin. We found an enormous increase in heme-oxygenase suggesting that at least you have the machinery to make more bilirubin.

GARTNER: I would like to ask Dr. Landaw whether there is increased production of CO during the newborn period?

LANDAW: If we normalize the amount of CO that is produced to body weight, there is twice as much CO produced in the newborn as in the adult. We have just completed a study in the rat, in which we found that the life span of red cells labeled in utero was markedly reduced. The one study that was done with

N-15 glycine does seem to indicate that the early labeled peak is relatively increased in magnitude. Thus we have evidence for shortened red cell survival and an increased early labeled peak as two possible reasons for the increased carbon monoxide production.

TOTAL BODY HANDLING OF BILIRUBIN

Paul D. Berk

National Institute of Arthritis, Metabolism and Digestive Diseases, National Institutes of Health

Bethesda, Maryland 20014

In a symposium at which Professor Rudi Schmid has given an elegant overview of bilirubin metabolism, and at which each individual step in the production and disposition of bilirubin has been or will be the subject of a detailed presentation by an equally distinguished expert, I am at somewhat of a loss as to the proper content of a talk covering "Total Body Handling of Bilirubin". I believe it may be most helpful if I introduce the concept of clearance, already familiar to you in the context of renal disease, and indicate the value of measurements of bilirubin clearance in the evaluation of the patient with hyperbilirubinemia.

Non-volatile metabolic waste products, as well as exogenously administered drugs and chemicals, are cleared from the plasma and excreted primarily by the liver and kidneys. If both the quantity of a substance excreted per unit time and its plasma concentration can be measured, then the volume of plasma cleared of the substance per unit time can be calculated from the simple expression indicated in equation (1).

$$(1)\ \text{Clearance (ml/min)} = \frac{\text{amount excreted per unit time (mg/min)}}{\text{plasma concentration (mg/ml)}}.$$

While this equation is equally applicable to materials removed from plasma by both the liver and kidneys, in practice, application of the clearance concept has largely been restricted to the assessment of renal function. This stems in large part from the technical problems involved in accurately quantitating the excretion rates of materials eliminated in the feces. Accordingly, I shall first describe a technique for calculating hepatic bilirubin clearance from measurements made entirely in the plasma, thus avoiding the need for chemical measurement of fecal metabolites.

Following the intravenous injection of a tracer dose of unconjugated radiobilirubin, blood samples are obtained for a period of 24-48 hours. The unconjugated bilirubin is extracted from the plasma by the solvent partition method of Weber and Schalm (1) and counted in a liquid scintillation counter. The resulting plasma disappearance curve of unconjugated radiobilirubin in a typical normal volunteer is shown in Fig. 1, in which the experimental data have been fitted by digital computer to a sum of 3 exponential functions. Such curves have now been obtained on more than 150 occasions in both normal volunteers and patients with a wide variety of disease states. Although the rate at which the isotope is removed from the plasma varies with the state of hepatic function, in every instance the mathematical form of P(t), the curve fitting the data, was identical: namely, a sum of 3 exponentials.

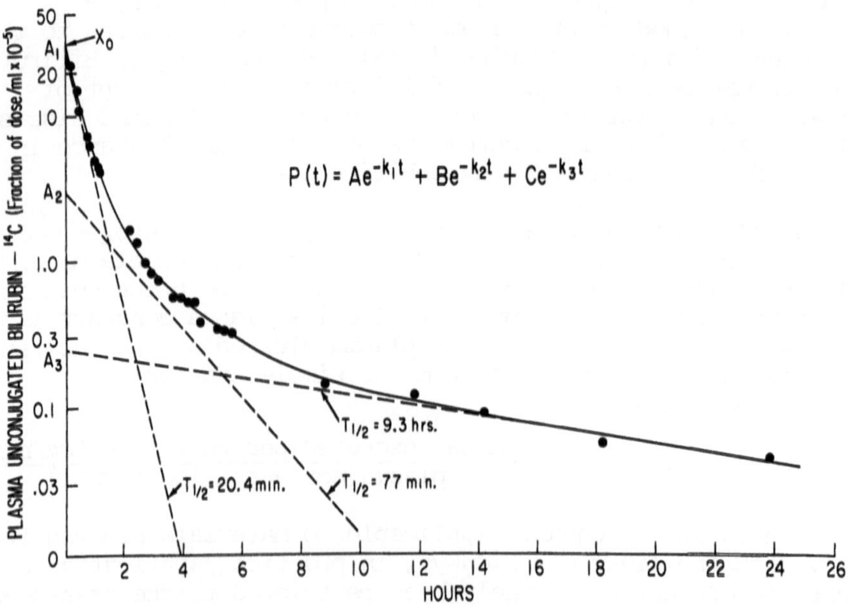

Fig. 1. The clearance of unconjugated radiobilirubin from the plasma of a normal volunteer. The solid curve represents a computer fit of the data to a sum of 3 exponential functions. Dashed lines are the individual exponential components. X_o is the extrapolated value of the curve at zero time.

This particular mathematical function facilitates direct calculation of several parameters of physiologic interest. From the injected dose of radiobilirubin and the computer-extrapolated value of the plasma curve at zero time, one can calculate VDBR - the initial distribution volume of the injected radiobilirubin, as indicated by equation (2).

(2) Volume of Distribution of Radiobilirubin (VDBR) =

$$\frac{\text{injected radiobilirubin (dpm)}}{\text{dpm/ml plasma at zero time}}$$

This space has been found to correspond almost exactly to the plasma volume as determined with ^{131}I-labeled albumin (2,3).

Next, using standard methods for the analysis of isotope tracer data, it can be shown that the fraction of VDBR irreversibly cleared of bilirubin per minute, designated k_e, is equal to the reciprocal of the area under the plasma disappearance curve (2). This area is calculated by integrating the 3-exponential disappearance function, P(t), from zero to infinity. That is:

(3) $k_e \equiv$ Fraction of VDBR cleared of unconjugated bilirubin per minute

(4) $$k_e = \frac{1}{\text{area under plasma radiobilirubin curve}} = \frac{1}{\int_0^\infty P(t)\,dt}$$

If we know VDBR, the volume in which the plasma unconjugated bilirubin pool is distributed, and k_e, the fraction of that pool irreversibly cleared of bilirubin per minute, then hepatic bilirubin clearance, in ml/min, is calculated simply as the product of VDBR and k_e.

(5) HEPATIC BILIRUBIN CLEARANCE $(C_{BR}) = k_e \times$ VDBR.

Finally, if the volume of plasma cleared of bilirubin per unit time and the unconjugated bilirubin content of the plasma, $\overline{BR}$, are both known, then the mass of unconjugated bilirubin extracted from the plasma per unit time may also be calculated by means of equation (6).

(6) $$\text{PLASMA BILIRUBIN TURNOVER(mg/day)} = C_{BR}\text{(ml/min)} \times \frac{\overline{BR}\text{(mg/100 ml)}}{100} \times 1440 \text{ (min/day)}$$

In the steady state, the rate at which bilirubin is removed from the plasma equals the rate at which newly synthesized bilirubin enters. We have called this quantity the daily plasma bilirubin turnover, or BRT. It appears on both theoretical and experimental grounds that BRT provides a close approximation of total bilirubin production (BRP).

If the above formulation is correct, both bilirubin turnover (BRT) and bilirubin clearance (C_{BR}) can be calculated in a perfectly straightforward manner from the plasma radiobilirubin disappearance curve and the plasma unconjugated bilirubin concentration ($\overline{BR}$). Measurement of bilirubin clearance appears to be a useful tool for the initial evaluation and serial assessment of patients with hepatic disease, and particularly in the evaluation of patients with unconjugated hyperbilirubinemia (4). Furthermore, compartmental analysis of plasma radiobilirubin disappearance curves provides estimates of a number of additional parameters of hepatic function not readily measurable in man by other techniques (2,4,5). However, before proceeding with the physiological and diagnostic implications of equation (6), it may be worthwhile to review the evidence that the data derived from this equation are valid and meaningful.

During the catabolism of heme, one molecule of bilirubin and one molecule of carbon monoxide are formed for each molecule of heme degraded. Hence, measurements of bilirubin production and CO production should provide essentially equivalent data when both are expressed as molar quantities. Measurements of daily plasma bilirubin turnover in normal adults - 6.6 ± 1.1 (S.D.) µMoles/kg/day, agree very closely with measurements of CO production which averaged 6.6 ± 1.3 (6), 6.6 ± 0.9 (7) and 7.0 ± 2.1 (8) µMoles/kg/day in three independent studies. Furthermore, simultaneous measurements of plasma bilirubin turnover and CO production in our laboratory, performed in 37 individuals with a wide range of heme turnover values, have also shown excellent agreement (9), as illustrated in Fig. 2. The slope of the regression line relating these two parameters was 1.0, and the correlation coefficient 0.994. Since these two parameters are measured by entirely independent techniques, their agreement tends to support the validity of both methods.

Although the calculation of hepatic bilirubin clearance and bilirubin turnover from plasma disappearance curves merely represents a new application of a well established mathematical technique widely used in other areas, it is useful to compare the results of this approach with values for bilirubin clearance calculated from independent data using the standard clearance formula presented in equation (1). Use of this equation requires a knowledge of the daily bilirubin excretion rate. Direct measurement of fecal bilirubin excretion is of no value since, as the result of bacterial action within the gut, little bilirubin, as such, appears in the feces. Furthermore, as we have shown in a previous publication, quantitative measurements of fecal urobilin (stercobilin) excretion consistently underestimate bilirubin production (10). The following

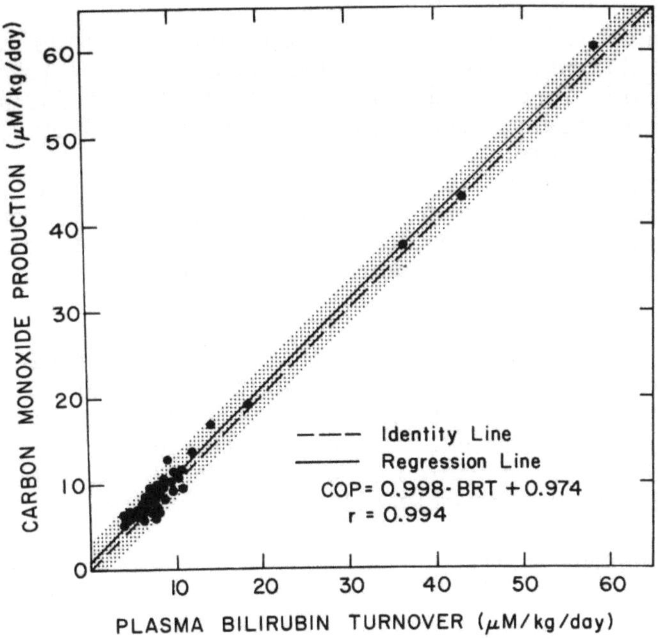

Fig. 2. Comparison of simultaneous measurements of carbon monoxide production (COP) and plasma bilirubin turnover (BRT) in 37 patients and normal volunteers. Stippled area represents two standard errors of the estimate about the regression line.

approach to the calculation of bilirubin excretion was suggested to us by Dr. Samuel Schwartz, and is based on the observation that virtually all of the isotope injected into normal subjects in the form of radiobilirubin is recovered in the feces within seven days. Under these circumstances, if one collects feces for a sufficient period of time after injection of radiobilirubin to obtain complete recovery of the administered isotope, then the amount of bilirubin excreted during this time period may be calculated from the injected dose, in dpm, and the specific activity of the bilirubin isolated from the pooled feces (11).

$$\text{(7) Bilirubin excreted(mg)} = \frac{\text{injected dose (dpm)}}{\text{specific activity of excreted "bilirubin" (dpm/mg)}}.$$

While the bilirubin specific activity cannot be obtained directly, it can be calculated from the specific activity of stercobilin, which is readily crystallized from the pooled fecal sample. Once the excretion rate of bilirubin is known, hepatic bilirubin clearance is readily calculated from equation (1).

Application of this fecal isotope dilution technique to the calculation of bilirubin production and clearance in 4 patients with normal hepatic function is shown in Table I. As illustrated, the results are virtually identical to those obtained by analysis of plasma radiobilirubin disappearance curves. While the fecal isotope dilution technique is an example of the classical approach to clearance measurements, and represents an essential reference method, the requirement for prolonged collection of feces and for chemical extraction and purification of stercobilin sharply curtails its clinical usefulness.

I have indicated in equation (6) that plasma bilirubin turnover may be calculated from the product of hepatic bilirubin clearance, C_{BR}, and the plasma concentration of unconjugated bilirubin, $\overline{BR}$. If equation (6) is solved for $\overline{BR}$, we see that the plasma concentration of unconjugated bilirubin varies linearly with plasma bilirubin turnover, and inversely with hepatic bilirubin clearance.

$$(8)\quad \overline{BR} = \text{Constant} \times \frac{BRT}{C_{BR}}$$

Note, further, that for any particular value for plasma bilirubin turnover, the plasma unconjugated bilirubin concentration and hepatic bilirubin clearance are related by an equation of the form X times Y equals a constant, which is the equation of a rectangular hyperbola. Fig. 3 illustrates three such rectangular hyperbolae, depicting the relationship between hepatic bilirubin clearance and the plasma concentration of unconjugated bilirubin which would be observed at rates of bilirubin turnover representing 100%, 200% and 400% of the mean normal value.

Several important relationships are illustrated by Fig. 3. First, as suggested by equation (8), for any particular value of hepatic bilirubin clearance, doubling the rate of bilirubin turnover will result in a doubling of the plasma unconjugated bilirubin concentration. Similarly, for any particular value of bilirubin turnover, a 50% reduction in hepatic bilirubin clearance will also result in a doubling of the plasma concentration of unconjugated bilirubin. It is important to note that while the fractional change in plasma bilirubin concentration is always equal to the fractional change in either plasma bilirubin turnover or in hepatic bilirubin clearance, the absolute magnitude of the change in plasma bilirubin concentration will depend greatly on the baseline value for clearance. For example, if one doubles plasma bilirubin turnover from 3.9 to 7.8 mg/kg/day in a typical normal subject, the plasma unconjugated bilirubin concentration will increase by only about 0.45 mg%, and may, therefore, remain in the normal range. A 50% reduction in hepatic bilirubin clearance will also produce an increment of only 0.45 mg% in the plasma unconjugated bilirubin concentration.

TABLE I

COMPARISON OF METHODS FOR CALCULATION OF HEPATIC BILIRUBIN CLEARANCE

Study	Bilirubin Production Rate (BRP)* (mg/day)	Plasma Bilirubin Turnover (BRT)† (mg/day)	Hepatic Bilirubin Clearance (ml/min)		
			(A) Calculated From BRP	(B) Calculated From BRT	B/A
A	364	377	57.6	59.4	1.032
B	164	148	45.6	41.1	0.903
C	361	344	71.6	68.2	0.953
D	428	455	49.8	52.9	1.063
B/A = 0.99 ± 0.03 (Mean ± S.E.M.)					

* Determined by fecal isotope dilution technique

† Calculated from plasma radiobilirubin disappearance curves

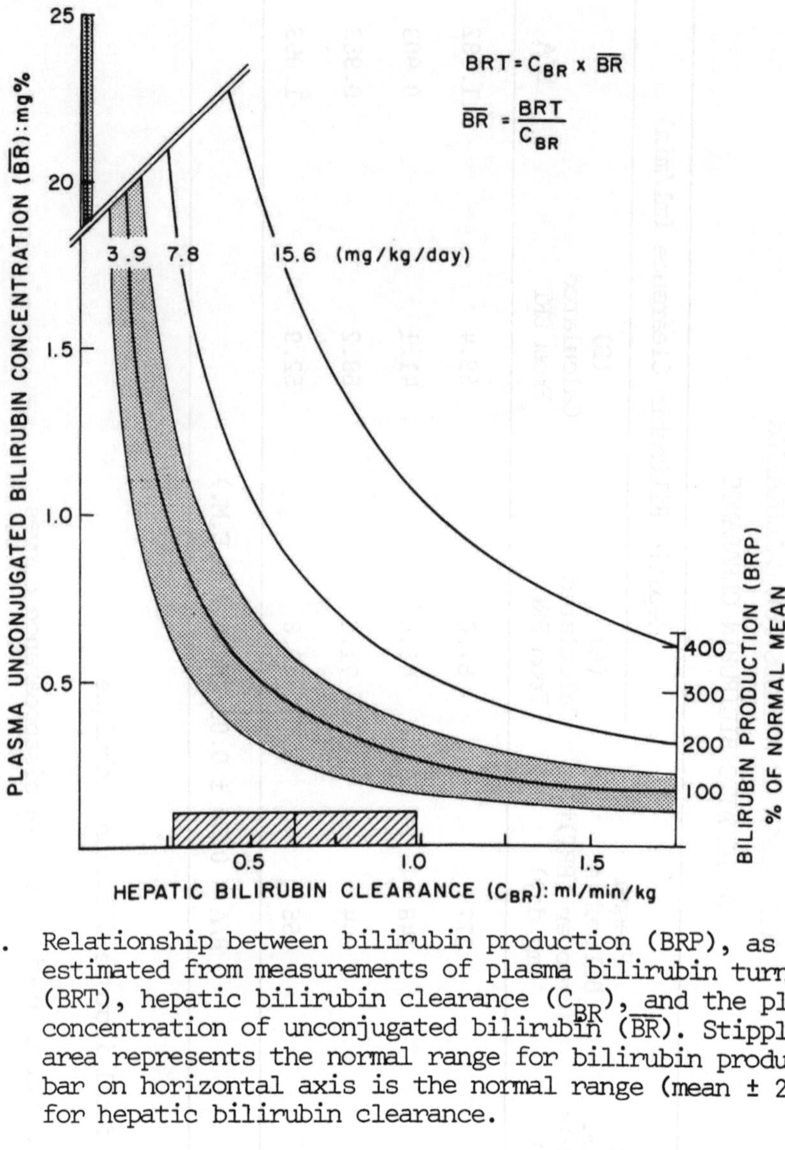

Fig. 3. Relationship between bilirubin production (BRP), as estimated from measurements of plasma bilirubin turnover (BRT), hepatic bilirubin clearance (C_{BR}), and the plasma concentration of unconjugated bilirubin ($\overline{BR}$). Stippled area represents the normal range for bilirubin production; bar on horizontal axis is the normal range (mean ± 2 S.D.) for hepatic bilirubin clearance.

On the other hand, if the patient's baseline clearance rate is only 0.1 ml/min/kg, an identical increase in bilirubin turnover, or a further 50% reduction in bilirubin clearance, will produce an increment of about 2.5 mg% in the plasma bilirubin concentration.

The relationships between plasma bilirubin turnover, bilirubin clearance and plasma bilirubin concentration are identical to the relationships between the rate of urea production, urea clearance and the blood urea nitrogen concentration. However, the applicability of these basic relationships to the liver is not widely appreciated.

From equation (8) it is apparent that an elevated plasma concentration of unconjugated bilirubin can result from an increase in plasma bilirubin turnover, a reduction in bilirubin clearance, or some combination of the two. The availability of a method for calculating both bilirubin turnover and bilirubin clearance should make it possible to establish precisely the responsible mechanism in any patient with unconjugated hyperbilirubinemia. As an example of the value of this technique, let us consider the problem of constitutional hepatic dysfunction, or Gilbert's syndrome.

Gilbert's syndrome may be defined as chronic or recurrent mild unconjugated hyperbilirubinemia which occurs in the absence of other biochemical or morphologic evidence of liver disease (4,12). Patients with demonstrable hemolysis are usually excluded from this diagnostic category because of the presumption that the hyperbilirubinemia in these cases results entirely from bilirubin overproduction.

We have now performed plasma radiobilirubin disappearance studies in 14 patients who meet the classical clinical, biochemical and histologic criteria for Gilbert's syndrome (4,12,13). As illustrated in Fig. 4, the curves in these patients have a characteristic pattern, which is easily distinguished from normal. As shown in Table II, neither red cell survival nor plasma bilirubin turnover in these 14 patients with classical Gilbert's syndrome (Table II: Gilbert's Syndrome, Group I) differed significantly from the corresponding values in 23 normal volunteers. On the other hand, retention of isotope in the plasma at four hours was markedly increased. The increase in the plasma concentration of unconjugated bilirubin in these patients is entirely attributable to a reduction in hepatic bilirubin clearance to less than 1/3 of normal. In contrast, the degree of unconjugated hyperbilirubinemia observed in a group of 13 patients with uncomplicated hemolysis (Table II: Hemolysis) was found to precisely parallel the extent to which plasma bilirubin turnover was increased (4). Both 4 hour isotope retention and hepatic bilirubin clearance were entirely normal in the group with pure hemolysis.

Gilbert's syndrome appears to be a relatively common abnormality, which is being recognized with increasing frequency. Since hemolytic anemia is also relatively common, it should not be surprising to find the simultaneous occurrence of both the hepatic lesion of Gilbert's syndrome and a shortened red cell lifespan in some patients. We have also had the opportunity to perform radiobilirubin clearance studies in 12 patients with hemolysis in whom the degree of hyper-

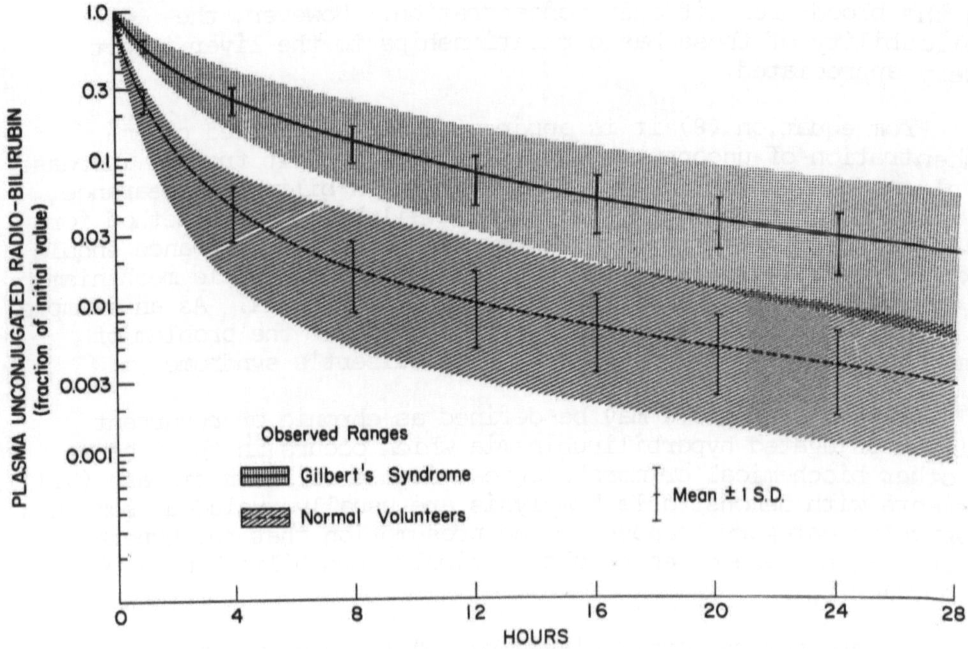

Fig. 4. Observed ranges of plasma radiobilirubin disappearance curves in patients with Gilbert's syndrome and in healthy, young adult volunteers. The average curve for each group was calculated by computer from the mean values for that group of the parameters of a compartmental model of bilirubin metabolism. There is no overlap between the two groups for the first sixteen hours after injection.

bilirubinemia was greater than expected for the rate of red cell destruction. Liver biopsies in these patients showed no evidence of hepatic disease, and liver function tests, except for the plasma unconjugated bilirubin concentration, were normal. In these patients (Table II: Gilbert's Syndrome, Group II) plasma retention of radiobilirubin at 4 hours and hepatic bilirubin clearance were identical to the values observed in the group with "classical Gilbert's syndrome." Plasma bilirubin turnover was increased in proportion to the rate of hemolysis. These patients appear to have the hepatic defect of Gilbert's syndrome as well as hemolysis. These studies therefore confirm the earlier observations of Powell, Billing and Williams, who deduced the simultaneous occurrence of Gilbert's syndrome and hemolytic anemia from measurements of plasma bilirubin concentration and chromium^{51} red cell survival (14). To date, the radiobilirubin clearance pattern indicative of Gilbert's syndrome has been observed in patients with congenital spherocytosis, glucose-6-phosphate dehydrogenase deficiency, and a variety of

TABLE II

RESULTS OF RADIO-BILIRUBIN CLEARANCE STUDIES IN NORMAL CONTROLS, PATIENTS WITH HEMOLYSIS AND PATIENTS WITH GILBERT'S SYNDROME

	^{51}Cr RBC Half-life (days)	Plasma Unconjugated Bilirubin Concentration (mg/100 ml)	4 Hour Retention (%)	C_{BR} (ml/min/kg)	BRT (mg/kg/day)
Gilbert's Syndrome Group I (n=14)	28 ± 2	1.6 ± 0.5	26.9 ± 6.7	0.19 ± 0.04	4.3 ± 1.2
Group II (n=12)	17 ± 6	3.9 ± 1.9	27.4 ± 9.7	0.20 ± 0.08	9.4 ± 5.7
Normal Controls (n=23)	29 ± 3	0.44 ± 0.10	5.2 ± 1.9	0.65 ± 0.18	3.9 ± 0.7
Hemolysis (n=13)	15 ± 5	1.3 ± 0.8	4.6 ± 1.9	0.68 ± 0.15	12.9 ± 8.9

uncharacterized non-spherocytic hemolytic anemias (11). We believe that the simultaneous occurrence of hemolysis and Gilbert's syndrome is a chance occurrence, and does not imply any causal relationship between the two conditions.

In passing, note that the ability to quantitate both BRT and C_{BR} permits a precise classification of patients with unconjugated hyperbilirubinemia into (a) those with increased bilirubin production (as reflected by an increased BRT), (b) those with decreased bilirubin clearance, and (c) those in whom both factors play a role. No other approach permits the ready identification of group (c).

Before going on to the next topic, it will be useful to return briefly to equation (8). It is a well recognized, empirical clinical fact that chronic hemolysis, alone, does not produce elevations of the plasma bilirubin concentration in excess of 4 mg%. A variety of explanations, mostly incorrect, have been proposed for this observation. The real explanation is evident from equation (8). For a given individual with a constant value for C_{BR}, or for a population of individuals, such as the normal population, whose values for C_{BR} lie within a restricted range, the plasma concentration of unconjugated bilirubin ($\overline{BR}$) will vary in a linear fashion with BRT. i.e.:

(9) $\overline{BR}$ = Constant x BRT.

In Fig. 5, values for $\overline{BR}$ are plotted as a function of BRT in individuals with normal values for C_{BR}, and individuals with reduced C_{BR} due to Gilbert's syndrome. A regression line ± 2 standard errors of the estimate has been drawn through the points representing individuals with normal hepatic function, and this line represents the rate at which the plasma bilirubin concentration will increase with an increasing bilirubin load due to, e.g., hemolysis. It is well known that the maximal rate of hemoglobin synthesis by the bone marrow, in response to hemolysis, is no more than 8 times baseline. This implies that, since bilirubin is derived principally from hemoglobin, in steady state hemolytic anemias the maximal rate of bilirubin production cannot exceed eight times normal, or about 40 mg/kg/day. If we extrapolate the regression line in Fig. 5 to 40 mg/kg/day, we see that this corresponds to a plasma unconjugated bilirubin concentration of 3.5 - 4.0 mg%. Hence, it is the limited ability of the bone marrow to produce hemoglobin, coupled with the relationship between bilirubin turnover and bilirubin concentration, which explains why chronic, steady state hemolysis does not elevate the bilirubin above 4 mg% in the presence of normal hepatic bilirubin metabolism. Since bilirubin production may briefly be much greater than eight times normal in acute hemolytic crises, such as occur in sickle cell disease, glucose-6-phosphate dehydrogenase deficiency, or paroxysmal nocturnal hemo-

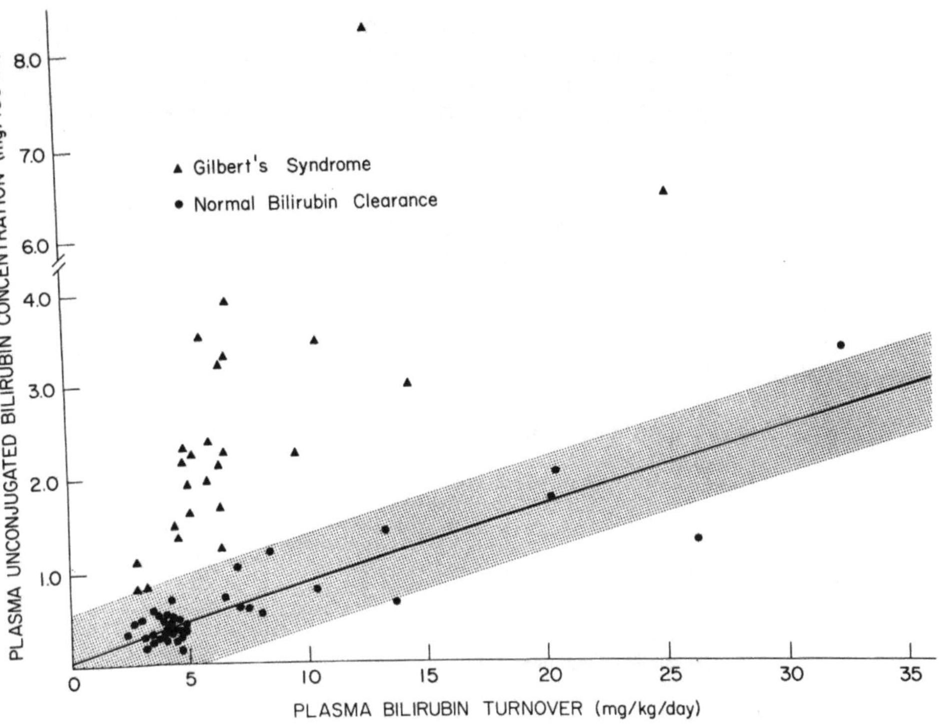

Fig. 5. Relationship between plasma bilirubin turnover and the plasma concentration of unconjugated bilirubin. When hepatic bilirubin clearance is within the relatively narrow normal range, the plasma unconjugated bilirubin concentration will increase linearly with increasing rates of bilirubin production, as indicated by the regression line. Stippled area represents two standard errors of the estimate about the regression line. Extrapolation of the regression line to the maximum achievable rate of bilirubin production, or approximately 40 mg/kg/day, indicates the highest value for the plasma unconjugated bilirubin concentration which can occur as the result of sustained hemolysis in an individual with normal hepatic bilirubin clearance, corresponding to 3.5 - 4.0 mg%.

globinuria, the 4 mg% limit does not apply to these transient, non-steady state situations.

Although we have concentrated until now on measurements of hepatic bilirubin clearance and plasma bilirubin turnover, it is possible to obtain considerable additional information from studies with radio-bilirubin. Two approaches are possible. One may correlate calculated values for bilirubin clearance with independent measurements of some other aspect of hepatic physiology. This is illustrated in Fig. 6, in which values for bilirubin clearance in patients with Crigler-Najjar syndrome, Gilbert's syndrome, normal volunteers, and phenobarbital treated controls are plotted against measurements of hepatic UDP-bilirubin glucuronyl transferase activity in corresponding groups of patients. The bilirubin clearance data in this figure are from Bethesda, while the enzyme assay values are largely from papers by Black and Billing, in London (15,16). The excellent correlation between these parameters strongly suggests that changes in glucuronyl transferase activity are important determinants of the differences in bilirubin clearance observed between groups.

Alternatively, one can make the assumption that the unconjugated

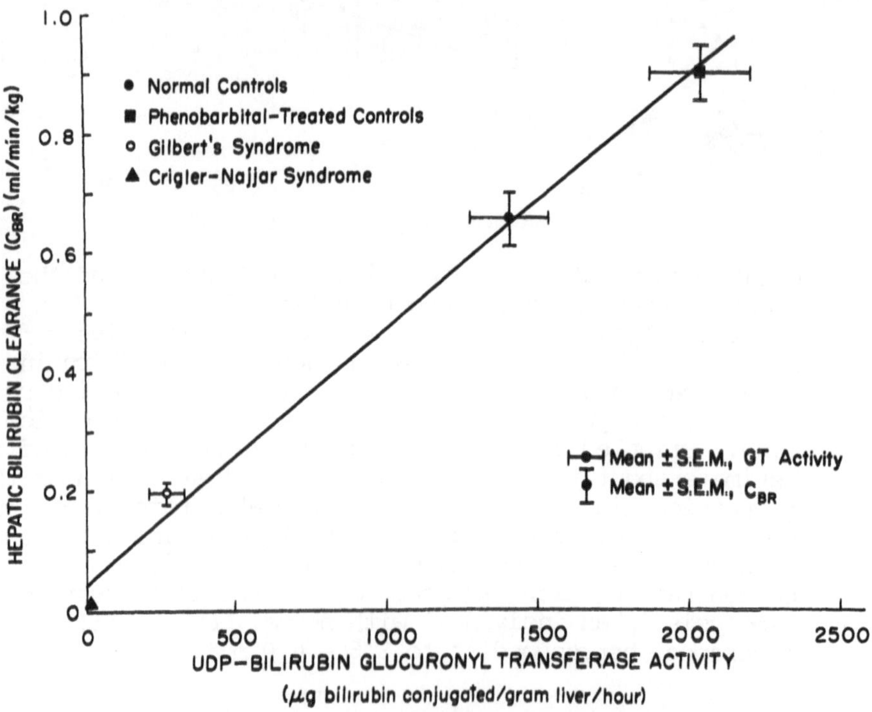

Fig. 6. Mean values (± S.E.M.) of hepatic bilirubin clearance in patients with the Crigler-Najjar syndrome, Gilbert's syndrome, healthy normal controls, and healthy phenobarbital-treated controls, plotted as a function of hepatic bilirubin-UDP glucuronyl transferase activity in corresponding groups of patients. Bilirubin clearance measurements are from Bethesda, while enzyme assays are from the published data of M. Black and B.H. Billing, in London (15,16).

bilirubin within the body is compartmentalized, and that the shape of the plasma radiobilirubin disappearance curve results from the transfer of bilirubin from the plasma into and out of the various other compartments which exchange with plasma. It can be shown mathematically, from the fact that the plasma radiobilirubin disappearance curve consists of a sum of three exponential functions, that there must be at least two additional compartments exchanging with the plasma pool (2). From the many possible three compartment models, we have selected the model shown in Fig. 7 as being most compatible with our current concepts of bilirubin metabolism. In this model, plasma unconjugated bilirubin is thought to exchange with an extra-hepatic/extra-vascular pool and an intra-hepatic pool of unconjugated bilirubin. Bilirubin leaves this system via the liver pool, either by conjugation or some other form of biotransformation. Note that this model contains the implicit postulate that the exchange of bilirubin between liver and plasma is bidirectional.

This model can be expressed mathematically as a system of differential equations, which can be solved for the various model parameters using the data obtained from the plasma radiobilirubin disappearance curve (2). Hence, the experimental plasma radiobilirubin disappearance curve and the equations of the model make it possible to calculate values for a number of additional parameters of physiologic interest. These include:

(1) Size of the plasma, intrahepatic, and extrahepatic-extravascular pools of unconjugated bilirubin. From the sizes of the plasma and intrahepatic pools, the relative storage capacity of the liver for unconjugated bilirubin, S (mg/mg/100 ml), can be estimated.

(2) Fractional transfer rates (λ's) between pools. This permits calculation of fluxes between pools: e.g. hepatic bilirubin uptake.

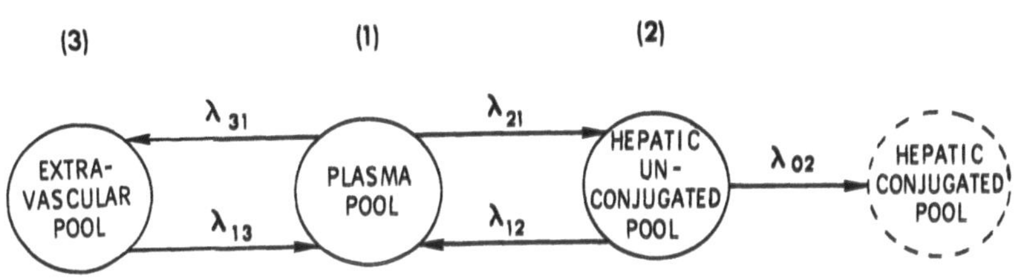

Fig. 7 A three compartment model of the metabolism of unconjugated bilirubin. Values for the λ's, which are the fractional transfer rates between compartments, and for the relative pool sizes are calculated from the plasma disappearance curve of unconjugated radiobilirubin.

(3) Radiobilirubin specific activity curves for the intrahepatic and extrahepatic-extravascular pools, as well as the cumulative curve for radiobilirubin conjugation.

(4) Estimate of the minimal intrahepatic bilirubin concentration and the liver:plasma concentration gradient.

The hypothesis that the bilirubin in the body is compartmentalized is logical, intuitively appealing, and clinically useful. It is, nevertheless, only a hypothesis, as is the selection of a particular compartmental model. Since the results derived by compartmental analysis are valid only to the extent that these hypotheses are valid, it is necessary to maintain a constructive skepticism about such results. I would like to mention briefly several of the lines of evidence which tend to support the validity of the model, and hence, of the experimental results derived from it. In particular, studies in normal volunteers indicate that, when compared to the direct experimental measurement of the corresponding parameter, analysis of plasma radiobilirubin disappearance curves in terms of the model: (a) accurately predicts the relative storage capacity of the liver for bilirubin; (b) accurately predicts the rate of excretion of conjugated radiobilirubin in the bile, following administration of unconjugated radiobilirubin; and (c) accurately predicts the proportion of the bilirubin-^{14}C, derived in the liver from the administration of δ-aminolevulinic acid-4-^{14}C, which will reflux from liver to plasma prior to its ultimate excretion in the bile.

Let us first consider the calculation of relative storage capacity. While the relative storage capacity of the liver for organic anions, such as BSP, is usually calculated from continuous infusion studies, Quarfordt and co-workers have recently described a method for calculation of this parameter from compartmental analysis of plasma BSP disappearance curves (17). The values for relative BSP storage capacity derived by this technique were generally in good agreement with the published values of Wheeler and co-workers, who used the standard infusion method (18). In Table III we have compared values for the relative bilirubin storage capacity in normal subjects, calculated by compartmental analysis of plasma radiobilirubin disappearance curves, with values obtained by Raymond and Galambos (19) using the standard infusion technique. The difference between the means is not statistically significant, and the observed ranges are virtually identical. Since the values for S are dependent on use of the model to calculate the size of the intrahepatic bilirubin pool, these results suggest the validity of this particular model-dependent calculation.

In the normal liver, conjugation of bilirubin is followed by the prompt biliary excretion of the conjugated material. Hence, if

TABLE III

RELATIVE STORAGE CAPACITY FOR BILIRUBIN IN NORMAL HUMAN VOLUNTEERS

	Compartmental Analysis (n=22)		Infusion Technique (n=10)*	
	(Mean ± S.E.M.)	(Range)	(Mean ± S.E.M.)	(Range)
S(mg/mg %)	41.8 ± 3.1	15 - 69	31.3 ± 7.0†	13 - 77

* Data of Raymond et Galambos: See reference 19.

† Student's t test: $p > 0.1$

the model-derived transfer rates for bilirubin between plasma and liver and from liver to bile are correct, then the hypothetical curve of cumulative radiobilirubin conjugation (calculated by the model from the plasma radiobilirubin disappearance curve) should reflect the cumulative excretion of conjugated radiobilirubin in T-tube drainage. Comparison of the two curves requires allowance of an appropriate time lag for passage of bilirubin through the biliary tract and the T-tube itself. In patients in whom the volume of the biliary tract and the rate of bile flow - and hence, the appropriate time lag - were accurately known, we have been able to show that the experimental curve of radiobilirubin excretion and the corresponding model-derived curve of cumulative conjugation are virtually superimposable (2).

As illustrated in Fig. 7, the proposed model of unconjugated bilirubin metabolism implies that the exchange of bilirubin between plasma and liver is bi-directional. As a consequence, unconjugated bilirubin within the hepatic pool may either undergo conjugation and subsequent biliary excretion, or may reflux to the plasma unconjugated bilirubin pool. During a visit to our laboratory, Dr. E. Anthony Jones used δ-aminolevulinic acid-^{14}C to selectively label the intrahepatic pool of unconjugated bilirubin. He was then able to demonstrate that some of the intrahepatic unconjugated bilirubin-^{14}C refluxed to the plasma, confirming that a bi-directional flux of bilirubin between liver and plasma in fact occurs (20). Furthermore, by mathematical technique known as deconvolution he was able to show that the fraction of this intrahepatic bilirubin-^{14}C which refluxed to plasma was similar to that predicted from compartmental analysis of a bilirubin-^{3}H disappearance curve which was obtained simultaneously. The three groups of experiments just summarized suggest that both the size of the intrahepatic unconjugated bilirubin pool, and the three fractional transfer rates into and out of this pool, can be accurately determined from compartmental analysis of plasma radiobilirubin disappearance curves.

I have focused, until now, on some of the evidence tending to support the validity of the proposed compartmental model of bilirubin metabolism. I should next like to provide an example of the type of physiologic data obtainable by this technique.

Because the exchange of unconjugated bilirubin between plasma and liver is bi-directional, there may be a considerable difference between the absolute rate at which bilirubin enters the liver cell, and net hepatic sequestration. Data on the absolute rate of hepatic bilirubin uptake, as well as the fraction of the material entering the liver which refluxes to plasma in normal subjects and patients with both Gilbert's and Crigler-Najjar syndromes are presented in Table IV. This table indicates, first of all, that the liver has the capacity to increase bilirubin uptake to at least 50 times the basal rate, indicating that the uptake mechanism

TABLE IV

HEPATIC BILIRUBIN UPTAKE AND REFLUX IN NORMAL VOLUNTEERS AND PATIENTS WITH UNCONJUGATED HYPERBILIRUBINEMIA

Group	Plasma Unconjugated Bilirubin Concentration (mg/100 ml)	Hepatic uptake (μg/min/kg)	Reflux/Uptake (%)
Normal volunteers (n=23)	0.44*	4.6	40
Gilbert's Syndrome (n=26)	2.7	16.0	59
Crigler-Najjar (n=4)	22.0	80 - 203	98

* Mean values

has a large reserve capacity. Furthermore, although the initial or absolute uptake rate appears to increase as the bilirubin concentration increases, independent of the subsequent fate of the molecule, in jaundiced patients most of the bilirubin entering the liver promptly refluxes to plasma. Hence, net hepatic bilirubin uptake is highly dependent on the integrity of subsequent metabolic pathways.

Although my topic is the "Whole Body Handling of Bilirubin", I have focused principally on the hepatic metabolism of unconjugated bilirubin because available methodologies currently restrict clinical

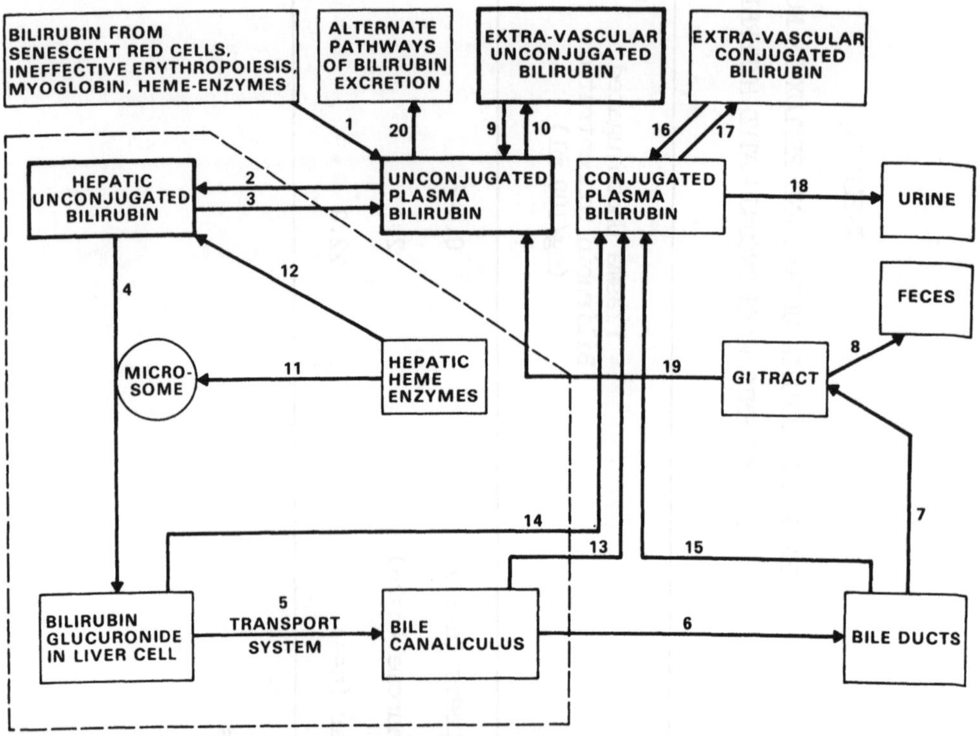

Fig. 8. Schematic compartmental model of total body bilirubin metabolism. For clarity, pathways representing the hepatic uptake and re-excretion of conjugated bilirubin have been omitted. If radiolabeled conjugated bilirubin were available, quantitative estimates of the transfer rates corresponding to many of these pathways could be obtained from the simultaneous injection of, e.g., unconjugated bilirubin-^{14}C and conjugated bilirubin-^{3}H.

studies to this aspect of the overall problem. In Fig. 8, I have illustrated a hypothetical compartmental model which would, in fact, encompass the Whole Body Handling of Bilirubin. In addition to the plasma, intrahepatic, and extravascular pools of unconjugated bilirubin already discussed in detail, this model includes the normal pathways for the excretion of conjugated bilirubin into the gastrointestinal tract and feces, as well as the various pathways by which conjugated bilirubin may find its way to the plasma. For the sake of clarity, the subsequent hepatic uptake and re-excretion of conjugated bilirubin has been omitted.

It is probable that in normal man there is virtually no conjugated bilirubin in the circulation, and that the 0.1 mg% or so of direct reacting bilirubin commonly measured in normal subjects is an artifact of the Van den Bergh reaction. Hence, many of the additional pathways present in this more detailed model would be operative to a measurable degree only in pathologic states. To date, the combination of non-invasive isotope tracer methodology with appropriate methods of data analysis permits a precise and quantitative localization of the abnormal process responsible for any instance of unconjugated hyperbilirubinemia. As methods for the isolation, purification and radiolabeling of conjugated bilirubin are developed, these techniques can be logically extended to permit detailed analyses of all aspects of the total body handling of bilirubin in normal man, and in patients with all types of hepato-biliary dysfunction.

SUMMARY

The major points presented can be summarized as follows:

(1) Clinical studies of radiobilirubin kinetics permit the accurate determination of hepatic bilirubin clearance (C_{BR}) and plasma bilirubin turnover (BRT).

(2) Measurement of C_{BR} appears to be a useful technique in the assessment of hepatic function, and simultaneous measurement of C_{BR} and BRT permits precise classification of patients with unconjugated hyperbilirubinemia.

(3) Compartmental analysis of plasma radiobilirubin disappearance curves permits calculation of several other important parameters of hepatic function. In general, values calculated by this technique have agreed with direct experimental measurements of the corresponding parameter. Although these early results appear promising, the validity of this approach continues to require independent experimental verification.

ACKNOWLEDGEMENTS

I would like to acknowledge the efforts of Drs. Joseph Bloomer, Terrence Blaschke and Nathaniel I. Berlin, each of whom has made a major contribution to the work presented today. In addition, thanks are due to Mrs. Beva Schellhase for the accurate preparation of the manuscript.

REFERENCES

1. WEBER AP, SCHALM L: Quantitative separation and determination of bilirubin and conjugated bilirubin in human serum. Clin Chim Acta 7: 805-810, 1962.

2. BERK PD, HOWE RB, BLOOMER JR et al: Studies of bilirubin kinetics in normal adults. J Clin Invest 48: 2176-2190, 1969.

3. BLOOMER JR, BERK PD, VERGALLA J et al: Influence of albumin on the hepatic uptake of unconjugated bilirubin. Clin Sci and Molec Med 45: 505-516, 1973.

4. BERK PD, BLOOMER JR, HOWE RB et al: Constitutional hepatic dysfunction (Gilbert's syndrome). Amer J Med 49: 296-305, 1970.

5. BARRETT PVD, BERK PD, MENKEN et al: Bilirubin turnover studies in normal and pathologic states using bilirubin-^{14}C. Ann Inter Med 68: 355-377, 1968.

6. COBURN RF, BLAKEMORE WS, FORSTER RE: Endogenous carbon monoxide production in man. J Clin Invest 42: 1172-1178, 1963.

7. COLTMAN CA Jr, DUDLEY GM III: The relationship between endogenous carbon monoxide production and total heme mass in normal and abnormal subjects. Amer J Med Sci 258: 374-385, 1969.

8. LYNCH SR, MOEDE AL: Variation in the rate of endogenous carbon monoxide production in normal human beings. J Lab Clin Med 79: 85-95, 1972.

9. BERK PD, RODKEY FL, BLASCHKE TF et al: Comparison of plasma bilirubin turnover and carbon monoxide production in man. J Lab Clin Med 83: 29-37, 1974.

10. BLOOMER JR, BERK PD, HOWE RB et al: Comparison of fecal urobilinogen excretion with bilirubin production in normal volunteers and patients with increased bilirubin production. Clin Chim Acta 29: 463-471, 1970.

11. BERK PD, BLOOMER JR, HOWE RB et al: Bilirubin production as a measure of red cell life span. J Lab Clin Med 79: 364-378, 1972.

12. FOULK WT, BUTT HR, OWEN CA et al: Constitutional hepatic dysfunction (Gilbert's disease): Its natural history and related syndromes. Medicine 38: 25-46, 1959.

13. BARTH RF, GRIMLEY PM, BERK PD et al: Excess lipofuscin accumulation in constitutional hepatic dysfunction (Gilbert's syndrome). Arch Pathol 91: 41-47, 1971.

14. POWELL LW, BILLING BH, WILLIAMS HS: An assessment of red cell survival in idiopathic unconjugated hyperbilirubinaemia (Gilbert's syndrome) by the use of radioactive diisopropylfluorophosphate and chromium. Austral Ann Med 16: 221-225, 1967.

15. BLACK M, BILLING BH: Hepatic bilirubin UDP glucuronyl transferase activity in liver disease and Gilbert's syndrome. N Eng J Med 280: 1266-1271, 1969.

16. BLACK M, PERRETT RD, CARTER AE: Hepatic bilirubin UDP-glucuronyl transferase activity and cytochrome P_{450} content in a surgical population, and the effects of pre-operative drug therapy. J Lab Clin Med 81: 704-712, 1973.

17. QUARFORDT SH, HILDERMAN HL, VALLE D et al: Compartmental analysis of sulfobromophthalein transport in normal patients and patients with hepatic dysfunction. Gastroent 60: 246-255, 1971.

18. WHEELER HO, MELTZER JI, BRADLEY SE: Biliary transport and hepatic storage of sulfobromophthalein sodium in the unanesthetized dog, in normal man and in patients with hepatic disease. J Clin Invest 39: 1131-1144, 1960.

19. RAYMOND GD, GALAMBOS JT: Hepatic storage and excretion of bilirubin in man. Amer J Gastroent 55: 135-144, 1971.

20. JONES EA, SHRAGER R, BLOOMER JR et al: Quantitative studies of the delivery of hepatic synthesized bilirubin to plasma utilizing δ-aminolevulinic acid-4-^{14}C and bilirubin-^{3}H in man. J Clin Invest 51: 2450-2458, 1972.

THE HEPATIC UPTAKE PROCESS: ITS IMPLICATIONS FOR BILIRUBIN TRANSPORT

Carl A. Goresky

The McGill University Medical Clinic in the Montreal General Hospital, Montreal, Quebec, Canada H3G 1A4

One of the fundamental aims of this symposium is to provide a framework upon which information concerning the handling of bilirubin can be knitted together, a framework which will prove useful both to the investigator concerned with fundamental phenomena and the clinician concerned with the care of a patient with jaundice. My task, within this framework, is to provide some insight into the kinetic processes involved in the uptake by the liver of substances like bilirubin. In order to attain this end I will present to you a general examination of the process of uptake at the hepatic cell surface. From this background, I will develop ideas concerning the manner in which the processes of biliary secretion or intracellular metabolic sequestration create steady state concentration gradients in the parenchymal cells distributed along the length of the sinusoids within each liver lobule. Finally, I will deal with the manner in which the lobular gradient phenomenon may account for the increase in the Tm for the biliary secretion of bilirubin which accompanies bile salt induced increments in bile flow.

THE UPTAKE PROCESS

The structural design of the liver is unique. From the point of view of the arrangement of the hepatic lobules in space, the liver has an ordered structure. Vascular input sources and output points are symmetrically arranged and, for adjacent sinusoids, the entrances and exits are coaligned. Flow in adjacent sinusoids is concurrent and there is no opportunity within the lobular structure for diffusible materials to shortcircuit the vascular pathway and exit prematurely.

In order to investigate the process of uptake in this structure, I have utilized the multiple indicator dilution technique. This consists of the rapid injection into the portal vein of blood containing a mixture of the labeled materials to be used in the study, and of the subsequent rapid collection of serial samples of hepatic venous blood (1). In each of the experiments described here three substances were injected: ^{51}Cr-labeled red blood cells, which serve as a reference substance for vascular flow; a second labeled reference substance, which has the same extracellular distribution pattern as would the substance under study, in the absence of an uptake process; and the tracer substance whose uptake pattern is under study. Ideally these studies are carried out against a background steady state concentration, in a situation in which the level of the unlabeled study substance is not changing.

The kinetic processes expected to be involved in the handling of materials entering cells are outlined in Fig. 1. Under ordinary circumstances the materials penetrate the sinusoidal lining freely, pass through the membrane by means of a carrier-mediated transport mechanism, and then either return to the extracellular space by the same mechanism or become sequestered by a metabolic process or by biliary secretion. In order to provide a broad picture of the kind of results found experimentally, we will examine the results of single studies illustrating, in sequence, the uptake of a substance not sequestered in the liver cells, the uptake of a substance partly sequestered in the liver cells by a metabolic process, and the uptake of a substance for which virtually all of the material entering liver cells is sequestered by secretion into bile, during a single passage.

1. Glucose, an exchanging material. The uptake of labeled D-glucose, when the steady state glucose level is 137 mg/100 ml, is shown in Fig. 2. At glucose levels above 90 mg/100 ml there will be virtually no net uptake of the labeled glucose, and the tracer glucose

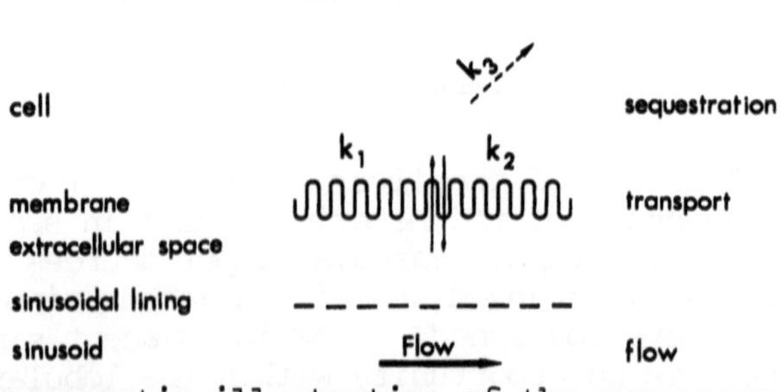

Fig. 1. A diagrammatic illustration of the processes involved in the handling of materials which enter cells and then are sequestered either by metabolic processes or biliary secretion. In this scheme k_1 is an influx coefficient; k_2, an efflux coefficient; and k_3, a sequestration coefficient.

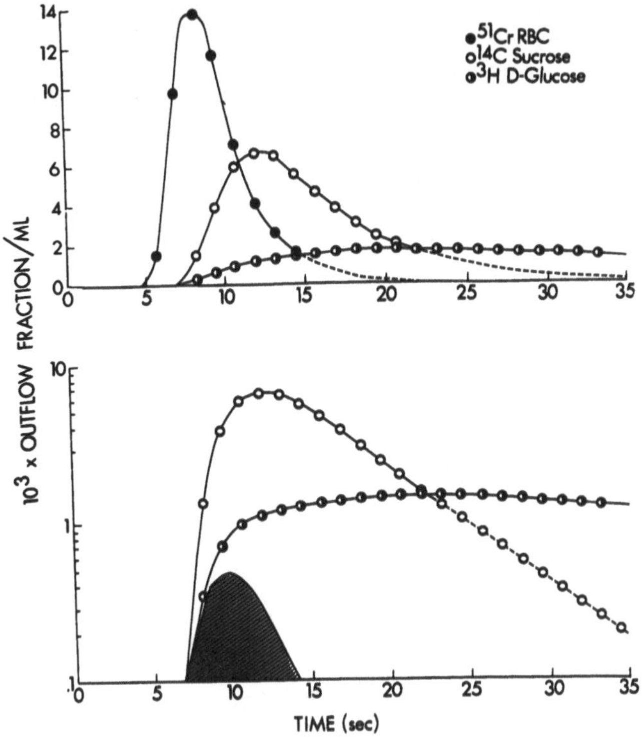

Fig. 2. The hepatic venous dilution patterns from a typical glucose experiment. The ordinate scale of the upper plot is linear; that of the lower, semilogarithmic. The time delay in the collecting system was 2.21 seconds. The dashed lines indicate the extrapolated correction of the labeled red cell and sucrose dilution curves for recirculation of label. (Reprinted with permission, from Goresky (3)).

molecules can be viewed as exchanging across the liver cell membrane, without being sequestered (2). In the illustration the ordinate value, for each of the indicators, is expressed as a fraction of the total amount of material injected per milliliter of blood. This normalizes the curves so that, if no indicator is lost during the passage of indicator through the liver, the area under the first passage curves of each of the tracers will be the same. For the three indicators utilized here, this proves to be true. In the figure the labeled red cells emerge first, their outflow fraction per ml reaches the highest and earliest peak, and then decays rapidly until recirculation occurs. The values for the second reference substance, labeled sucrose, are lower on the upslope, reach a peak which is lower and delayed with respect to that of the labeled red cell curve, and decay more slowly on the downslope.

The curve as a whole is displaced from the labeled red cell curve, in a fashion which may be shown to result from the flow-limited distribution of this labeled material out to the surface of the liver cells (1). The labeled glucose curve rises even more slowly to a peak which is later and substantially lower than that of the sucrose curve, and then slowly begins to drop. We have shown, by analysis, that the curve may be resolved into two components: a first or throughput component, which consists of material which has propagated along as a moving wave, adjacent to the hepatic cell surfaces, but which has not entered the liver cells and which therefore emerges within the envelope of the sucrose curve; and a second or exchanging component, which is delayed and which consists of material which has entered the liver cells, remained there for a period, and then returned to the circulation, to emerge in the hepatic venous blood, later in time (4). The lower panel of Fig. 2 illustrates the resolution of the tracer D-glucose curve into its two components. The throughput material is the darkly shaded early peak. It makes up the larger proportion of the early parts of the glucose profile, but contributes little to the later parts of the curve. The second component, the returning or exchanging material, represented by the difference between the throughput component and the total profile, dominates the later parts of the curve.

The resolution of the glucose outflow profile into its two components, in turn, leads to estimates for an influx coefficient, and for an efflux coefficient. The value of the former is, in this instance, 0.41 sec^{-1}; and that of the latter, 0.22 sec^{-1}. The former essentially represents a permeability surface product per volume accessible to the tracer outside the liver cells; and the latter, the same permeability surface product per volume of accessible intracellular space. The ratio of the two is the ratio of the cellular space to the total space accessible outside the cells, since glucose at equilibrium reaches identical concentration values in cell and plasma (5). The net uptake of the tracer glucose was found to be too small to be discerned, with the present technique. The rate constant for sequestration of this label is exceedingly small.

The glucose cellular entry process exhibits saturation kinetics (2). When the glucose concentration is raised the throughput component is found to form a greater part of the curve (that is, the proportion of the tracer entering the cells becomes smaller). The entry process is also stereospecific. The proportion of tracer L-glucose entering the cells during a single passage is very small. Almost all of this tracer emerges at the outflow as throughput material. These two characteristics, saturation kinetics and stereospecificity, are characteristic of carrier-mediated transport processes.

2. Galactose, a partly sequestered material. The second substance to be examined is D-galactose. Fig. 3 illustrates the set of hepatic venous outflow dilution curves from a typical experiment, in which the endogenous input portal venous plasma D-galactose concentration was 5 mg%. At this plasma concentration approximately 90% of the galactose is extracted from the blood (6). The tracer D-galactose curve showed a corresponding extraction. Only a very small proportion of the input material emerges at the outflow.

Galactose would be expected to be transported into the hepatic parenchymal cells, and then to undergo metabolic sequestration, by virtue of conversion to galactose-1-phosphate, which will not interact with the carrier transport mechanism. Early in time this

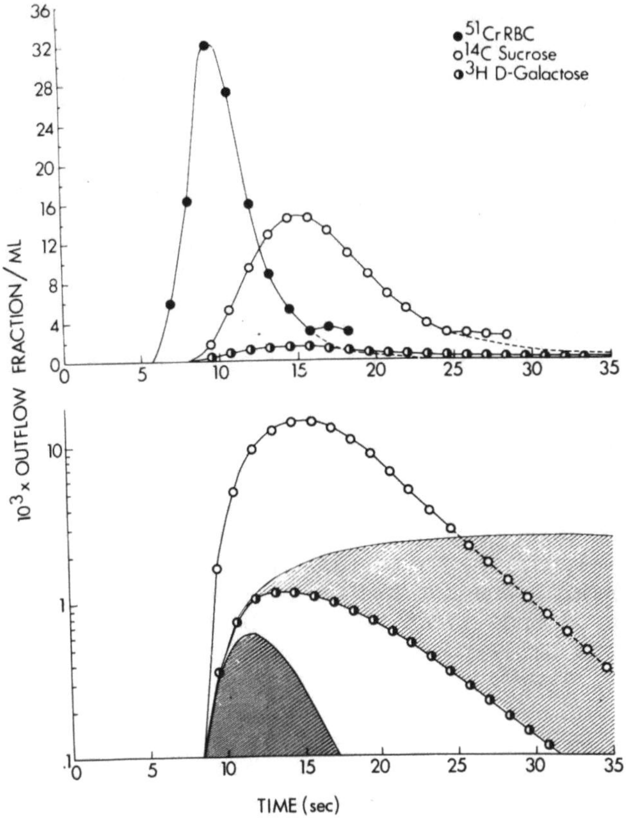

Fig. 3. The hepatic venous dilution patterns from a typical D-galactose experiment. The ordinate scale of the upper plot is linear; that of the lower, semilogarithmic. The time delay in the collecting system was 2.54 seconds. The dashed lines once again indicate the extrapolated correction of the labeled red cell and sucrose curves for recirculation of label. (Reprinted with permission, from Goresky (3)).

process can be regarded as one which sequesters labeled material, so that it cannot return to the circulation. A model analysis of this process (7) indicates that the outflow curve can once again be resolved into two components: an early throughput component, which consists of material which has not entered the hepatic parenchymal cells but which instead has propagated along as a moving wave, adjacent to the hepatic parenchymal cell surface; and returning material which, in this case, has entered the hepatic cells, escaped the process of metabolic sequestration, returned to the circulation, and emerged at the outflow. In Fig. 3 the two parts of the galactose profile are illustrated in the lower panel. The throughput material is the darkly shaded early peak; and the returning material, the difference between this and the total profile. The more lightly shaded area, later in time, marks out the outflow time pattern which the sequestered moiety would have added to the curve, if the metabolic removal process had not been taking place. As expected the shape of this total curve, with the additional final component, resembles very closely that for tracer D-glucose, illustrated in Fig. 2.

In this instance the resolution of the galactose profile into its three components leads to estimates for the three coefficients describing its kinetics. The value for the influx coefficient is 0.40 sec^{-1}; that for the efflux coefficient, 0.18 sec^{-1}; and that for the sequestration coefficient, 0.19 sec^{-1}. The sequestration coefficient is relatively large and the activity of the sequestration process leads to the removal of a fairly high proportion of the tracer material which has entered the liver cells.

Elevation of the plasma galactose level again leads to the appearance of saturation phenomena (7). The sequestration process saturates at very low values of plasma galactose (the Michaelis constant Km of the phosphorylation process is less than 20 mg%); and, with progressive elevation of the plasma galactose, saturation of the membrane carrier transport mechanism also becomes demonstrable. The entry process is once again found to be stereo-specific. The L-isomer enters the cells poorly and, once inside, is not phosphorylated.

3. Tracer sulfobromophthalein, where virtually all the entering material is sequestered. The hepatic handling of sulfobromophthalein has been thought to be similar to that of bilirubin. The compound is tightly bound to serum albumin, taken up by the liver, and excreted into the biliary tree by a system which saturates fairly readily. Some years ago I carried out an indicator dilution exploration of the kinetics of sulfobromophthalein uptake (8). In these experiments no preceding sulfobromophthalein infusion was utilized to provide background steady state concentration levels. Rather the sulfobromophthalein content of the injection bolus was varied.

Fig. 4 illustrates an experiment in which the injection mixture contained only high specific ^{35}S-labeled sulfobromophthalein, with no added carrier. The tracer sulfobromophthalein emerges at the outflow within the envelope of its appropriate extracellular reference substance, labeled albumin. The emerging sulfobromophthalein appears to be composed completely of throughput material, material which passed along the sinusoids without ever entering the cells. The influx coefficient in this experiment is found to be 0.07 sec^{-1} (see Table I). This value is substantially lower than the values found for the influx coefficient in the D-glucose and D-galactose experiments. The return of labeled material from the cells is exceedingly small, and this makes the process of ascertaining values for the efflux and sequestration coefficients somewhat uncertain. It does suggest, however, that the value of the sequestration coefficient is comparatively large.

When a higher dose of material was used in the injection mixture a smaller proportion of the single passage bolus was removed. A larger proportion of the material emerged at the outflow as throughput material. At the higher dose the outflow profile still shows little evidence of the return to the circulation of material which has entered the cells. In this experimental design the cellular space is empty of sulfobromophthalein, at the time of the beginning of the experiment, and consequently the binding sites on the intracellular binding proteins (9) and the biliary secretory transport mechanism for sulfobromophthalein (10) will not be saturated. These experiments therefore provided evidence of saturation of the membrane carrier transport mechanism without giving any insight into intracellular events. To provide the latter a different sort of experiment would be necessary, one in which the plasma level of sulfobromophthalein is set to various levels by a preceding steady infusion, and the indicator dilution bolus contains only tracer amounts of labeled sulfobromophthalein.

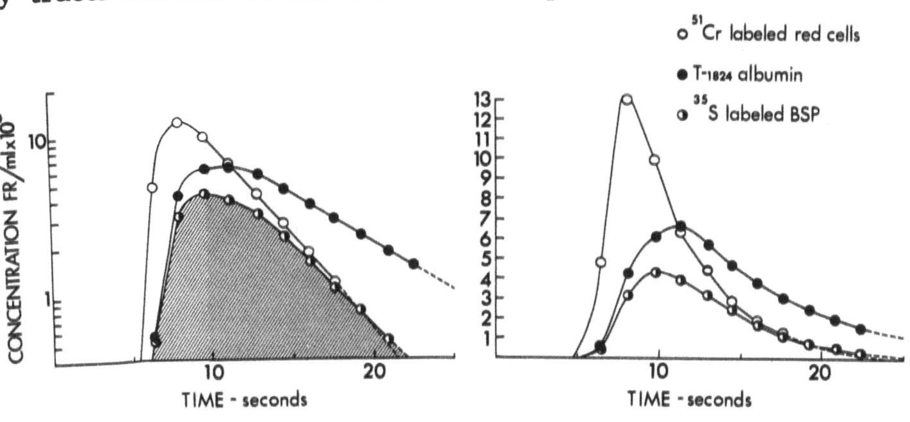

Fig. 4. The hepatic venous dilution patterns from a sulfobromophthalein experiment.

TABLE I
Transport and Sequestration Coefficients

Substance	Influx coefficient sec^{-1}	Efflux coefficient sec^{-1}	Sequestration coefficient sec^{-1}
Glucose	0.41	0.22	~ 0
Galactose	0.40	0.18	0.19
Sulfobromophthalein	0.07	?	?

4. The initial uptake of labeled bilirubin. Unless some new phenomena present themselves, the uptake of labeled bilirubin would be expected to conform, in a general way, to the preceding observations. The outflow labeled bilirubin curve would be expected to be lower than the corresponding points for its carrier molecule, labeled albumin, and thereafter the curve would be expected to diverge from the labeled albumin on a semilogarithmic plot, in the same fashion as was seen with sulfobromophthalein. Return of label to the circulation would be expected to be manifested by a later and lower component.

The outflow curves from a multiple indicator dilution study with labeled bilirubin are shown in Fig. 5. The experiment was

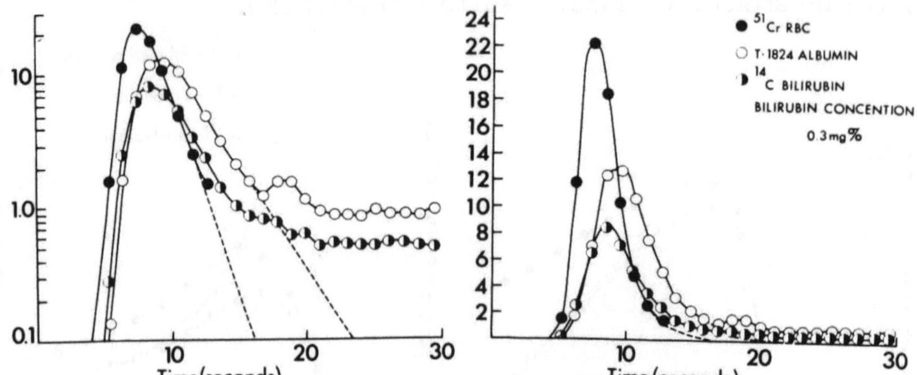

Fig. 5. The hepatic venous dilution patterns from a labeled bilirubin experiment, when the endogenous level of bilirubin was 0.3 mg%.

carried out in a dog in which the endogenous or background bilirubin concentration was 0.3 mg%. The labeled bilirubin was produced biosynthetically and its specific activity was relatively low and so, to avoid concentrations of bilirubin in the input mixture above the endogenous levels, the amount of labeled carbon injected was relatively small. A label for the carrier molecule, albumin, was therefore selected which avoids the problem of cross-over counting, the blue dye T-1824. In the outflow curves from this experiment a new phenomenon is seen. On the upslope the values for the labeled bilirubin are, unexpectedly, higher than those for its carrier molecule, albumin. Uptake then modifies the curve and, on the downslope, the labeled bilirubin curve progressively diverges from that of the labeled albumin, on the semilogarithmic plot, as expected. The upslope phenomenon is not due to displacement of T-1824 from its binding site on albumin. It is also found when ^{125}I-labeled albumin is utilized as the albumin carrier reference tracer.

The most logical explanation for the upslope phenomenon is that part of the label is being carried by red cells, that part of the labeled bilirubin is binding to the marker red cells in the injection mixture and, during the dilution study, is carried ahead of the albumin by the more rapidly advancing red cells (11). The presence of binding of bilirubin to red cells is easily documented in another way, by the incubation of red cells in a labeled bilirubin solution. Barnhart and Clarenberg (12) have carried out such experiments. Their data indicate that, in bovine blood, at a hematocrit of 0.39 and albumin concentration of 3 g/100 ml, and at normal bilirubin concentrations, approximately 11% of the bilirubin in this blood will have been taken up or bound by the red cells.

The presence of the red cell carriage phenomenon makes the task of securing influx, efflux, and sequestration constants from the bilirubin experiments more complex than was the case for the preceding experiments. The mathematical problems associated with this task have yet to be resolved.

When the serum bilirubin level is raised by infusion of a load of bilirubin in the few minutes preceding a dilution experiment, saturation of the uptake mechanism becomes evident. Such an experiment is illustrated in Fig. 6. There is still minor evidence of a red cell carriage phenomenon on the upslope of the curve, but now the labeled bilirubin curve does not diverge markedly from the labeled albumin curve on the downslope. At the higher plasma level the proportion of material removed from the plasma space has been markedly decreased.

The presence of a saturation phenomenon effectively precludes the existence of a passive non-carrier-mediated diffusion leak as a mechanism for the entry of bilirubin into liver cells. If the

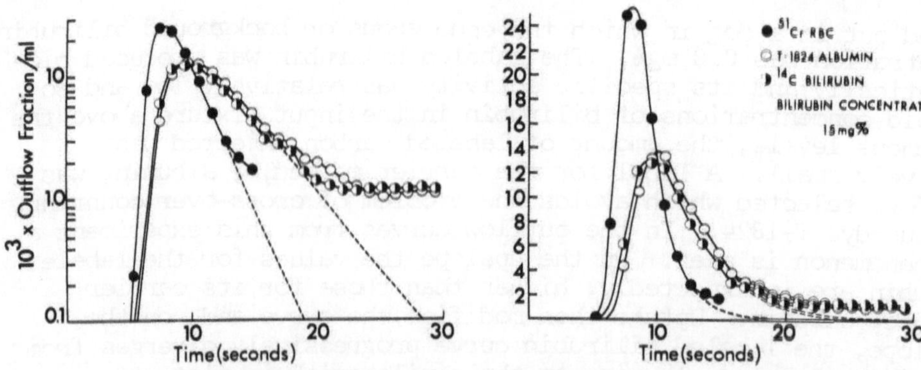

Fig. 6. The hepatic venous dilution patterns from a labeled bilirubin experiment, when the bilirubin level has been raised to 15 mg% by the preceding infusion of bilirubin.

mechanism had been a passive leak of this sort, no evidence of saturation of the uptake mechanism would have been found. If anything, as the labeled bilirubin was displaced from stronger binding sites on the carrier albumin by the load of unlabeled bilirubin, the uptake might have been expected to become proportionately larger.

These results appear to indicate that the uptake of labeled bilirubin displays no unique unexpected characteristics, apart from its complication by the presence of a minor red cell carriage phenomenon. The uptake process at the first or cellular surface appears to be carrier-mediated and to behave in a fashion analogous to the uptake mechanism for glucose and galactose.

LOBULAR CONCENTRATION GRADIENTS

The process of biliary secretion or metabolic sequestration will result in the removal of material from the hepatic parenchymal cells at each point along the length of the hepatic sinusoid. There will be, in consequence of this, a decline in the steady state concentration of material in these cells, from the site of input of blood to its site of egress. The decline in cellular concentrations in space, along the length of the sinusoids, will be expected to be approximately exponential (7). The process dominating the rate of decline will be the biliary secretory or metabolic removal process.

In our study of the hepatic uptake of labeled galactose we predicted that the lobular gradient, from portal triad to central vein, would be demonstrable. We therefore examined radioautographic sections of liver taken shortly after the administration of labeled galactose. One is displayed in Fig. 7. In this instance the liver

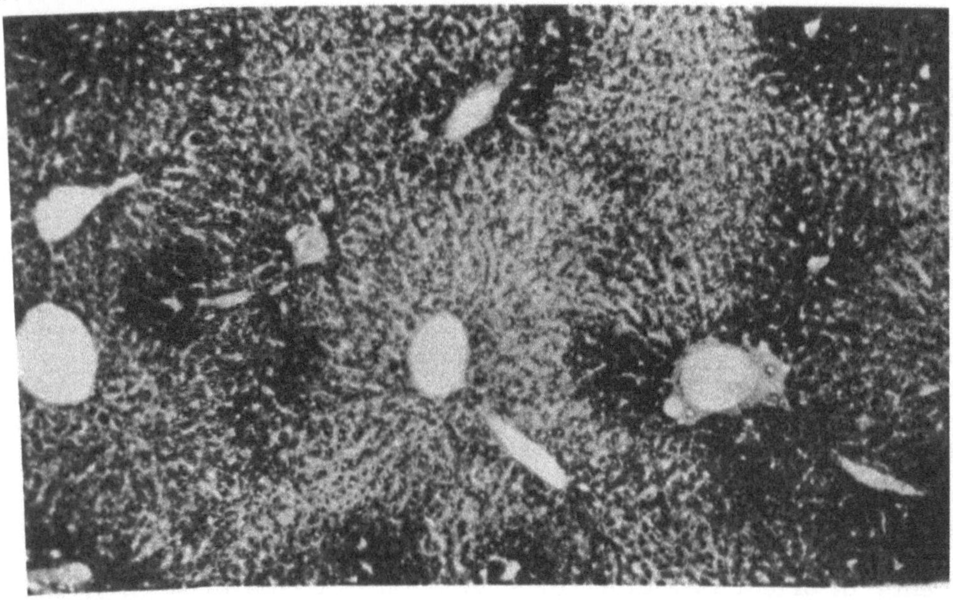

Fig. 7. The lobular intracellular concentration gradient. This radioautograph was prepared by Dr. Gary Bennett of the McGill University Department of Anatomy, to whom we express our appreciation. (Reprinted with permission, from Goresky, Bach and Nadeau (7)).

was removed two minutes after the administration of tritium-labeled galactose to a suckling mouse in trace dose. During this short period a portion of the labeled galactose entered the cell, was phosphorylated and isomerized to form galactose-1-phosphate, and was then incorporated into glycogen. During fixation of the tissue water-soluble hexoses and hexose phosphates were washed away and only the glycogen polymer remained. The slide was stained with periodic acid Schiff, which delineates glycogen as pink clumps (these show as grey areas) and a radioautograph was then developed in the overlying layer of emulsion. There is clearly a large concentration of radioactivity (the black material) in the areas surrounding the portal triads and this decreases in intensity in the direction of the central veins. The kind of gradient expected is present.

A similar gradient for bilirubin will be present and, perhaps, even more importantly, from the point of view of its biliary secretion as a conjugate, there will be a steeper and even more impressive gradient for bile acids. The effect of this gradient upon the linked secretion of bilirubin and bile acids will be explored in the next section.

THE BILIARY TRANSPORT MAXIMUM FOR BILIRUBIN

When bilirubin is infused intravenously in the dog, the biliary concentration of bilirubin rapidly increases, and the rate of excretion of bilirubin levels off at an apparent transport maximum or Tm. The biliary canalicular secretory mechanism for bilirubin becomes limiting under these circumstances, and further infusion of bilirubin results only in the elevation of the plasma levels.

Some years ago, O'Maille, Richards and Short demonstrated that the maximal rate for the biliary secretion of sulfobromophthalein, another organic anion, is increased by increasing the bile flow with taurocholate infusion (13). We hypothesized that a similar phenomenon would occur with bilirubin and we present here an experimental exploration of this hypothesis (14). The transport maximum for bilirubin secretion in bile was determined at various rates of taurocholate infusion. The data observed are portrayed in Fig. 8. The Tm for bilirubin increases with taurocholate-induced increments in bile flow, in a linear fashion. At low bile flows the bilirubin concentration in bile reaches very high values and, as a result, there is an apparent substantial value for the Tm on extrapolation to zero bile flow.

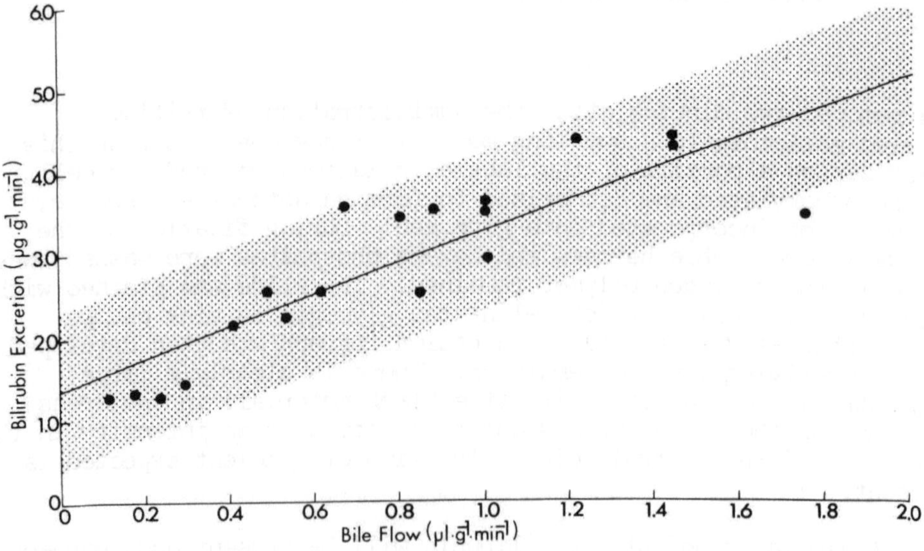

Fig. 8. The relation between maximal bilirubin excretion or Tm and bile flow, when the bile flow has been manipulated by taurocholate infusion. The shaded area corresponds to ± two standard errors of the estimate.

The change in the transport maximum with taurocholate-induced increments in bile flow may be accounted for in the following manner. When the plasma taurocholate concentrations are low, the extraction of this bile acid across the hepatic lobule is almost complete. Most of the canalicular secretion of the bile acid takes place in the periportal areas of the lobule and the bilirubin secretion accompanying this also appears to take place in the periphery. When the taurocholate concentration is raised, the extraction of taurocholate across the lobule becomes incomplete, more of the bile acid is delivered to the downstream areas, and increased secretion of the taurocholate into the biliary canaliculi in the more central areas provokes both a relatively larger increase in bile flow and in bilirubin excretion from these parts of the lobule. Thus the flattening of the bile acid gradient, with its resulting increase in centrolobular bile secretion, appears to underlie the increase in the maximum transport rate for bilirubin, with the increases in bile flow provoked by taurocholate.

The linkage between bilirubin and taurocholate excretion appears to depend more directly on a physiological or chemical effect, than on the change in bile flow itself, if we reason again by analogy with the handling of sulfobromophthalein. Barnhart and Combes (15) and Erlinger and Dumont (16) have demonstrated that, although theophylline increases canalicular bile flow, it does not change the Tm for sulfobromophthalein. The linkage must therefore exist either at the level of the canalicular transport surface itself or in the bile itself, or at both levels. No way of testing for the existence of an association at the first site has yet been devised. However, at the second site, there is firm evidence of a chemical association. Verschure and Mijnlieff (17) and Juniper (18) have both shown that when micelles are separated from bile in an ultracentrifugal field, virtually all of the bilirubin in the bile (this is almost wholly conjugated bilirubin) moves with the micelles. The micelles therefore appear to serve as an absorptive sink for conjugated bilirubin.

Thus the washout of the lobular concentration gradient for taurocholate, with infusion of taurocholate, appears to underlie the simultaneous increase in the biliary transport maximum for bilirubin and in canalicular bile flow, observed with infusion of taurocholate.

SUMMARY

We have presented an examination of three areas important for an appreciation of the kinetic events underlying the transport of bilirubin into bile: the uptake process at the cell membrane and its interaction with the biliary secretion process, the lobular intracellular gradient which develops as a result of the process of biliary secretion, and the linkage between bilirubin and bile salt secretion into bile, which underlies the increase in the biliary transport maximum for bilirubin which follows the infusion of taurocholate. The process of uptake for bilirubin was demonstrated to show saturation, one of the usual characteristics of a carrier-mediated transport process, and to be complicated by a minor phenomenon, the red cell carriage of a small proportion of the bilirubin. The initial passage of bilirubin across the cell membrane appeared to resemble, in great part, the kind of process underlying the entrance of glucose, galactose, and sulfobromophthalein. It was shown that the process of intracellular removal by biliary secretion would be expected to result in a lobular gradient in bilirubin concentration; and to result in a similar gradient for bile acids. It was hypothesized that the increase in the transport maximum for bilirubin observed after the infusion of taurocholate was the result of the flattening of the lobular profile for taurocholate, the increased delivery of taurocholate to the centrolobular areas, and the linkage between bilirubin and taurocholate secretion which results in an increased centrolobular secretion of both. Part of this linkage may reside in the adsorption of conjugated bilirubin by the micelles in bile.

ACKNOWLEDGEMENTS

These studies were supported by grants from the Medical Research Council of Canada and the Quebec Heart Foundation. The author wishes to express his appreciation to Mrs. Brita Nadeau, Mrs. Heather Kennedy, and Mrs. Denise Joubert for their superb technical assistance; and to Miss Margaret Mulherin for typing this manuscript.

REFERENCES

1. GORESKY CA: A linear method for determining liver sinusoidal and extravascular volumes. Am J Physiol 204: 626-640, 1963.

2. GORESKY CA, NADEAU BE: Uptake of materials by the intact liver: the exchange of glucose across the cell membrane. J Clin Invest 53: 634-646, 1974.

3. GORESKY CA: The lobular design of the liver: its effect on uptake processes, in Regulation of Hepatic Metabolism, edited by LUNDQUIST F, TYGSTRUP N, Copenhagen, Munksgaard, 1974, p 808-822.

4. GORESKY CA, BACH GG: On the uptake of materials by the intact liver: the concentrative transport of rubidium-86. J Clin Invest 52: 975-990, 1973.

5. CAHILL GF, Jr, ASHMORE J, EARLE AS, ZOTTU S: Glucose penetration into liver. Am J Physiol 192: 491-496, 1958.

6. TYGSTRUP N, WINKLER K: Kinetics of galactose elimination. Acta Physiol Scand 32: 354-362, 1954.

7. GORESKY CA, BACH GG, NADEAU BE: On the uptake of materials by the intact liver: the transport and net removal of galactose. J Clin Invest 52: 991-1009, 1973.

8. GORESKY CA: Initial distribution and rate of uptake of sulfobromophthalein in the liver. Am J Physiol 207: 13-26, 1964.

9. LEVI AJ, GAITMAITAN Z, ARIAS IM: Two hepatic cytoplasmic protein fractions, Y and Z, and their possible role in the hepatic uptake of bilirubin, sulfobromophthalein, and other organic anions. J Clin Invest 48: 2156-2167, 1969.

10. WHEELER HO, EPSTEIN RM, ROBINSON RR et al: Hepatic storage and excretion of sulfobromophthalein sodium in the dog. J Clin Invest 39: 236-247, 1960.

11. GORESKY CA, BACH GG, NADEAU BE: Red cell carriage of label: its limiting effect on the exchange of materials in the liver. Circ Res. In Press.

12. BARNHART JL, CLARENBERG R: Binding of bilirubin to erythrocytes. Proc Soc Biol Med 142: 1101-1103, 1973.

13. O'MAILLE ERL, RICHARDS TG, SHORT AH: Factors determining the maximal rate of organic anion secretion by the liver and further evidence of the hepatic site of action of the hormone secretin. J Physiol 186: 424-438, 1966.

14. GORESKY CA, HADDAD HH, KLUGER WS et al: The enhancement of maximal bilirubin excretion with taurocholate-induced increments in bile flow. Can J Physiol Pharmacol 52: 389-403, 1974.

15. BARNHART J, RITT D, WARE A et al: A comparison of the effects of taurocholate and theophylline on BSP excretion in dogs, in The Liver - Quantitative Aspects of Structure and Function, edited by PAUMGARTNER G, PREISIG R, Basel, S. Karger, 1973, p 315-325.

16. ERLINGER S, DUMONT M: Influence of canalicular bile flow on sulfobromophthalein transport maximum in bile in the dog, in The Liver - Quantitative Aspects of Structure and Function, edited by PAUMGARTNER G, PREISIG R, Basel, S. Karger, 1973, p 306 - 314.

17. VERSCHURE JCM, MIJNLIEFF PF: The dominating macromolecular complex of human bile. Clin Chim Acta 1: 154-166, 1956.

18. JUNIPER K: Physicochemical characteristics of bile and their relation to gallstone formation. Am J Med 39: 98-107, 1965.

PROTEIN BINDING AND CONJUGATION OF BILIRUBIN IN THE LIVER CELL

Irwin M. Arias and Peter Jansen

Liver Research Center, Albert Einstein College of Medicine

Bronx, New York 10461

For over 40 years, it has been known that following injection of "physiologic" amounts of bilirubin and a variety of other organic anions, a large proportion of the injected dose is recovered within the liver in a matter of minutes. Complete elucidation of the mechanism responsible for this rapid and seemingly selective transfer from plasma into the liver remains unknown; however, experimental studies suggest several hypotheses; (i) bilirubin is noncovalently bound to plasma albumin and enters the liver by pinocytosis as a pigment: albumin complex; (ii) "unbound" bilirubin in plasma is transferred across the plasma membrane of the liver cell by non-ionic diffusion and net uptake flux is determined by intracellular binding and/or subsequent metabolism and biliary excretion; (iii) a plasma membrane carrier system exists with relative specificity for bilirubin; (iv) net hepatic uptake of bilirubin is largely determined by hepatic blood flow and a high extraction ratio of the bile pigment, and (v) an active transport system for bilirubin and other organic anions exists in the portion of the plasma membrane of the parenchymal liver cells which faces the sinusoid.

None of these hypotheses has been studied to a degree that conclusively explains specificity for hepatic uptake of bilirubin from plasma. It is clear that the plasma albumin concentration and, in particular, the number of available binding sites on albumin influence the net hepatic bilirubin flux. Several studies demonstrate that bilirubin enters the liver cell at a faster rate than does plasma albumin thereby excluding the pinocytosis theory. Hepatic uptake of bilirubin is unaffected by inhibitors of intermediary metabolism, protein synthesis and cellular respiration, and plasma: liver concentration gradients for bilirubin do not suggest an active transport system for bilirubin. Hepatic blood flow is a major factor influencing hepatic uptake of compounds having a high extraction ratio; however, definitive studies with respect to bilirubin are lacking. Carrier molecules in plasma membranes of liver cells have been identified for various hormones and peptides; however, the state of the art is currently limited with respect to preparation of that part of the plasma membrane facing the sinusoid, which is the first step in attempting to identify a "bilirubin" carrier. Therefore, studies of bilirubin transport into liver have concerned competition between various compounds for hepatic uptake measured either as disappearance from plasma or, in the case of Dr. Goresky's elegant studies, to "throughput" comparisons with substances of known distribution.

My colleagues and I have been studying the role of hepatic cytoplasmic proteins in facilitating the net flux of bilirubin and other organic anions from plasma into the liver. To date these investigations have resulted in identification, purification and partial characterization of Y and Z, two organic anion binding proteins in liver, as well as studies regarding their function. Our working hypothesis is that Y and Z influence the net flux of organic anions from plasma into the liver specifically by determining efflux from the cell back into the plasma. It seems obvious that there is no way in which a substance in plasma can know what is in the liver and, therefore, influx into the cell must be independent of cytoplasmic binding proteins. Several important by-products of these studies have been development of immunologic methods for quantitating Y and Z, immunofluorescent methods for determining their cellular localization, and detailed binding studies using circular dichroism and equilibrium dialysis. Y and Z proteins have been found in tissues other than liver, particularly in kidney and small intestinal mucosa. A variety of phylogenetic, ontogenetic, induction and inhibition studies have been performed to investigate the function of these proteins.

In 1968, we determined that approximately 80% of intrahepatic bilirubin is associated with the 100,000 x g supernatant fraction of liver after radioactive bilirubin was injected into a rat. Fractionation of supernatant by gel filtration revealed that radiobilirubin was found in two non-albumin containing peaks which were called Y and Z. In subsequent years, a specific Y and a specific Z protein were purified and shown to account for at least 85% of bilirubin binding in the Y and Z fractions. The following paragraphs summarize current knowledge and controversy regarding these two proteins.

Y protein is the major organic anion binding protein in rat and human liver. When isolated homogenously from rat liver, it is a basic protein (pI 9.0) of 46,000 daltons consisting of two apparently identical subunits of 23,000 daltons connected by a disulphide bridge. The dimer is required for organic anion binding and one mole of Y binds one mole of the several organic anions studied including bilirubin. Addition of monospecific anti-Y IgG, but not control IgG, removes up to 90% of various organic anions, including bilirubin, bound to the protein *in vivo* or *in vitro*. Immunoquantitation by the Mancini diffusion technique and recently by radioimmunoassay, reveals an unusually large concentration of Y protein in the liver. Y accounts for 6% of all cytoplasmic protein in liver and is present only in two other organs. In the kidney, Y accounts for 2% of cytoplasmic protein and in the small intestinal mucosa, it accounts for 2% of cytoplasmic protein. No other tissue or fluid tested contains Y as measured by these sensitive and specific techniques. Immunofluorescent studies localize Y to all parenchymal liver cells, proximal tubule cell of the kidney and the non-goblet mucosal cells of the small intestine. Following tissue injury, Y disappears from liver cells but has not been detected in plasma or bile.

The concentration of Y in liver is subject to several important control mechanisms. For example, following pulse-labeling with guanadino ^{14}C-arginine and serial purification, Y has a half-life of 2 days. In addition, administration of several drugs and chemicals such as phenobarbital, DDT, dieldrin, methyl cholanthrene, benzpyrene and AIA increase synthesis of Y to a new steady-state when Y constitutes up to 11% of hepatic cytoplasmic protein. In the absence of thyroid hormone, Y is stabilized (i.e. degradation of Y is markedly reduced). To illustrate the magnitude of these changes, administration of phenobarbital to a thyroidectomized rat results in this single protein constituting as much as 20% of hepatic cytoplasmic protein!

In 1970, Ketterer, Litwack and our group at Einstein discovered that Y is identical to the cortisol metabolite binding protein I (Litwack) and the azocarcinogen binding protein (Ketterer). The name "Ligandin" was agreed upon because it designates a binding protein and does not commit specific function either in terms of steroid binding, carcinogenicity or organic anion transport. More recently it was claimed that ligandin is a GSH-transferase which catalyzes formation of the GSH conjugate of 2,3-dichloronitrobenzene. Homogenous ligandin from rat and human liver lacks catalytic activity with this substrate. Better than 99% of catalytic activity with this substrate is eluted from another portion of the column used to purify ligandin. In addition, Jakoby has purified to homogenicity five GSH transferases in liver supernatant. Each of these enzymes are dimers of 46,000 daltons which differ in amino acid composition, immunospecificity and isoelectric point (pI). The crude preparation originally utilized to study this question was contaminated with all five GSH transferases. Nevertheless, competitive data and the fact that GSH binds to ligandin warrants further investigation of the possible catalytic role of the protein in GSH metabolism. A large number of ligands bind to ligandin whether they are injected in vivo or added in vitro to liver supernatant prior to fractionation. The current list is presented in Table I and includes various dyes, porphyrins, bilirubin, cholecystographic agents, fatty acids, thyroid hormones and others as well as several conjugates. Specificity in vitro is indicated by the fact that several organic anions do not bind to ligandin including free and conjugated bile salts and pyruvate. Organic cations do not bind to ligandin. Circular dichroism study of homogeneous rat liver ligandin reveals an ordered structure of the protein with about 40% α helix. Bilirubin binds at one major site with a calculated affinity constant of 10^{-6}. Various organic anions added in vitro compete with bilirubin for binding at the major binding site and include BSP, ICG and others. Other organic anions added at equimolar concentrations to ligandin

TABLE I

Compounds bound to Ligandin (Y protein) in vivo and in vitro

I. Covalently bound
- azodye carcinogen
- methylcholanthrene metabolite

II. Noncovalently bound
- azodye GSH conjugate
- corticosteroids and metabolites
- bilirubin
- bilirubin glucuronide
- BSP, ICG, Rose Bengal, DBSP
- BSP glutathione
- glutathione
- hematin
- phylloerythrin
- cholecystographic agents
- tri- and tetra-iodo thyronine
- methyl cholanthrene
- various sulfonamides
- various fatty acids
- probenecid
- penicillin
- vasoflavine
- cephalothin
- cephalex
- tetracyclines
- nitrofurantin
- ethacrynic acid

and bilirubin fail to displace bilirubin although at higher concentrations displacement is observed. GSH appears to bind at a different site by a different mechanism. Transfer of ligands, including bilirubin, from rat serum albumin to rat liver ligandin has been demonstrated as the affinity constants for binding are almost equal in this system.

We have proposed that ligandin is a determinant of the efflux of organic anion from the liver into the plasma. What is the evidence in support of this hypothesis particularly in view of the fact that such flux has not, as yet, been determined directly on a cellular level?

(i) Phyllogenetic studies reveal absence of Y and Z in liver of elasmobranches and teleosts which are species in which selective hepatic uptake of bilirubin and BSP do not occur. Amphibia lack Y and Z as well as selective hepatic organic anion uptake during aquatic life but develop both processes during metamorphosis. All reptiles, birds and mammals studied, including man, have abundant hepatic Y and Z proteins and manifest relatively selective hepatic organic anion uptake when this was studied.

(ii) Ontogenetically in guinea pig, monkey and man, Y is virtually absent in the late fetus and rapidly matures during the first 5-10 days of life. Maturation of Y correlates with maturation of plasma disappearance of various organic anions including bilirubin and may be an important pathophysiologic aspect of the "physiologic" jaundice of human and monkey neonates.

(iii) Following induction of ligandin by administration of several drugs such as phenobarbital, plasma disappearance and hepatic accumulation bound to Y of bilirubin, indocyanine green and BSP are increased.

(iv) In Gunn rats, bilirubin bound to Y retards plasma disappearance, hepatic uptake and binding of other organic anions such as BSP, tri-iodothyronine and others.

(v) Results of various studies of competition in vivo for hepatic organic anion uptake between different organic anions can be accounted for on the basis of the known binding constants for the ligand and ligandin.

(vi) Studies with renal ligandin demonstrate that renal organic anion excretion of probenecid, penicillin and BSP can be predicted on the basis of the competitive binding of these compounds to homogenous rat renal ligandin in vitro.

The strongest argument against this hypothesis is the finding that the primary binding affinity of ligandin for bilirubin or BSP is less than the primary binding constants for these ligands and serum albumin. The differences are relatively small: 4×10^{-6} for bilirubin and rat ligandin and 8×10^{-6} for bilirubin and rat serum albumin after defatting. We have been able to model hepatic bilirubin uptake using the derived binding constants and large amount of ligandin present within the cell.

Our hypothesis probably represents an oversimplification and one cannot ignore effects of blood flow and possible membrane carrier transport proteins. We have no evidence to suggest that Y is in the plasma membrane of the liver cell but this has not been exhaustively studied. It is unlikely that the large number of potential ligands act as substrates for ligandin as an enzyme; however, storage of intracellular GSH is a possible alternative role for the protein. We are slowly beginning to appreciate the relationship between bilirubin binding to albumin and ligandin and the presence of transport processes in the plasma membrane of the hepatocyte.

Z is an acidic (pI 5.2) protein of 12,000 daltons which has an ordered structure as studied by circular dichroism. Z has been purified to homogeneity from rat and human liver and can be measured quantitatively by Mancini immunodiffusion and radio-immunoassay. Initially we observed that bilirubin and virtually all organic anions on Table I bind to Z in vitro and usually in vivo. After saturation of binding to ligandin by bilirubin or BSP, binding to Z occurs. Initially Z was detected only in liver and supernatant from the small intestine mucosa; however, with development of better techniques and realization that long chain fatty acids bind to Z with high affinity, Z was detected in kidney, myocardium, skeletal muscle and fat cell. Mishkin at Einstein and Ockner in San Francisco found that fatty acid binding to Z increases with chain length and decreases with unsaturation. Ockner termed Z "Fatty Acid Binding Protein" (FABP) and suggested that it functions in esterification of fatty acids within the gut. Mishkin recently found that CoA derivatives of fatty acids bind with higher affinity to Z than the fatty acids themselves, further suggesting a possible role in esterification. Ockner observed that rats fed a high fat diet have increased Z when compared with rats fed a low fat diet. We have demonstrated that Z is the same as Ockner's FABP in that monospecific anti-Z IgG, but not control IgG, removes fatty acid binding from liver supernatant Z fraction. Z is different from Y with respect to composition, pI, sedimentation velocity, Stoke's radius and turnover. In addition, Z is not induced by phenobarbital and other drugs, develops at a different rate, and is not stabilized in the absence of thyroid hormone. Thus far, Z has been localized to the supernatant fraction. We postulate that Z participates in organic anion uptake unrelated to binding by unsaturated fatty acids and their CoA derivatives. For example, flavaspidic acid-n-methyl-glucaminate, which is derived from male fern, retards net hepatic uptake of bilirubin and BSP in rabbits, man and rats; this organic anion is bound selectively to Z with high affinity in the supernatant of rat liver and displaces bilirubin and BSP *in vivo* and *in vitro*. Schmid and Hammaker showed that flavaspidic acid in perfused Gunn rat liver displaces radio-bilirubin from the liver. Our studies indicate that this displacement affects Z protein. Similar results have been obtained using BSP and cholecystographic agents as ligands. In addition, hepatic uptake or esterification of labeled oleate are not reduced by flavaspidic acid administration although BSP uptake and binding are abolished by male fern extract and oleate binding to Z is obliterated. This phenomenon may contribute to the pathogenesis of unconjugated hyperbilirubinemia after fasting in man, Gunn rats, and horses. Increased bilirubin production resulting from induced heme oxygenase activity has been proposed but there is controversy regarding quantitation of CO excretion as a product of this reaction in fasted individuals. Because the changes occur in Gunn rats, it seems unlikely that altered UDP glucuronyl transferase is responsible. Furthermore, the unconjugated hyperbilirubinemia develops slowly during several days in fasted man and over 5 days in fasted horses; nevertheless, the serum bilirubin concentration returns to normal within hours after institution of carbohydrate feeding. These observations suggest that an inhibitor of bilirubin binding to Y and/or Z may be released in starvation and limit the net efflux of bilirubin and other organic anions from the liver cell. Fatty acids and perhaps lactic acid, which also bind avidly to Z, may be responsible and contribute to the pathogenesis of this condition. Other studies in fasted rats indicate that both the synthesis of Y and its rapid degradation, with respect to total liver protein, are reduced during fasting.

Many efforts have been made to demonstrate that binding of bilirubin to Y or Z confers some special property with respect to subsequent biotransformation and/or excretion. Thus far, equimolar amounts of Y, Z or albumin enhance bilirubin glucuronidation in a microsomal system. Anti-Y-IgG does not alter UDP glucuronyl transferase or reconstituted cytochrome P-450 activities *in vitro*. Albumin within the liver cell is compartmentalized and not available for cytoplasmic binding. Y and Z may serve as intracellular binding proteins analagous to the binding of albumin in the plasma. Relatively lipid soluble compounds, such as bilirubin, might not react normally with the conjugation mechanism if there were no binding protein available. Ockner has proposed a similar role for Z in the intestinal mucosal cell as regards fatty acid esterification.

Bilirubin in man is ultimately excreted in bile largely, if not exclusively, as an acyl glucuronide conjugate although complex sugar and sulfate conjugates have also been described. All bilirubin

TABLE II

COMPOSITION OF HUMAN BILE

Azopigments Identified	Amount	Hydrolysis: Alkali	Hydrolysis: β-glucuronidase	Hexuronic acid	Other Sugar	Chemical Identification	Prominent Pigment in bile of:
A. Heirwegh et al							
α_o	11.1%	-	-	No	No	Azodipyrrole	
α_2	1.2%	+	-	No	Yes	Azodipyrrole-xyloside	Dogs, chickens
α_3	3.5%	+	-	No	Yes	Azodipyrrole-glucoside	Dogs, alligators, cats, chickens, horses, rabbits, snakes
$\beta_{1,2};\gamma_{1,2}$	9.4%	+	-	Yes	?	Unidentified; after treatment with acid, delta-like pigments are formed	Alligators, armadillos, cats
δ	75.4%	+	(77-95%)	Yes	No	Azodipyrrole-glucuronide	All species studied except alligators, armadillos and snakes

TABLE II (cont'd)

COMPOSITION OF HUMAN BILE

Azopigments Identified	Amount	Hydrolysis: Alkali	Hydrolysis: β-glucuronidase	Hexuronic acid	Other Sugar	Chemical Identification	Prominent Pigment in bile of:
B. Kuenzle et al							
A_1	++++	-	-	No	No	Azodipyrrole	
A_2	+	?	-	No	No	unidentified non-polar ester	
B_1	+	-	-	?	Yes	? conjugated at the vinyl group	
B_2	+	+	?	?	Yes	not further characterized	
B_3	+	+	?	?	Yes	not further characterized	
B_4	++	+	-	Yes	Yes	mixture of 3 azo-dipyrrole-glucuronosyl-glucosides	
B_5	++++	+	+	Yes	No	azodipyrrole-glucuronosyl-glucuronide	
B_6	++++	+	+	Yes	Yes	azodipyrrole-glucosyl-glucuronide	

conjugates are more polar than unconjugated bilirubin and have different stereo conformation. Bilirubin is a rigid molecule probably due to four intramolecular hydrogen bonds. Esterification of the carboxyl groups of the two propionic acid side-chains permits the two dipyrrole-halves to rotate about the central methylene bridge. As a result bilirubin conjugates are labile making study of their structure difficult. Most studies have been performed with azo derivatives which are relatively stable and easily separated chromatographically; however, it is difficult to reconstruct original structures from azopigment mixtures. Despite these chemical difficulties, knowledge of bilirubin conjugates has increased and several new concepts have been introduced by Heirwegh and Kuenzle and their associates.

The findings of these two groups of investigators are compared in Table II. The validity of such comparison is questionable as each group used different diazo reagents, reaction conditions, and pH, and obtained significantly different recoveries. Heirwegh worked at a micro scale and reported high recovery of azopigments. Kuenzle worked at a macro scale with recovery of about 4.5%. In contrast to the traditional view that bilirubin is mainly excreted as an alkali-labile, β glucuronidase-hydrolysable glucuronide conjugate, the findings of each group revealed that a considerable fraction of human "T-tube" bile consists of β-glucuronidase-resistant, sugar conjugates. Almost all analysed conjugates had conjugating groups attached by alkali-labile ester bonds to the carboxyl group of the propionic acid side-chain. A large amount of mono-conjugates was found in bile.

Kuenzle has claimed that B_5 and B_6, which are glucuronosyl-glucuronide and glucuronosyl-glucoside conjugates respectively, are the main bilirubin conjugates in human bile rather than a simple glucuronide. If Kuenzle is correct, B_5 should be identical with delta and B_6 could be identical with α_3. The B_4 pigments are likely candidates for the unidentified disaccharides containing β and γ pigments.

To establish possible clinical importance of these findings, Fevery analyzed bile from patients with cirrhosis, hepatitis or obstructive jaundice. In general, all cases showed an increase in β and γ (possible disaccharide-containing) conjugates at the expense of the simple glucuronide conjugates. No diagnostic specificity was observed. Similar results were observed in rat bile after bile duct ligation.

The biosynthetic mechanism responsible for formation of disaccharide-containing bilirubin conjugates is unclear. Glucose and xylose conjugates have been identified after incubation of liver homogenate, bilirubin and UDP glucose or UDP xylose. In several species, there is little relationship between the ability to form sugar conjugates in vitro and their presence in bile. For example, glucose and xylose conjugates are not found in rat bile under physiologic conditions, where abundant glucose and xylose conjugates are formed in vitro. Glucose, xylose and glucuronic acid conjugates of bilirubin are not formed by homogenates of Gunn rat liver nor are they present in bile from Gunn rats or patients with UDP glucuronyl transferase deficiency (Type I).

The general properties of UDP glucuronyl transferase have been extensively studied; however, purification has not been successful. The enzyme is bound to endoplasmic reticulum membrane and solubilization usually results in inactivation. Treatment of microsomal vesicles with phospholipase A produced an unstable glucuronyl transferase with increased activity at V_{max} but decreased binding affinity. Furthermore, the enzyme lost specificity for UDP glucuronic acid and several other UDP-sugars were able to bind to the active site. The effect of phospholipase A can be mimicked in vivo by means of a protein-free diet which increased membrane lysophosphatide content as well as UDP glucuronyl transferase activity. Addition of lysophosphatidylcholine in vitro had the same effect.

These studies reveal that allosteric effectors, such as UDP N-acetyl-glucosamine and perturbation of microsomal membranes, profoundly influence activity and specificity of glucuronyl transferase. The appearance of different bilirubin conjugates in bile during pathological conditions may reflect altered phospholipid enzyme-protein relations in microsomal membranes.

Enzymatic reactions involved in bilirubin diglucuronide synthesis were recently studied by Jansen who found that the two glucuronyl groups are separately attached to the bilirubin molecule. In addition, the pH optima for the enzymatic catalysis of the two glucuronidation steps differed considerably. A similar finding was reported by Fevery for attachment of the first and second xylosyl groups. These findings suggest that two enzymes may be involved in the formation of diconjugates. One enzyme may require bilirubin and the second may require bilirubin monoglucuronide as natural substrates. Despite considerable experimental studies, possible multiplicity of glucuronyl transferases - or varied substrate affinity - remains uncertain. The major problem appears to be the current technical handicap in solubilizing and purifying membrane-bound enzymes. A methodologic breakthrough is required to solve this problem.

SUMMARY

This presentation has reviewed speculations concerning the mechanism of transfer of bilirubin from plasma into the liver cell.

The hypothesis is presented that the binding proteins, ligandin (Y) and Z protein, regulate the efflux of organic anions from the liver cell into the plasma and thus determine the net uptake of these materials by the liver. The multiplicity and purification of UDP glucuronyl transferase, and the nature, biosynthesis and possible functional importance of nonglucuronide conjugates of bilirubin were also discussed.

ACKNOWLEDGEMENTS

Research in the author's laboratories was supported by grants from NIH (AM 0291, 5384, 16281), the New York Heart Association and Heart Fund, Inc., Gail I. Zuckerman Foundation and the Sara Chait Memorial Foundation.

REFERENCES

1. LEVI AJ, GATMAITAN Z, ARIAS IM: The role of two hepatic cytoplasmic proteins (Y and Z) in the transfer of sulphobromophthalein (BSP) and bilirubin from plasma into the liver. J Clin Invest 48: 2156-2167, 1969.

2. LEVI AJ, GATMAITAN Z, ARIAS IM: Deficiency of hepatic organic anion binding protein, impaired organic anion uptake by liver and "physiologic" jaundice in newborn monkeys. New Eng J Med 284: 1136-1139, 1970.

3. LEVI AJ, GATMAITAN Z, ARIAS IM: Deficiency of hepatic organic anion binding protein: a possible cause of non-hemolytic unconjugated hyperbilirubinemia in the newborn. Lancet 297: 139-140, 1969.

4. REYES H, LEVI AJ, GATMAITAN Z, ARIAS IM: Organic anion-binding protein in rat liver: Drug induction and its physiologic consequence. Proc Nat Acad Sci 64: 168-170, 1969.

5. REYES H, LEVI AJ, ARIAS IM: Studies of Y and Z, two hepatic cytoplasmic organic anion-binding proteins: effect of drugs, chemicals, hormones and cholestasis. J Clin Invest 50: 2242-2252, 1971.

6. REYES H, LEVINE R, LEVI AJ et al: Bilirubin: a model for studies of drug metabolism in man. Ann NY Acad Sci 179: 520-528, 1971.

7. FLEISCHNER G, ROBBINS J, ARIAS IM: Immunologic studies of Y, a major cytoplasmic organic anion-binding protein in rat liver. J Clin Invest 51: 677-684, 1972.

8. FLEISCHNER G, ARIAS IM: Recent advances in bilirubin formation, transport, metabolism and excretion. Am J Med 49: 576-589, 1970.

9. LITWACK G, KETTERER B, ARIAS IM: Ligandin: An abundant liver protein which binds steroids, bilirubin, carcinogens and a number of exogenous anions. Nature 234: 466-467, 1971.

10. ARIAS IM: Pathogenesis of "physiologic" jaundice of the newborn: a re-evaluation. In Birth Defects, edited by D. Bergsma, Baltimore, Williams and Wilkins, 1970. Volume VI, pp. 55-59.

11. ARIAS IM: Transfer of bilirubin from blood to bile. Seminars of Hematology 9: 55-70, 1972.

12. KAMISAKA K, LISTOWSKY I, ARIAS IM: Circular dichroism studies of Y protein (Ligandin), a major organic anion binding protein in liver, kidney, and small intestine. Annals NY Acad Sci 226: 148-153, 1973.

13. KAMISAKA K, LISTOWSKY I, BETHEIL J, ARIAS IM: Competitive binding of bilirubin, sulfobromophthalein, indocyanine green and other organic anions to human and bovine serum albumin. Biochem Biophys Acta (in press) 1975.

14. KAPLOWITZ N, PERCY-ROBB IW, JAVITT NB: Role of hepatic anion-binding protein in bromsulphthalein conjugation. J Exp Med 183: 483-487, 1973.

15. MISHKIN S, STEIN L, GATMAITAN Z, ARIAS IM: The binding of fatty acids to cytoplasmic proteins: binding to Z protein in liver and other tissues of the rat. Biochem Biophys Res Comm 47: 997-1003, 1972.

16. OCKNER R, MANNING J, PAPPENHAUSEN R, HO W: A binding protein for fatty acids in cytosol of intestinal mucosa, liver myocardium and other tissues. Science 177: 56-58, 1972.

17. MISHKIN S, STEIN L, GATMAITAN Z, ARIAS IM: Studies on the possible role of Z protein and other cytoplasmic proteins in the hepatic uptake of long-chain fatty acids. J Clin Invest 1975.

18. HEIRWEGH KPM, VAN HEES GP, LEROY P et al: Heterogeneity of bile pigment conjugates as revealed by chromatography of their ethyl anthranilate azopigments. Biochem J 120: 877-890, 1970.

19. COMPERNOLLE F, JANSEN FH, HEIRWEGH KPM: Mass-spectrometric study of the azopigments obtained from bile pigments with diazotized ethyl anthranilate. Biochem J 120: 891-894, 1970.

20. COMPERNOLLE F, VAN HEES GP, FEVERY J, HEIRWEGH KPM: Mass-spectrometric structure elucidation of dog bile azopigments as the acyl glycosides of glucopyranose and xylopyranose. Biochem J 125: 811-819, 1971.

21. FEVERY J, VAN HEES GP, LEROY P et al: Excretion in dog bile of glucose and xylose conjugates of bilirubin. Biochem J 125: 803-810, 1971.

22. KUENZLE CC, WEIBEL MH, PELLONI RR: The reaction of bilirubin with diazomethane. Biochem J 133: 357-368, 1973.

23. KUENZLE CC: Bilirubin conjugates of human bile. Chapter in Metabolic Conjugation and Hydrolysis. Ed. WH Fishman, vol. III, Academic Press, New York & London, 1973.

24. CORNELIUS CE, KELLEY KC, HIMES JA: Heterogeneity of bilirubin conjugates in several animal species. J Vet Res (in press) 1975.

25. FEVERY J, VAN DAMME B, MICHIELS R et al: Bilirubin conjugates in bile of man and rat in the normal state and in liver disease. J Clin Invest 51: 2482-2492, 1972.

26. GRAHAM AB, WOODCOCK BG, WOOD GC: The phospholipid-dependence of uridine diphosphate glucuronyltransferase. Effect of protein deficiency on the phospholipid composition and enzyme activity of rat liver microsomal fraction. Biochem J 137: 567-574, 1974.

27. ZAKIM D, GOLDENBERG J, VESSEY DA: Influence of membrane lipids on the regulatory properties of UDP-glucuronyltransferase. Eur J Biochem 38: 59-63, 1973.

28. VESSEY DA, ZAKIM D: Regulation of microsomal enzymes by phospholipids. II. Activation of hepatic uridine diphosphate-glucuronyltransferase. J Biol Chem 246: 4649-4656, 1971.

29. JANSEN PL: The isomerisation of bilirubin monoglucuronide. Clin Chim Acta 49: 233-240, 1973.

30. JANSEN PL: The enzyme-catalyzed formation of bilirubin diglucuronide by a solubilized preparation from cat liver microsomes. Biochim Biophys Acta 338: 170-182, 1974.

DISCUSSION OF PAPERS ON BILIRUBIN THROUGHPUT

CHAIRMAN: H.O. WHEELER

ARIAS: Dr. Berk, since you have defined the kinetic abnormalities so clearly in Gilbert's syndrome, can you make a statement about the actual underlying mechanism. In other words, is the relative deficiency of glucuronyl transferase the sole underlying defect or does the kinetic analysis provide indication of an uptake defect?

BERK: To answer this question several things need to be considered. First, utilizing the most widely used and certainly the most reproduceable method for assaying glucuronyl transferase activity in human liver, all patients with Gilbert's syndrome are found to have reduced values. That having been said, if we give phenobarbital to patients with Gilbert's syndrome, we can totally correct the kinetic abnormality in bilirubin metabolism. However, in the very limited number of studiés published to date, virtually no change is found in the enzyme assay. So one has to ask whether or not that assay, as measured in vitro, with manipulation of co-factors and a variety of other things, is relevant to what is happening in vivo. Secondly, if we try to analyze our kinetic data in terms of the model, the model tells us that patients with Gilbert's syndrome have a very marked reduction in hepatic bilirubin uptake as well as a modest but still statistically significant reduction in conjugation rate. The predominant defect seems to be uptake, but conjugation also occurs at a lower rate. If one looks at the uptake of other anions which are not conjugated with glucuronic acid, there is a subpopulation of patients who, clinically and in terms of bilirubin kinetics, are identical to typical

Gilbert's syndrome, but who also have a clear-cut uptake defect for sulfobromophthalein and indocyanine green. Thus there is clearly a subgroup which has an uptake defect for two anions which are not processed by glucuronyl transferase.

GORESKY: I would like to comment about Gilbert's syndrome. One of the fundamental problems in this area is to determine what process is limiting. This information cannot be obtained from a tracer experiment but it could be obtained from a load experiment. Experiments of this kind were reported several years ago from Klatskin's laboratory (Tisdale, Klatskin, Kinsella; Am J Med 26: 214-227, 1959) and we have repeated them, with similar findings. An exogenous load of bilirubin, administered intravenously to a patient with Gilbert's syndrome, remains in the plasma compartment for a very long time, for days, and virtually none of the bilirubin in the plasma becomes conjugated. I think that this indicates that the more fundamental defect is that in conjugation.

ARIAS: One of my problems in understanding the postulate that Gilbert's disease is specifically related to a defect in glucuronide formation, secondary to a deficiency of glucuronyl transferase activity, is the fact that when the enzyme activity in liver biopsies taken from pheno-typically normal anicteric heterozygous carriers, the parents of children with Gilbert's disease, is assayed by the method of Black and Billing, one finds an approximately 40% reduction in enzyme activity. Yet this is not associated with hyper-bilirubinemia. There also is the curious phenomenon that, in patients with Wilson's disease, similar reductions in activity are found, for unexplained reasons. That doesn't mean that I think that the method is not of interest and possibly of some importance. I think it focuses on a point that Dr. Javitt mentioned earlier today, that we may very well be dealing with a much more complex situation than that related to the quantitative amount of enzyme that is there. There are allosteric and other changes, which affect the activity in both this assay and the patient.

ROBINSON: Dr. Berk reported that a total of 12 out of his 26 patients with Gilbert's syndrome had significant hemolysis. This proportion seems to me to be a little beyond the limits of coincidence.

BERK: The coincidence is now 27 out of 55. I think that what we are seeing here is a case finding situation. The patient who has pure hemolytic disease with a bilirubin of 2 mg% or a patient who has pure Gilbert's syndrome with a bilirubin of 2 mg% are both very likely to go through life undetected. However, a patient who has both, with a bilirubin of 4 or 5 mg% is going to be found and sent to us for evaluation. We have now seen a large number of patients who have both spherocytosis and Gilbert's syndrome and we have been able to do family studies on some of them. We have been able to show that the two abnormalities entered the family pedigree independently and that they segregate totally independently. There are members of the family who have Gilbert's syndrome, members of the family who have spherocytosis, members who have both, and members who have neither. There doesn't seem to be any real linkage between the two conditions in large kindreds in which both exist.

ROBINSON: Do you think the coincidence has anything to do with the extremely high incidence of the Gilbert's abnormality, if it is even an abnormality?

BERK: I would say that of the last 300 college students who were admitted to the National Institutes of Health as normal volunteers in various studies about 7% had Gilbert's syndrome. So there are millions of people in North America who have Gilbert's syndrome. In these days of routine screening it is no longer a textbook abnormality and I'm not at all surprised that, just by chance and because hemolysis adds to the detectability of Gilbert's syndrome, we should see a fairly high incidence of hemolysis in a population with Gilbert's syndrome. Again, this does not imply any physiologic relationship between the two. As physicians we shouldn't be carried away by the autoanalyzer and I don't think we should investigate these patients unless we are carrying out investigative studies.

ROBINSON: I think that your explanation makes sense. You mentioned an upper limit of 4 mg% for unconjugated bilirubin, in patients with hemolysis, and yet I think, as a hematologist, that we not infrequently see patients who have hemolysis as their primary abnormality and yet have serum bilirubins which sporadically, although not chronically, go as high as 6 or 7 mg%, virtually all unconjugated. Something else is going on at the time. They are usually febrile and frequently more anemic at the time. We have some evidence that in some there may be at this time an ineffective erythropoiesis component superadded to peripheral hemolysis. It is also possible that with intercurrent infection there is decreased hepatic bilirubin clearance. I wonder if you know something about the mechanism of this sporadic increase beyond 4 mg% in some patients with hemolysis.

BERK: In the steady state situation the limiting factor is the ability of the marrow to produce hemoglobin. Nevertheless we have certainly seen unconjugated bilirubin levels as high as 10 or 12 mg%, during a hemolytic crisis in sickle cell disease, in paroxysmal nocturnal hemoglobinuria, or in any sort of acute intravascular hemolytic crisis. The rate of bilirubin production temporarily reaches a value many times normal. It also appears that during fever and during a variety of other complications, the bilirubin clearance may fall temporarily. We have demonstrated very clearly that pyrogen induced fever in normal volunteers produces dramatic reductions in sulfobromophthalein clearance and I think the same would be true for bilirubin. If you see a bilirubin greater than 4 mg% I think the inference is that either there is a non-steady state excessive increase in bilirubin production which is usually not being compensated by the marrow since, as you pointed out, the patients usually become more anemic at that point, or for whatever reason, there is a temporary reduction in hepatic function.

JABBARI: It has been mentioned here that sulfobromophthalein retention is elevated in some patients with Gilbert's syndrome. What percentage of the patients exhibited this? We usually utilize the sulfobromophthalein retention to rule out the presence of intrahepatic disease. With Gilbert's syndrome, we expect it to be normal.

BERK: Twenty percent of our patients who have otherwise typical Gilbert's syndrome, documented with enzyme assays and morphologic examination of liver biopsies, had abnormal sulfobromophthalein metabolism. However, we are essentially a referral center and most of those patients were, in fact, sent to us because a physician in practice was puzzled and concerned by the fact that he had found a patient who seemed to have abnormal sulfobromophthalein retention, with otherwise typical Gilbert's syndrome. I assume that the incidence of this concurrence in the general population would be much lower.

SCHMID: I have a question for Dr. Arias. When you originally described the role of Y and Z proteins in the uptake of organic anions, particularly sulfobromophthalein and bilirubin, you found the Y fraction to be present in such larger amounts that it would be expected to play a much bigger role than the Z fraction. Now, if one gives all sorts of compounds which are also picked up by the Y fraction, one might expect a priori, a competition for bilirubin uptake and/or perhaps an increase in the bilirubin level. That is, one ought to produce a mild unconjugated hyperbilirubinemia. The only compound which does this is flavaspidic acid and it invariably does so both in patients and in experimental animals. What you now show is that flavaspidic acid displaces bilirubin only from the Z fraction and not from the Y fraction. This, to me, is a discrepancy between the in vivo and the in vitro findings. I wonder whether you can clarify it.

ARIAS: The effect of flavaspidic acid is unique and occurs only with respect to Z. We have now defined the effect more closely in terms of affinity constants. There are two responses to your question. One is that these compounds and the organic anions undoubtedly have other effects. For instance, there may be competition for binding sites on serum albumin. The other is that two factors are important intracellularly: both the affinity constants and the total amount of binding protein present. Both determine total binding. For instance, tri-iodothyronine binds to ligandin. When its binding sites are blocked there is an impairment in its removal. One would hardly consider that the amounts of tri-iodothyronine present physiologically would be able to interfere with bilirubin transport. On the other hand, a compound which binds to ligandin with an affinity almost equal to bilirubin, if present for a long period of time, could conceivably produce hyperbilirubinemia. This type of compound has not yet been observed. It is precisely because such a large number of compounds do bind to these proteins that we feel it is extremely important to ascertain both binding constants and the sites of binding. Glutathione, for example, appears to bind to ligandin by a totally different mechanism and at a different site than the organic anions. We will have to proceed from the qualitative stage to the quantitative stage.

FORKER: This question is for Dr. Arias. Particular compounds, such as Evans Blue, bind to the anion binding proteins very tightly, yet are taken up by the liver slowly. This indicates that binding to the intracellular proteins may not be crucial to the uptake process.

ARIAS: This is an excellent example of the problem that I alluded to earlier. It is true that administration of Evans Blue to the rat was not associated with its presence in the liver when we subsequently fractionated the liver at 10 minutes, yet it binds very tightly. Part of the explanation may come from studies in which we have been using circular dichroism (Kamisaka, Listowsky, Arias; Ann N.Y. Acad Sci 226: 148-161, 1973) to determine the binding affinity of Evans Blue to serum albumin. It is enormously great, relative to that of the other anions that we have been studying. On the other hand, it is equally possible that there is another barrier that is involved, most probably the plasma membrane.

PRINCIPLES OF BILIARY SECRETION

Henry O. Wheeler

University of California, San Diego School of Medicine

University Hospital, San Diego, California 92103

INTRODUCTION

Bile is a transparent, colored, single-phase solution containing substantial quantities of organic as well as inorganic solutes, and produced continuously by the liver with great variations in rate of flow and composition. Although technically an "external" secretion, the great bulk of its constituents is destined for intestinal reabsorption and is returned to the liver via the so-called enterohepatic circulation. Although bile is primarily a digestive fluid the biliary tract also serves as a route of excretion for a variety of substances, and for a few (e.g. bilirubin) it is practically the sole excretory pathway. Heretofore, the study of bile formation has necessitated at least temporary diversion of bile to the exterior by various unphysiological maneuvres, and hence interruption of the enterohepatic circulation. Newer techniques such as those devised by Dowling and his associates (1) for study of the rhesus monkey have permitted the examination of the flow and composition of bile in conscious animals with either minimal or controlled interruption of the enterohepatic circulation. The following remarks will summarize some of our present knowledge of the flow, pressure, composition, regulation and mechanisms of bile formation. For more detailed information particular attention is called to the excellent recent review by Erlinger and Dhumeaux (2). Despite the comparative inaccessibility of bile its flow and composition have been a source of fascination and interest for centuries. The important work prior to 1937 was beautifully summarized in Sobotka's classic monograph (3).

BILE COMPOSITION

Despite great variations in composition bile is nearly always approximately isotonic with respect to plasma (4,5,6) and its osmolality rather faithfully mirrors changes in plasma osmolality (4,5). It may be slightly hypotonic during choleresis induced by rapid bile acid secretion (7) and slightly hypertonic during choleresis induced by secretin (7,8). The reasons for these deviations are not known.

The principal organic solutes of bile are the conjugated bile acids (sometimes referred to as "bile salts"), phospholipids (principally lecithin in man), cholesterol (which is entirely unesterified) and the bile pigments (principally conjugated bilirubin). Typical concentrations for these constituents in human hepatic bile as reported in the studies of Thureborn (9), for example, are: bile acids 140 to 2230 mg% or 3 to 45 mEq/L (up to 53% of total biliary solids by weight), lecithin 140 to 810 mg%, cholesterol 97 to 320 mg% and bilirubin 12 to 70 mg% (i.e. no more than 2% of total solids). Protein concentrations in bile are remarkably low, reported values ranging from 30 to 300 mg% in human bile (10,11,12,9), and serum albumin is usually the most abundant protein.

The concentrations of inorganic cations in bile are roughly proportional to those in interstitial fluid so that sodium is always the dominant cation. Since the conjugated bile acids are relatively strong acids they are dissociated at biliary pH, and therefore inorganic cations are required to balance the total charge of the bile acids as well as the inorganic anions. Moreover, since the bile acids are largely aggregated into osmotically inactive micelles the total cationic concentration must necessarily be higher than that in plasma in order for the bile to be isotonic. Thus typical cationic concentrations recorded in human bile under various circumstances (9,13,14) are as follows (expressed in mEq/L): Na^+ 146 to 165, K^+ 2.7 to 4.9, Ca^{++} 2.5 to 4.8, Mg^{++} 1.4 to 3.0. Inorganic anionic concentrations are much more variable: Cl^- 88 to 115, HCO_3^- 27 to 55. As already noted the bile acids themselves represent the other major anionic constituent. The particularly high bicarbonate concentration observed under some circumstances suggests that this anion may be actively secreted (see below).

Many of the data on bile composition in the literature are based upon analyses of bile aspirated from the gallbladder. This bile, of course, is not representative of the bile which is secreted by the liver since it has already been subjected to concentration by active absorption of water and inorganic electrolytes. Thus the concentrations of all of the organic constituents and of the cations tend to be much higher than those cited above, whereas the concentrations of chloride and bicarbonate tend to be much lower.

BILIARY SECRETORY MECHANISMS

A. Fluid Movement and Secretory Pressure

Every secretory process requires a source of energy and must include mechanisms for translation of that energy into the mechanical work involved in moving the secreted fluid against opposing resistance, and into the chemical work involved in the creation of a solution whose composition differs from that in the compartment of origin. In the kidney, for example, the original mechanical energy for glomerular filtration is supplied by cardiac contraction and chemical modification is accomplished by active transport processes in the tubules. In the biliary system, on the other hand, there is no structural counterpart to the renal glomerulus and since bile can be secreted against opposing pressures of the order of 20 mm Hg (15,16,17,18,19,20), pressures appreciably higher than the usual hepatic sinusoidal pressures (and demonstrably higher than the external perfusing pressure in an isolated perfused liver system (18)) it is clear that hydrostatic filtration can play little or no role in initiating bile formation. Thus all of the energy for bile formation must be derived from local energy sources via active transport mechanisms. Active transport of water per se has not ever been satisfactorily demonstrated in any biological system and in view of the extremely high permeability of most membranes to water (21) and the very high ratio of water molecules to solute particles in isotonic solutions (approximately 180 to 1) this would be a very inefficient means of generating movement of solution. Therefore, active solute transport appears to be the most attractive mechanism for secretion of solution.

If a solute were actively transported into a relatively confined region (e.g. bile canaliculi, or the intercellular spaces of gallbladder, intestinal or renal tubular epithelium) this in turn would create an osmotic gradient favoring passive movement of water and other diffusible solutes into the same region according to models described in detail by Curran (22,23), Diamond (24,25) and others (26,27,28). It has been estimated that the surface area of the bile canaliculi is of the order of 10 m^2 for a whole human liver (29), and because the bile canaliculi consist of a network of long narrow pores the "standing gradient" model of Diamond (24) may be particularly applicable. In this model solute is actively transported across the wall into the lumen of a long narrow tube. In response to the osmotic gradient water moves passively across the wall generating hydrostatic pressure for movement of solution down the tube. During this passage further osmotic water movement occurs until virtually complete osmotic equilibration is achieved by the time fluid reaches the distal end of the tube. If other small solutes are permitted to cross the wall by diffusion or "solvent drag" then an additional volume of solution will be generated in response to each mole of actively transported solute (29). The hypothesis that active solute transport actually provides the driving force for bile production was first proposed by Sperber (30,31) who pointed out that many organic solutes appear indeed to be actively transported into the bile, particularly a wide variety of organic anions, and that many of these can, in fact, be shown to produce a choleresis. In order to understand the mechanisms of bile formation it is therefore necessary to examine the active secretion of various solutes into the bile.

B. Active Solute Secretion

Mechanisms of bile pigment secretion are discussed in detail in other parts of this symposium. In addition to bile pigments many other organic compounds are excreted in bile in such high concentrations that the assumption of active secretory transport is inescapable (32). The best known of these are organic acids such as phenolphthalein derivatives (30,33), some hippuric acid derivatives (34,35), several sulfonamides (36), penicillin (34), erythromycin (37), ampicillin (38), cyanine dyes (39,40), phlorhizin (41), chlorothiazide (42), and of course the bile acids themselves (43,44,45). Except for those organic acids which are extremely firmly bound to plasma albumin (e.g. bilirubin, sulfobromophthalein, rose bengal and indocyanine green) it is interesting that most of these compounds appear to be actively secreted by the renal tubule as well as the bile canaliculus (30). There also appears to be competition for biliary secretion among a number of compounds of this class (31,35,36,42,46,47). These observations have suggested the existence of a possible common anion transport carrier which is present both in the bile canaliculi and the renal tubules (30,32). If such a carrier exists, however, there is good reason to believe it is not shared by the bile acids since these compounds are not secreted by the renal tubule (48) and since bile acids may actually enhance rather than compete with the maximal biliary secretory capacity of other anionic compounds under some circumstances (49,50,51,52,53,54,55, 56,57). Moreover, the demonstration by Alpert (43) that mutant Corriedale sheep, which have markedly depressed transport capacity for sulphobromophthalein, bilirubin and a variety of other anions, have a perfectly normal secretory capacity for taurocholate strongly suggests the existence of a separate pathway for bile acid secretory transport.

In addition to the foregoing organic acids there is a small group of quaternary ammonium cations, of which procaine amide ethobromide (PAEB) is the best characterized, which are also actively transported into bile by what appears to be a separate active transport carrier (32,58,59).

A third group of apparently actively transported organic compounds are electrically neutral. These include several cardiac glycosides (60), ferrioxamine derivatives (61) and, in the chicken, low molecular weight polyethylene glycol (PEG-1500) (62).

C. Clearance Techniques for Estimation of Canalicular Bile Flow

Measurement of the biliary clearances of inert solutes such as mannitol and erythritol has permitted an estimation of the rate of fluid movement into the bile canaliculi (63,64,65,66). The principle is quite comparable to that involved in the use of inulin clearance for the estimation of glomerular filtration rate. Erythritol and mannitol equilibrate rapidly between plasma and liver cell water (64,66,67,68,69) so that their steady state biliary "clearance" (e.g. biliary excretion rate/plasma concentration) should therefore be a function of the rate at which water moves into the bile canaliculi. In the dog (66) the clearances of mannitol and erythritol are nearly identical over a very wide range suggesting that either compound provides a measure of the rate of canalicular water production. In the guinea pig (64,70) erythritol clearance is appreciably higher than mannitol clearance although both are proportional to bile flow when the latter is varied by varying the rates of bile acid secretion. This suggests that the movement of at least the larger of the two solutes, mannitol, across the canalicular wall is restricted. In the rat the clearance of mannitol is only slightly less than that of erythritol (65).

If the biliary clearance of an inert solute is to be usable for estimating the rate of canalicular bile production it must be assumed not only that there is unrestricted movement of the substance from plasma to canalicular lumen (analogous to the movement of inulin into the renal glomeruli), but also that the ductal structures distal to the canaliculi must be virtually impermeable to the test solute. The evidence for the satisfaction of the latter criterion is admittedly indirect, but consists of the observations that the clearances of mannitol and erythritol are not influenced by secretin-induced choleresis (64,71,72) (whose mechanism is presumed to reside in the bile ducts).

In view of the foregoing limited evidence, and lacking the sort of direct micropuncture analyses which are available to the

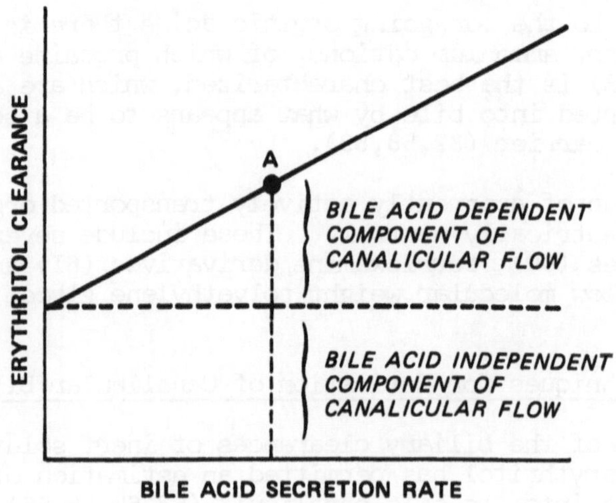

Fig. 1: Relationship between biliary erythritol clearance and bile acid secretion rate. The solid line is generated by actual observations of erythritol clearance over a wide range of bile acid secretion rates. By extrapolation of this line to the vertical axis an estimate is obtained of the "bile acid independent" component of canalicular flow. The total canalicular flow (i.e. erythritol clearance) at any given point A is the sum of the bile acid independent component plus a bile acid dependent component as illustrated.

renal physiologists, it has been tacitly assumed that erythritol clearance (and in the dog, mannitol clearance also) provides a reasonable estimation of canalicular bile flow. On this basis the clearance technique has been used to deduce the level at which various mechanisms operate to change the flow of bile.

D. Bile Acid Dependent and Independent Canalicular Bile Production

In every species in which the foregoing techniques have been applied thus far a relationship comparable to that illustrated in Fig. 1 is found between bile acid secretion rate and canalicular bile production (as estimated by erythritol clearance (63,66,73, 74,75). There appears to be a linear relationship between erythritol clearance and bile acid secretion rate, but extrapolation of this relationship leads to a positive intercept on the vertical axis suggesting that an appreciable component of canalicular bile production would exist even if bile acid secretion could be completely "turned off". The latter component has come to be referred to as the "bile acid independent" or "non-bile acid

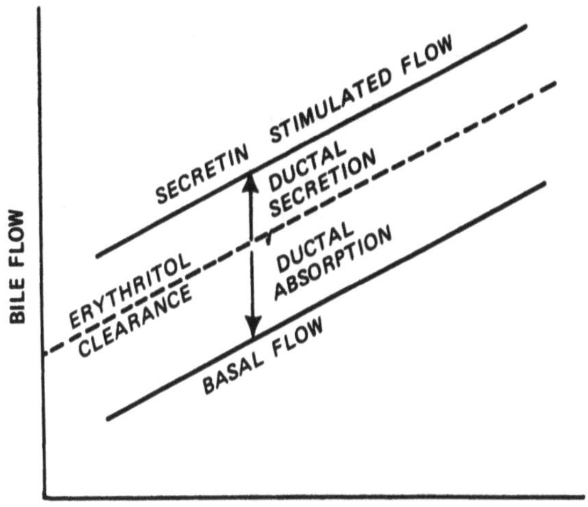

Fig. 2: Behavior of ductal system as illustrated by relationship between bile flow, erythritol clearance and bile acid secretion rate. The erythritol clearance (dashed line) is reproduced from Fig. 1. Values below this line (e.g. points on the solid line labeled "basal flow") are indicative of ductal absorption of fluid. Values above the line, as in secretin stimulated bile flow, provide evidence for ductal secretion of fluid.

dependent" component of canalicular bile flow. The increment in flow above this level which is related to the rate of bile acid secretion is referred to as the "bile acid dependent" component of canalicular bile flow. In other words, the positive relationship between bile acid secretion and erythritol clearance, which exists in all species studied so far, corroborates Sperber's (30) original views of the importance of bile acid secretion in the initiation of bile formation. However, it is now clear that there is also a completely independent component which is presumably due to inorganic ion (possibly sodium ion) transport into the canalicular lumen. In fact, it has been shown that some known inhibitors of sodium transport (e.g. ethacrynic acid, cardiac glycosides) (63,74) can reduce or eliminate the "bile acid independent" component without affecting the slope of the relationship between canalicular flow and bile acid secretion.

E. Bile Duct Activity

Structures distal to the canaliculi (that is, distal to the sites in which erythritol clearance is affected by water movement) are lumped together as "ductal" structures, but as yet it has not been possible to differentiate between mechanisms located in the small ductules, in the larger intrahepatic ducts and in the common bile duct. Studies of the sort illustrated schematically in Fig. 2, however, illustrate that at some times and in some species (e.g. during basal bile production in the cholecystectomized dog) there must be substantial reabsorption of fluid and electrolytes from the bile at some level of the ductal system. When the bile flow is appreciably less than the erythritol clearance, as illustrated by the line labeled "basal flow" the difference between the two lines must represent the volume of fluid reabsorbed between the canaliculi and the distal end of the common bile duct. Stated in another way, substances like erythritol and mannitol may, at times, be concentrated as much as threefold in canine bile as compared to plasma (66). In species such as the rabbit (63) and the rat (69) bile-to-plasma ratios are generally only slightly greater than unity so that it is as yet unclear if the bile ducts of species other than the dog engage in very active reabsorption of fluid.

The hormone secretin is a fairly potent choleretic agent which has been shown to enhance bile flow without affecting the clearance of mannitol or erythritol (64,66). This finding, plus other evidence (76), supports the view that secretin-induced choleresis is an example of ductal secretion of fluid and electrolyte. This phenomenon is illustrated by the line labeled "secretin stimulated flow" in Fig. 2. Secretin choleresis is also accompanied by a marked increase in bicarbonate concentration and secretion (7, 77, 78,79). Moreover an abrupt electronegativity of the bile duct lumen has been demonstrated during secretin choleresis (80). It seems very likely, therefore, that secretin stimulation causes active transport of anions (predominantly bicarbonate) into the lumen of some portion or portions of the bile duct system.

F. Summary of Biliary Secretory Mechanisms

Based upon the foregoing lines of evidence a minimum of four distinct mechanisms appear to be involved in the production and modification of hepatic bile: 1) Active organic solute secretion (principally bile acid secretion) with resultant passive movement of water and small solutes into the lumen. 2) Active inorganic solute secretion (possibly sodium ion), also accompanied by movement of water and other solutes. 3) Ductal water and electrolyte reabsorption. 4) Ductal secretion of electrolytes and water, with bicarbonate as the most important anion. The secretion of bile acids is presumably directly dependent upon their availability and this will be predominantly related to the state of the enterohepatic circulation at any given time. Ductal secretion must be under the control of endogenous secretin but also possibly other factors. Beyond this, however, the physiological regulation of these processes remains to be elucidated. The foregoing phenomena are illustrated in Fig. 3 in which the passive movement of water and solutes in response to active canalicular solute secretion is shown, and in which the small arrow labeled with a question mark serves to emphasize the possiblity of a preferential "shunt" pathway, conceivably via the intercellular spaces, for water and small solutes which has been proposed by Forker (81,82).

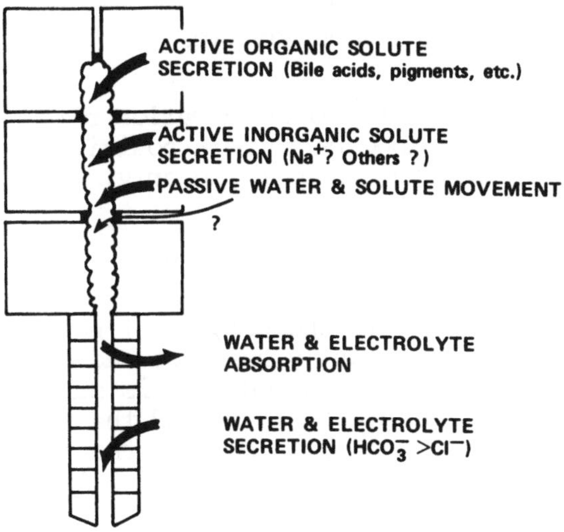

Fig. 3: Summary of biliary secretory mechanisms. Active transport of organic solutes, principally bile acids, leads to passive movement of water and small solutes into the lumen (the "bile acid dependent" component). Active inorganic solute secretion (e.g. Na^+ or other ions) also pulls water and other solutes into the lumen (the "bile acid independent" component). It is possible that some passive water and small solute movement may occur by a preferential shunt pathway (e.g. between cells) as illustrated by the narrow arrow labeled with a question mark. In the ducts there is evidence for water and electrolyte absorption, and under other circumstances (e.g. secretin choleresis) evidence for water and electrolyte secretion in which bicarbonate is characteristically the dominant anion.

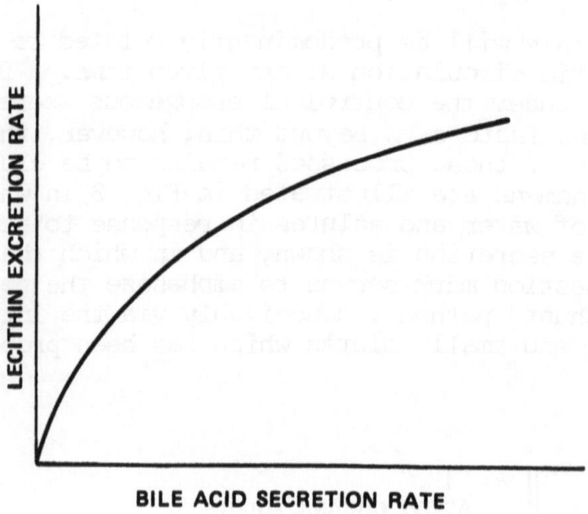

Fig. 4: Relationship between lecithin excretion rate and bile acid secretion rate. This appears to be a positive hyperbolic relationship which extrapolates through the origin.

BILIARY LIPID EXCRETION

In view of its importance to the problem of gallstone formation much attention has recently been focused on biliary lipid excretion. A detailed discussion of this subject and of the solubilization of cholesterol is beyond the scope of this paper, but the important relationships between the excretion of biliary lipid components need to be emphasized. As in the case of water and small solute excretion, the excretion of lecithin and, apparently to a somewhat lesser extent, of cholesterol is intimately dependent upon the active transport of bile acids into the bile canaliculi. Although there are marked quantitative differences between species, the general behavior of lecithin excretion with respect to bile acid excretion is well illustrated for most species by the relationship shown in Fig. 4. There is a strong positive relationship between lecithin excretion and bile acid secretion which appears to start at the origin and rise in hyperbolic fashion (83,84,85,86,87,88). It has been suggested (85,86) that such a relationship would be consistent with the view that the availability of bile acid micelles is responsible for the movement of lecithin into bile. Although the slope of this relationship is positive, there is a trend toward a plateau. As a consequence the lecithin-to-bile acid ratio actually diminishes as bile acid secretion increases (Fig. 5) despite the increase in absolute lecithin excretion rate.

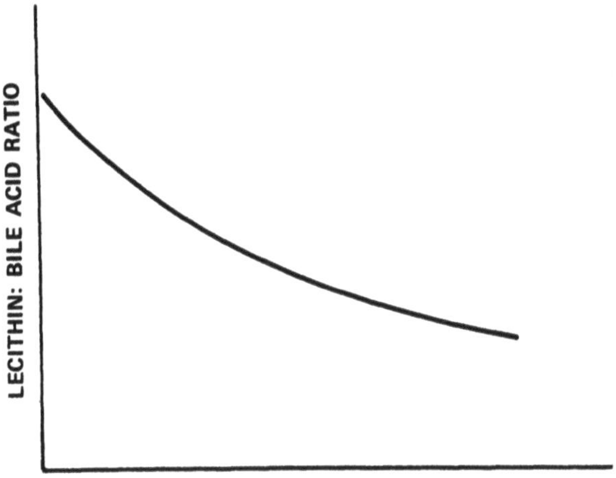

Fig. 5: Lecithin to bile acid ratio at various bile acid secretion rates. Because of the shape of the lecithin excretion rate curve (Fig. 4) the highest ratio is seen at low bile acid secretion rates even though the absolute rate of lecithin excretion increases with increasing bile acid secretion rates.

The relationship between cholesterol excretion rate and bile acid secretion rate is qualitatively similar except that it tends to be somewhat flatter and it is by no means clear that the curve can be extrapolated to the origin. Some indirect evidence in the dog (86) seemed to suggest that the behavior of cholesterol excretion at the lower end of the curve was attributable to a lecithin-independent, but bile acid dependent special cholesterol secretory mechanism. This would be illustrated by the dashed line labeled "a" in Fig. 6. On the other hand, evidence in man (89) suggests that there may be a very poor correlation between cholesterol excretion and bile acid secretion, consistent with the view that there is very likely a "bile acid independent" mechanism for cholesterol excretion. This could be illustrated by the dashed line labeled "b" in Fig. 6. Based upon the relationships shown in Fig. 6 the cholesterol to bile acid ratio (Fig. 7) is qualitatively similar to the lecithin to bile acid ratio (Fig. 5) but much steeper at low rates of bile acid secretion.

The cholesterol to lecithin ratio (Fig. 8) is particularly interesting because it suggests, at least in the dog (86) and the rat (85) that there may be a very close coupling between cholesterol and lecithin excretion at higher rates of bile acid secretion.

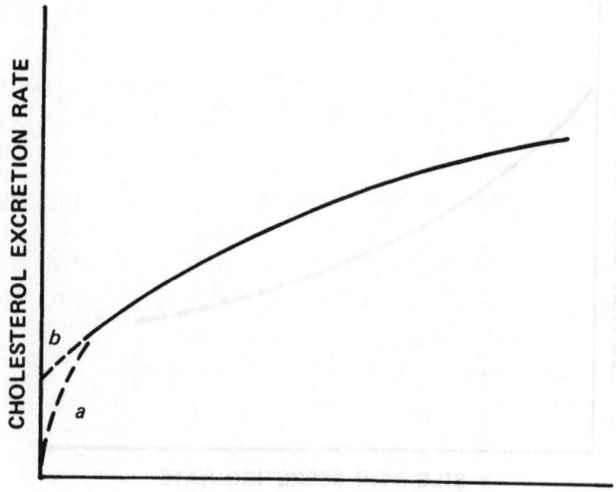

Fig. 6: Relationship between cholesterol excretion rate and bile acid secretion rate. The relationship is very similar to that shown for lecithin (Fig. 4) but the curve tends to be flatter in most species. Extrapolation of the lower end is dubious. In the dog there is some indirect evidence that the curve may dip to the origin as shown by a line "a" (i.e. that all cholesterol excretion is "bile acid dependent"). However, in other species such as man there is reason to believe that a "bile acid independent" cholesterol excretion process exists as illustrated by line "b".

This might suggest that these two lipids actually enter the bile in association with each other and then join the bile acids to form mixed micelles and are thereby carried in an aqueous solution. As anticipated by the earlier figures, the close apparent "coupling" between cholesterol and lecithin breaks down at low levels of bile acid secretion where the dominant mechanism for cholesterol excretion is a component which is clearly independent of lecithin excretion and may even be independent of bile acid secretion.

While much has been learned about the physical chemistry of cholesterol solubilization in recent years it is obvious that an understanding of the pathophysiology of gallstone formation can only be achieved when there is a much better understanding of the two or more mechanisms involved in transport of cholesterol from the liver cell into the hepatic bile.

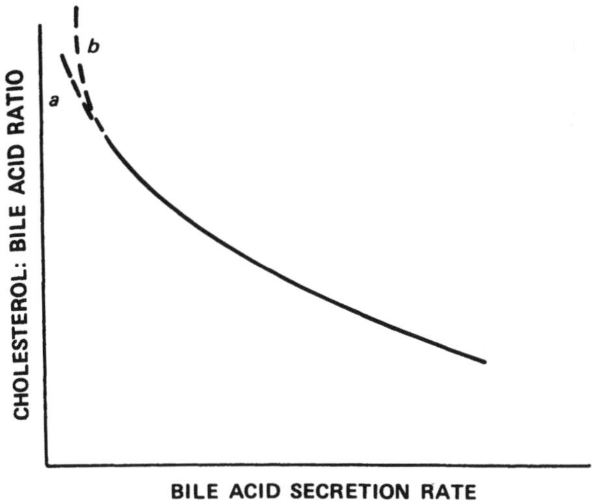

Fig. 7: Relationship between cholesterol to bile acid ratio and bile acid secretion rate. This is very similar to the relationship shown in Fig. 5 except that it is much steeper at low bile acid secretion rates. The differences between lines "a" and "b" are explained in the legend for Fig. 6.

SUMMARY

Bile is an approximately isotonic solution which contains mixed bile acid-lecithin-cholesterol micelles, bile pigments, small amounts of numerous other organic compounds and inorganic electrolytes. The driving force for bile formation clearly must be provided by active transport of solute into the lumen, followed by passive movement of water and smaller solutes. The major mechanisms appear to include a bile acid-dependent component and a bile acid independent component of canalicular secretion, ductal reabsorption and ductal secretion. The excretion of the biliary lipids lecithin and cholesterol is directly related to the secretion rate of bile acids. However, these relationships are curvilinear so that the highest relative concentrations of these constituents are found at low rates of bile acid secretion. Cholesterol excretion in particular appears to involve two processes: one is directly related to lecithin excretion suggesting the possibility of coupled entry of cholesterol and lecithin into the canaliculi. At low bile acid secretion rates, however, the dominant mechanism for cholesterol secretion appears to be entirely independent of lecithin excretion and possibly also independent of bile acid secretion. Elucidation

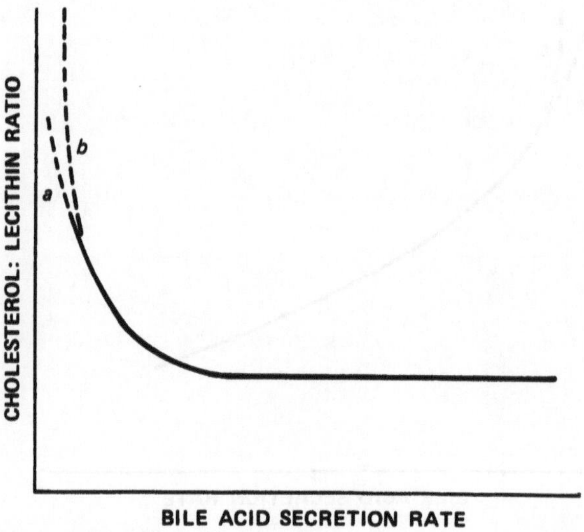

Fig. 8: Relationship between cholesterol to lecithin ratio and bile acid secretion rate. Over a wide range of high bile acid secretion rates the ratio is quite constant, suggesting that there may be a close coupling between cholesterol and lecithin excretion over this range. At low bile acid secretion rates, however, cholesterol excretion appears to be dominated by a process which is independent of lecithin, and possibly even of bile acids. The differences between lines "a" and "b" are explained in the legend of Fig. 6.

of the mechanisms of cholesterol gallstone formation must depend upon a more complete understanding of the mechanisms of cholesterol excretion in hepatic bile.

REFERENCES

1. DOWLING RH, MACK E, PICOTT J, et al: Experimental model for study of the enterohepatic circulation of bile in rhesus monkeys. J Lab Clin Med 72: 169-176, 1963.

2. ERLINGER S, DHUMEAUX D: Mechanisms and control of secretion of bile water and electrolytes. Gastroenterology 66: 281-304, 1974.

3. SOBOTKA H: Physiological Chemistry of the Bile. Baltimore, Williams and Wilkins, 1937,

4. CHENDEROVITCH J, PHOCAS E, RAUTUREAU M: Effects of hypertonic solutions on bile formation. Am J Physiol 205: 863-867, 1963.

5. GILMAN A, COWGILL GR: Osmotic relations between blood and body fluids. IV. Pancreatic juice, bile and lymph. Am J Physiol 104: 476-479, 1933.

6. WHEELER HO, RAMOS OL: Determinants of the flow and composition of bile in the unanesthetized dog during constant infusions of sodium taurocholate. J Clin Invest 39: 161-170, 1960.

7. PREISIG R, COOPER HL, WHEELER HO: The relationship between taurocholate secretion rate and bile production in the unanesthetized dog during cholinergic blockade and during secretin administration. J Clin Invest 41: 1152-1162, 1962.

8. HARDISON WGM, NORMAN JC: Effect of secretin on bile osmolality. J Lab Clin Med 73: 34-41, 1969.

9. THUREBORN E: Human hepatic bile. Composition changes due to altered enterohepatic circulation. Acta chir scand Suppl 303: 1-63, 1962.

10. HARDWICKE J, RANKIN JG, BAKER KJ et al: The loss of protein in human and canine hepatic bile. Clin Sci 26: 509-517, 1964.

11. ROSENTHAL WS, KUBO K, DOLINSKI M, et al: The passage of serum albumin into bile in man. Am J Dig Dis 10: 271-283, 1965.

12. RUSSELL IS, FLECK A, BURNETT W: The protein content of human bile. Clin Chim Acta 10: 210-213, 1964.

13. FINK S: Studies on hepatic bile obtained from a patient with an external biliary fistula; its composition and changes after diamox administration. N Eng J Med 254: 258-262, 1956.

14. WAITMAN AM, DYCK WP, JANOWITZ HD: Effect of secretin and acetazolamide on the volume and electrolyte composition of hepatic bile in man. Gastroenterology 56: 286-294, 1969.

15. BARBER-RILEY G: The rate of biliary secretion during flow up vertical cannulas of different bore. Experientia 20: 639-645, 1964.

16. BARBER-RILEY G: Measurement of the capacity of the biliary tree. In The Biliary System, edited by Taylor W, Oxford, Blackwell, 1965. pp 90-97.

17. BRAUER RW: Hepatic blood supply and the secretion in bile. In The Biliary System, edited by Taylor W, Oxford, Blackwell, 1965. pp. 41-67.

18. BRAUER RW, LEONG GF, HOLLOWAY RJ: Mechanics of bile secretion: The effect of perfusion pressure and temperature on bile flow and bile secretion pressure. Am J Physiol 177: 103-112, 1954.

19. RICHARDS TG, THOMSON JY: The secretion of bile against pressure. Gastroenterology 40: 705-707, 1961.

20. STRASBERG SM, DORN BC, REDINGER RN, et al: Effects of alteration of biliary pressure on bile composition - A method for study: primate biliary physiology V. Gastroenterology 61: 357-362, 1971.

21. MAFFLY RH, LEAF A: The potential of water in mammalian tissues. J Gen Physiol 42: 1257-1275, 1959.

22. CURRAN PF, McINTOSH JR: A model system for biological water transport. Nature (Lond) 193: 347-348, 1962.

23. OGILVIE JT, McINTOSH JR, CURRAN PF: Volume flow in a series membrane system. Biochim Biophys Acta 66: 441-444, 1963.

24. DIAMOND JM, BOSSERT WH: Standing-gradient osmotic flow. J Gen Physiol 50: 2061-2083, 1967.

25. TORMEY J McD, DIAMOND JM: The ultrastructural route of fluid transport in rabbit gallbladder. J Gen Physiol 50: 2031-2060, 1967.

26. PATLAK CS, GOLDSTEIN DA, HOFFMAN JF: The flow of solute and solvent across a two-membrane system. J Theor Biol 5: 426-442, 1963.

27. KAYE G, WHEELER HO, WHITLOCK RT, et al: Fluid transport in the rabbit gallbladder. A combined physiological and electron microscopic study. J Cell Biol 30: 237-268, 1967.

28. WHITLOCK RT, WHEELER HO: Coupled transport of solute and water across rabbit gallbladder epithelium. J Clin Invest 43: 2249-2265, 1964.

29. WHEELER HO: Water and electrolytes in bile. In Handbook of Physiology, Sect 6, Alimentary Canal, vol 5. Edited by Code CF, Washington, Amer Physiol Soc, 1968. pp 2409-2431.

30. SPERBER I: Secretion of organic anions in the formation of urine and bile. Pharm Rev 11: 109-134, 1959.

31. SPERBER I: Biliary secretion of organic anions and its influence on bile flow. In The Biliary System, edited by Taylor W, Oxford, Blackwell, 1965, pp 457-467.

32. SCHANKER LS: Secretion of organic compounds in bile. In Handbook of Physiology, Sect 6, Alimentary Canal, vol 5. Edited by Code CF, Washington, Amer Physiol Soc, 1968. pp 2433-2449.

33. HART LG, SCHANKER LS: The chemical forms in which phenol red is secreted into the bile of rats. Proc Soc Exp Biol Med 123: 433-435, 1966.

34. COOK DL, LAWLER CA, CALVIN LD, et al: Mechanisms of bile formation. Am J Physiol 171: 62-74, 1952.

35. DESPOPOULOS A: Congruence of excretory functions in liver and kidney: hippurates. Am J Physiol 210: 760-764, 1966.

36. DESPOPOULOS A, SONNENBERG H: Congruence of excretory functions of liver and kidney: sulfonamides. Am J Physiol 212: 1117-1122, 1967.

37. TWISS JR, BERGER WV, GILLETTE L, et al: The biliary excretion of erythromycin (Ilotycin). Surg, Gynec Obstet 102: 355-357, 1956.

38. AYLIFFE GAJ, DAVIES A: Ampicillin levels in human bile. Brit J Pharmacol 24: 189-193, 1965.

39. CHERRICK GR, STEIN SW, LEEVY CM, et al: Indocyanine green: observations on its physical properties, plasma decay and hepatic excretion. J Clin Invest 39: 592-600, 1960.

40. WHEELER HO, CRANSTON WI, MELTZER JI: Hepatic uptake and biliary excretion of indocyanine green in the dog. Proc Soc Exp Biol Med 99: 11-14, 1958.

41. JENNER FA, SMYTH DH: The excretion of phlorhizin. J Physiol (Lond) 146: 563-571, 1959.

42. HART LG, SCHANKER LS: Active transport of chlorothiazide into bile. Am J Physiol 211: 643-646, 1966.

43. ALPERT S, MOSHER M, SHANSKE A, et al: Multiplicity of hepatic excretory mechanisms for organic anions. J Gen Physiol 53: 238-247, 1969.

44. O'MAILLE ERL, RICHARDS TG, SHORT AH: Acute taurine depletion and maximal rates of hepatic conjugation and secretion of cholic acid in the dog. J Physiol (Lond) 180: 67-79, 1965.

45. O'MAILLE ERL, RICHARDS TG, SHORT AH: The influence of conjugation of cholic acid on its uptake and secretion: hepatic extraction of taurocholate and cholate in the dog. J Physiol (Lond) 189: 337-350, 1967.

46. SCHOENFIELD LJ, FOULK WT: Studies of sulfobromophthalein sodium (BSP) metabolism in man. II. The effect of artificially induced fever, norethandrolone (Nilevar) and iopanoic acid (Telepaque). J Clin Invest 43: 1419-1423, 1964.

47. GOETZEE AE, RICHARDS TG, TINDALL VR: Experimental changes in liver function induced by probenecid. Clin Sci 19: 63-78, 1960.

48. WEINER IM, GLASSER JE, LACK L: Renal excretion of bile: taurocholic, glycocholic, and cholic acids. Am J Physiol 207: 964-970, 1964.

49. BARNHART J, RITT D, WARE A, et al: A comparison of the effects of taurocholate and theophylline on BSP excretion in dogs. In The Liver, Quantitative Aspects of Structure and Function. Edited by Paumgartner G, Preisig R, Basel, Karger, 1973. pp. 315-325.

50. BOYER JL, SCHEIG RL, KLATSKIN G: The effect of sodium taurocholate on the hepatic metabolism of sulfobromophthalein sodium (BSP). The role of bile flow. J Clin Invest 49: 206-215, 1970.

51. ERLINGER S, DUMONT M: Influence of canalicular bile flow on sulfobromophthalein transport maximum in bile in the dog. In The Liver. Quantitative Aspects of Structure and Function. Edited by Paumgartner G, Preisig R, Basel, Karger, 1973. pp. 306-314.

52. FORKER EL, GIBSON G: Interaction between sulfobromophthalein (BSP) and taurocholate. In The Liver. Quantitative Aspects of Structure and Function. Edited by Paumgartner G, Preisig R, Basel, Karger, 1973. pp. 326-336.

53. O'MAILLE ERL, RICHARDS TG, SHORT AH: Factors determining the maximal rate of organic anion secretion by the liver and further evidence on the hepatic site of action of the hormone secretin. J Physiol (Lond) 186: 424-438, 1966.

54. RITT DJ, COMBES B: Enhancement of apparent excretory maximum of sulfobromophthalein sodium (BSP) by taurocholate and dehydrocholate. J Clin Invest 46: 1108, 1967 (Abstract).

55. BERK RN, GOLDBERGER LE, LOEB PM: The role of bile salts in the hepatic excretion of iopanoic acid. Invest Radiol. (in press).

56. DUNN CR, BERK RN: The pharmacokinetics of telepaque metabolism: The relation of blood concentration and bile flow to the rate of hepatic excretion. Am J Roentgenol 114: 758-766, 1972.

57. MOSS AA, AMBERG JR, JONES RS: Relationship of bile salts and bile flow to biliary excretion of iopanoic acid. Invest Radiol 7: 11-15, 1972.

58. SCHANKER LS: Hepatic transport of organic cations. In The Biliary System, edited by Taylor W, Oxford, Blackwell, 1965. pp 469-480.

59. SCHANKER LS, SOLOMON HM: Active transport of quaternary ammonium compounds into bile. Am J Physiol 204: 829-832, 1963.

60. KUPFERBERG HJ, SCHANKER LS: Biliary secretion of ouabain-H^3 and its uptake by liver slices in the rat. Am J Physiol 214: 1048-1053, 1968.

61. MEYER-BRUNOT HG, KEBERLE H: Biliary excretion of ferrioxamines of varying liposolubility in perfused rat liver. Am J Physiol 214: 1193-1200, 1968.

62. SPERBER I: Biliary excretion and choleresis. In Proceedings First International Pharmacological Meeting. Oxford, Pergamon Press, 1963. vol 4, pp. 137-143.

63. ERLINGER S, DHUMEAUX D, BERTHELOT P et al: Effect of inhibitors of sodium transport on bile formation in the rabbit. Amer J Physiol 219: 416-422, 1970.

64. FORKER EL: Two sites of bile formation as determined by mannitol and erythritol clearance in the guinea pig. J Clin Invest 46: 1189-1195, 1967.

65. FORKER EL, HICKLIN T, SORNSON T: The clearance of mannitol and erythritol in rat bile. Proc Soc Exp Biol Med 126: 115-119, 1967.

66. WHEELER HO, ROSS ED, BRADLEY SE: Canalicular bile production in dogs. Am J Physiol 214: 866-874, 1968.

67. CAHILL GF Jr, ASHMORE J, EARLE AS, et al: Glucose penetration into liver. Am J Physiol 192: 491-496, 1958.

68. SACKS J, BAKSHY S: Insulin and tissue distribution of pentose in nephrectomized cats. Am J Physiol 189:339-342, 1957.

69. SCHANKER LS, HOGBEN CAM: Biliary excretion of inulin, sucrose, and mannitol: analysis of bile formation. Am J Physiol 200:1087-1090, 1968.

70. FORKER EL: Bile formation in guinea pigs: analysis with inert solutes of graded molecular radius. Am J Physiol 216: 56-62, 1968.

71. FRIEDMAN MHF, SNAPE WJ: Comparative effectiveness of extracts of intestinal mucosa in stimulating the external secretions of the pancreas and the liver. Fed Proc 4: 21-22, 1945.

72. CRIGLER JF, Jr, NAJJAR VA: Congenital familial nonhemolytic jaundice with kernicterus. Pediatrics 10: 169-179, 1952.

73. BERTHELOT P, ERLINGER S, DHUMEAUX D, et al: Mechanism of phenobarbital-induced choleresis in the rat. Am J Physiol 219: 809-813, 1970.

74. BOYER JL: Canalicular bile formation in the isolated perfused rat liver. Am J Physiol 221: 1156-1163, 1971.

75. BOYER JL, KLATSKIN G: Canalicular bile flow and bile secretory pressure: Evidence for a non-bile salt dependent fraction in the isolated perfused rat liver. Gastroenterology 59: 853-859, 1970.

76. WHEELER HO, MANCUSI-UNGARO PL: Role of bile ducts during secretin choleresis in dogs. Am J Physiol 210: 1153-1159, 1966.

77. HARDISON WG, NORMAN JC: Electrolyte composition of the secretin fraction of bile from the perfused pig liver. Am J Physiol 214: 758-763, 1968.

78. JONES RS, GROSSMAN MI: Choleretic effects of secretin and histamine in the dog. Am J Physiol 217: 532-535, 1969.

79. ZATERKA S, GROSSMAN MI: The effect of gastrin and histamine on secretion of bile. Gastroenterology 50: 500-505, 1966.

80. LONDON CD, DIAMOND JM, BROOKS FP: Electrical potential differences in the biliary tree. Biochim Biophys Acta 150: 509-517, 1968.

81. FORKER EL: The effect of estrogen on bile formation in the rat. J Clin Invest 48: 654-663, 1969.

82. FORKER EL: Hepatocellular uptake of inulin, sucrose and mannitol in rats. Am J Physiol 219: 1568-1573, 1970.

83. SWELL L, ENTENMAN C, LEONG GF, et al: Bile acids and lipid metabolism: IV. Influence of bile acids on biliary and liver organelle phospholipids and cholesterol. Am J Physiol 215: 1390-1396, 1968.

84. NILSSON S, SCHERSTEN T: Importance of bile acids for phospholipid secretion into human hepatic bile. Gastroenterology 57: 525-532, 1969.

85. HARDISON WGM, APTER JT: Micellar theory of biliary cholesterol excretion. Am J Physiol 226: 61-67, 1972.

86. WHEELER HO, KING KK: Biliary excretion of lecithin and cholesterol in the dog. J Clin Invest 51: 1337-1350, 1972.

87. DOWLING RH, MACK E, SMALL DM: Biliary lipid secretion and bile composition after acute and chronic interruption of enterohepatic circulation in the rhesus monkey. IV. Primate biliary physiology. J Clin Invest 50: 1917-1926, 1971.

88. NILSSON S, SCHERSTEN T: Influence of bile acids on the synthesis of biliary phospholipids in man. Europ J Clin Invest 1: 109-111, 1970.

89. GRUNDY SM, METZGER AL, ADLER RD: Mechanisms of lithogenic bile formation in American Indian women with cholesterol gallstones. J Clin Invest 51: 3026-3043, 1972.

PHYSIOLOGICAL CONSIDERATIONS IN THE PLANNING OF STUDIES OF CHOLESTASIS

SM Strasberg, RG Ilson, KA Siminovitch

Medical Sciences Building, Room 7252
University of Toronto, Toronto, Ontario

INTRODUCTION

Cholestasis has been classically characterized by features unrelated or indirectly related to the processes of bile flow. Recent advances in the physiology of bile production may eventually allow definition of different forms of cholestasis in terms of their alteration of the specific processes involved in bile formation, particularly in their effect on the components of bile flow.

We have encountered difficulty in planning experiments of extrahepatic obstruction because of the incomplete characterization of normal processes, and the inability to resolve certain important differences in experimental findings in previous experiments. These are described below.

Wheeler demonstrated, in the fasting dog, that bile flow varied considerably at a steady bile salt secretion rate (1). This variability could be eliminated by the administration of anticholinergic agents (2). Under these conditions, good linear correlation between bile flow and bile salt secretion could be demonstrated; there was little or no bile flow at low bile salt secretion rates (i.e. there was little or no demonstrable bile salt independent flow). Dowling also demonstrated good linear correlation between bile flow and the bile salt secretion rate, in fed monkeys, not receiving anticholinergic agents. But, at low bile salt secretion rates, there was considerable bile salt independent flow (3). Nahrwold infused bile salts (as bile) into the duodenum of fasted dogs, not receiving anticholinergic agents, and although the bile salt secretion rate increased, there was no increase in bile flow (4).

It is not apparent why anticholinergic agents are required to demonstrate correlation between the two variables in the dog, but not the monkey, or why the bile salt independent flow is low in the dog but not the monkey. Do these results reflect a difference in species or experimental design? Nahrwold's experiment in fasted dogs suggests that bile salt secretion does not always influence bile flow and seems to cast some doubt on the observations of Wheeler and Dowling. Planning and interpretation of experiments of cholestasis are difficult indeed when one does not know how to choose experimental animals or how to compare results between different species. Should the animals be fasted or fed? Should the investigator use anticholinergic agents to stabilize bile flow? May one infer causal relationships between simultaneous changes in bile flow and bile salt secretion?

Even if these questions are resolved there remains the necessity to obtain a method to quantify the components of bile flow. The present study was undertaken in an attempt to clarify the reasons for the experimental differences cited above, and to obtain a method to confirm and quantify the components of bile flow. A resumé of the methods and results of these experiments will be presented. The full details may be obtained elsewhere (5,6,7).

STUDY I

Group I: Fasting Primates Receiving Intraduodenal Bile Salt Infusions

Methods: Five female rhesus monkeys were each prepared with a total external biliary fistula, a tube duodenostomy and a functional cholecystectomy, as described by Dowling (3). During the recovery period (3 weeks), the biliary tract dead space was measured (8) and the enterohepatic circulation was maintained by intraduodenal bile salt infusion.

In the experimental period, the animals were fed at 4-5 p.m. and two hours later any remaining food was removed. A bile salt or saline infusion was then started and continued throughout the night and the next day, at a constant rate. Sampling was started at 8.00 a.m. and continued to 4.00 p.m., when the animal was fed again and a new infusion rate established. Sodium cholate, sodium taurocholate, previously collected monkey bile, and normal saline were the infusions used. Each bile salt solution was infused in at least three animals at three different rates (3 days). Saline was infused for one day.

Results: There was a large variation in bile flow during each experimental day and a lesser variation in the bile salt secretion rate. Bile flow was plotted against the bile salt secretion rate.

Bile flow increased with increasing bile salt secretion rates, and the linear correlation coefficients were significant; however there was considerable scatter of the data (Fig. 1). This picture was

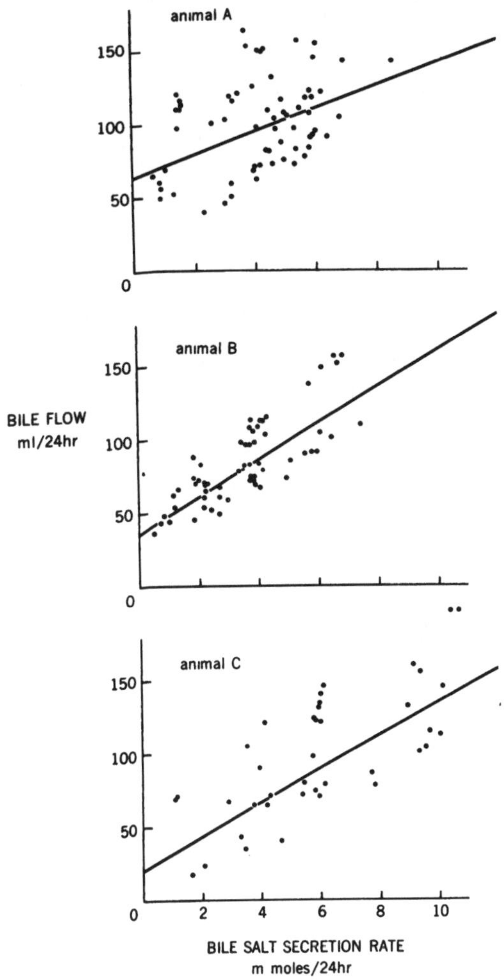

Fig. 1. Bile flow vs bile salt secretion rate in fasting monkeys receiving intraduodenal sodium cholate infusion. Note increasing flow with increasing bile salt secretion but with a large scatter in the data. Linear correlation coefficients were significant. Slopes and Y axis intercepts are not meaningful since the scatter of the data is large (i.e. other independent variables are present) and because 10% of the bile salt secreted was sodium cholate.

found in all three types of bile salt infusion, in all animals tested. These findings indicate that bile salt secretion is a determinant (independent variable) of bile flow (dependent variable) in the fasting primate but not the sole determinant. The other determinants (independent variables) have an inconsistent effect on bile flow in the fasting primate; this is reflected in the large scatter of the data. The findings in this group of animals are somewhat similar to those in fasting dogs described by Wheeler (1).

Group 2: Fed Primates Receiving Intraduodenal Bile Salt Infusions

Method: Four of the animals from group 1 were used in this experiment. The methods were similar to group 1, except that the animals were fed continually throughout the day, and only sodium cholate or saline was infused.

Results: There was considerably less variability in bile flow on each experimental day. Bile flow was increased at bile salt secretion rates comparable to group 1. Bile flow was plotted against bile salt secretion rate. Bile flow increased with increasing bile salt secretion rate, but the scatter in the data was eliminated (Fig. 2). The linear correlation coefficients were significant and also significantly greater than those in comparable experiments in the fasting group. This experiment also indicates that bile salt secretion is one independent variable affecting bile flow. The effect of other factors influencing bile flow is increased and stabilized by steady feeding.

COMMENT ON STUDY I

The findings in groups 1 and 2 demonstrated that:

a) bile flow is linearly related to bile salt secretion rate in fasted and fed primates;
b) other independent variable(s) affect bile flow in an inconsistent manner in the fasting primate. The effect of these variable(s) is increased and stabilized by constant feeding.

These findings substantially explained the differences in previous studies noted above. Dowling used a fed model and obtained results similar to group 2. Wheeler originally used a fasting model and found variable bile flow, at one bile salt secretion rate (as in group 1). When anticholinergic agents were administered, bile flow was stabilized and the linear regression line for bile flow vs bile salt secretion rate passed through the Y-axis at a point close to zero, i.e. effects on bile flow of independent variable(s), other than bile salt secretion, had been stabilized in this case by their elimination. The presence of high bile salt independent flow in Dowling's experiments, in the monkey, and the low bile salt independent flow in Wheeler's experiments, in the dog, do not represent a species difference but a difference in choice of a model. In the former,

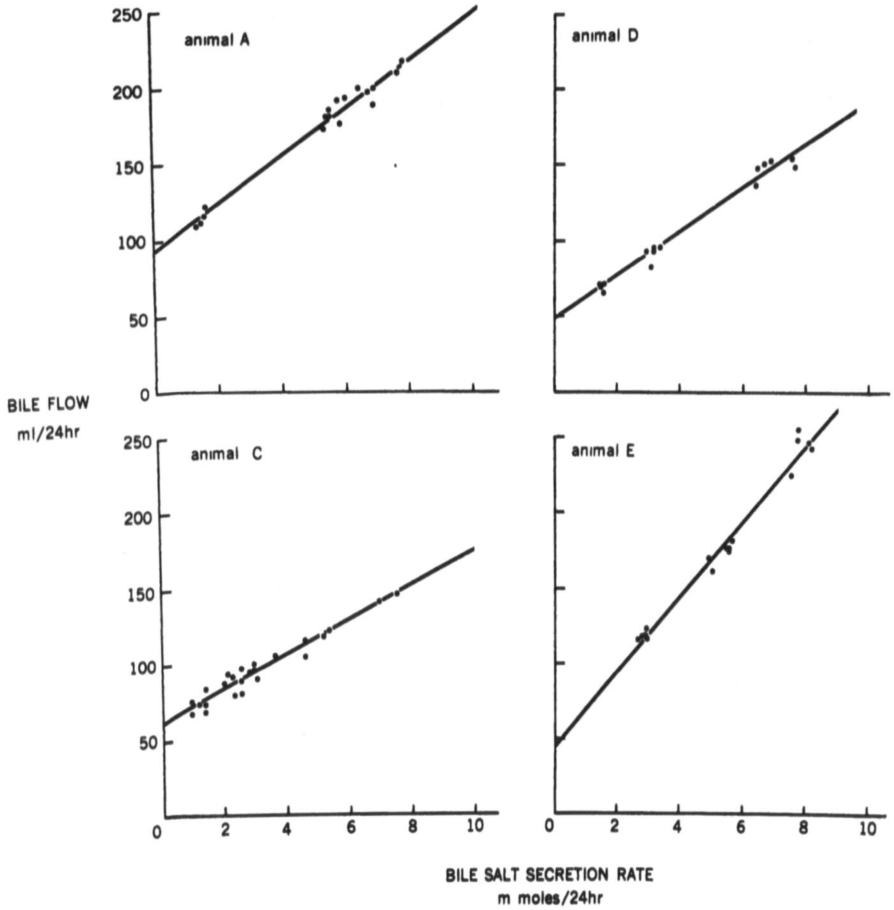

Fig. 2. As for Fig. 1 except that animals were fed throughout the day. The significant finding is the elimination of the scatter i.e. the effect on bile flow of independent variables (other than bile salt secretion) was stabilized by feeding. Again, slopes and Y axis intercepts are not meaningful because of the presence of some unconjugated bile salt.

feeding increased and stabilized independent variable(s) responsible for bile salt independent flow, and in the latter experiment these variable(s) had been eliminated by anticholinergic agents.

The results of group 1 also showed that there may be identical total bile flow in two paired samples, despite substantially different bile salt secretion rates. This is not surprising, and is due to the fact that, in fasting animals, the bile salt independent flow is extremely variable, so that the total bile flow in a sample with a high bile salt independent flow and a low bile salt dependent flow, may be equal to the total bile flow in a sample with a low bile salt independent flow and a high bile salt dependent flow. Nahrwold used fasting animals not receiving anticholinergic agents. He noted that an intraduodenal bile salt infusion did not affect bile flow even though the bile salt secretion rate increased. The intraduodenal bile salt infusion was in the form of bile, a liquid of slightly alkaline pH, capable of inhibiting secretin release from the duodenum. That inhibition of secretin release occurred is suggested by the marked drop in bile bicarbonate output which accompanied the intraduodenal bile infusion. This suggests that the increased bile salt secretion rate was indeed responsible for an increased bile salt dependent flow, but because bile salt independent flow was diminished, total bile flow remained unchanged.

The results of this study should be useful in planning studies of cholestasis. Food intake must be comparable in control and experimental periods. Since anorexia is commonly associated with intrahepatic or extrahepatic cholestasis, this may be difficult. If food intake does decrease, one may expect a variable reduction in bile flow which is only indirectly related to the cholestasis. One possible method of avoiding this problem is by the use of gastrostomy tube feedings in control and experimental periods. The use of anticholinergic agents to stabilize bile flow has been useful in physiological studies of bile flow in dogs. In studies of cholestasis their use is better avoided, since they eliminate a part of bile flow which may be altered by cholestasis.

STUDY 2

This study was undertaken in an attempt to define the independent variable(s) affecting bile flow in the fasting primate, and to find a method to quantify the components of bile flow.

Group 3: Fasting Primates Without a Small Intestine

Methods: Three rhesus monkeys were prepared as for group 1, except that the gastric antrum, duodenum, and small intestine were simultaneously excised. On the fourth post-operative day, sodium taurocholate was infused intravenously at three different rates. ^{14}C erythritol clearance and bicarbonate output were determined. As part of this experiment, it was shown that ^{14}C erythritol clearance is a canalicular and not a ductular function. This had been already demonstrated in the dog (9) and in other species (10). It was also determined that ^{14}C erythritol clearance was a passive process exclusively, i.e. active transport was ruled out.

Results: Bile flow was plotted against the bile salt secretion rate. The correlation coefficient of the linear regression line was highly significant; the line passed through the Y axis at a point close to zero and there was little scatter in the data points from the linear regression line. Therefore, resection of the antrum and small intestine in the monkey had a similar effect to the administration of anticholinergic agents to the dog (Fig.3). The linear regression line for bile flow vs bile salt secretion rate was parallel to that for ^{14}C erythritol clearance vs bile salt secretion rate. This indicates that, in the monkey, as suggested in the dog (9), ^{14}C erythritol clearance was quantitatively equal to canalicular flow, and that there was a constant amount of ductular reabsorption at all bile salt secretion rates, i.e. bile salt independent canalicular flow minus ductular reabsorption was a constant at all bile salt secretion rates (Fig.3).

The bicarbonate secretion rate was plotted against the bile salt secretion rate and it was shown by linear correlation-regression that net bicarbonate secretion in this preparation was totally dependent

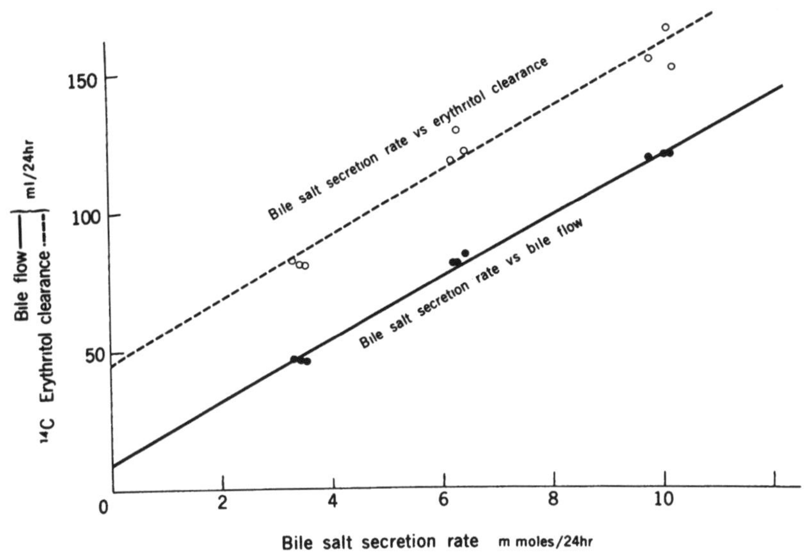

Fig.3. Bile flow vs bile salt secretion rate and ^{14}C erythritol clearance vs bile salt secretion rate in one of three animals showing similar results. Linear correlation coefficients were highly significant and the regression lines were parallel. Position of Y-axis intercepts and parallel slopes indicate that in this species ^{14}C erythritol clearance and canalicular flow are equal and that a constant amount of canalicular bile salt independent flow is reabsorbed in the ductules at all bile salt secretion rates.

on bile salt secretion, as in the dog receiving anticholinergic agents (2). There were 0.39 mEq bicarbonate secreted/mmole bile salt secretion.

Group 4: Primates Receiving Intraduodenal Sodium Taurocholate

Methods: This experiment was identical to group 1 except that only sodium taurocholate was infused for three days at three different rates, and these rates were repeated on three days in the second week of the experiment. ^{14}C erythritol clearance (for three days only) and bicarbonate secretion rates were also measured and at the end of the experimental day the animals were fed and several post-prandial samples of bile taken.

Results: Bile flow was plotted against the bile salt secretion rate (Fig.4). The results were identical to group 1 i.e. there was linear correlation between bile flow and bile salt secretion rate with

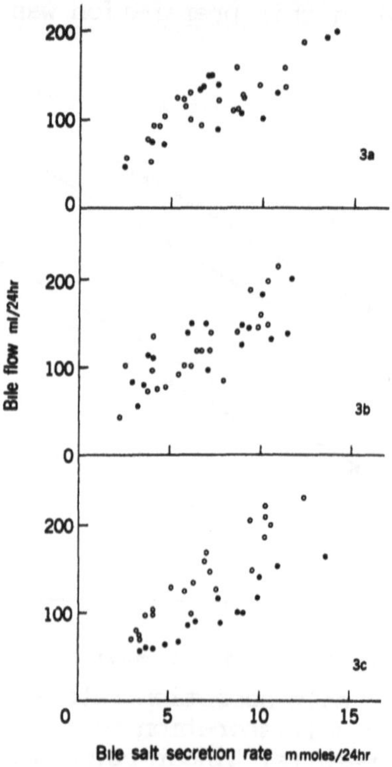

Fig. 4. Bile flow vs bile salt secretion rates in animals receiving intraduodenal sodium taurocholate infusion. Solid dots indicate samples in which ^{14}C erythritol clearance was simultaneously determined.

considerable scatter, indicating the presence of other fluctuating independent variable(s) affecting bile flow. There was little scatter in the plot of ^{14}C erythritol clearance (canalicular flow) vs bile salt secretion rate. This indicates that the variable(s) affecting bile flow did not act by causing a fluctuation in canalicular bile salt independent flow (Fig. 5).

The difficulty in analyzing these data was due to the fact that there was more than one independent variable affecting bile flow. When one independent variable is affecting a dependent variable in a linear fashion the equation $y = kx + b$ is applicable, where y is the dependent variable, x is the independent variable, k is a constant which expresses the magnitude of the effect of x on y, and b is the effect on y of another factor which is constant and may be zero.

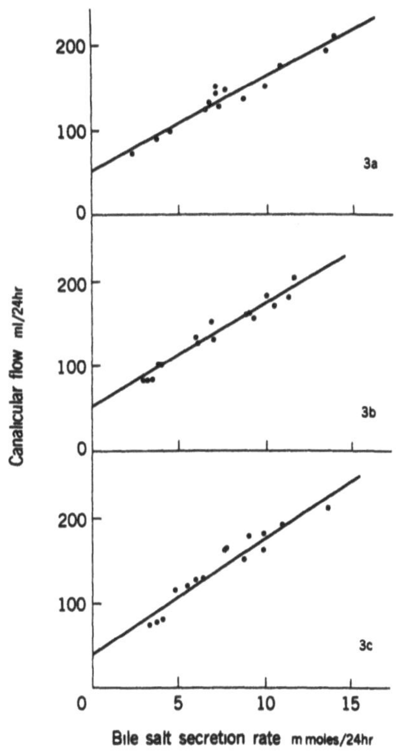

Fig. 5. ^{14}C erythritol clearance (canalicular flow) vs bile salt secretion rate in the same animals as in Fig. 4. Note the absence of scatter, which indicated that variation in canalicular bile salt independent flow was not responsible for the variation in total bile flow.

When more than one independent variable is present the equation becomes

$$y = k_1x_1 + k_2x_2 + \dots\dots\dots\, k_nx_n + b$$

where x_1, x_2, to x_n are the independent variables and k_1 to k_n constants which describe the effect of the corresponding independent variable on y.

Providing that y and x_1 to x_n are measurable and that x_1 to x_n are independent of each other this equation may be analyzed by multivariate linear regression analysis to obtain:

1) A value which indicates the ability of the chosen model to account for the fluctuations in the dependent variable i.e. the goodness of fit of the data to the model ($M\text{-}R^2$).
2) All values for k_1 to k_n and b.
3) The significance of the values k_1 to k_n i.e. whether each is different from zero.

On the basis of our previous experiments the following model was chosen for testing:

$$BF = BSSRk_1 + DBSRk_2 + k_3$$

where BF is bile flow
BSSR is bile salt secretion rate
DBSR is "ductular bicarbonate secretion rate" (see below)
k_3 is the constant difference between bile salt independent canalicular flow and ductular reabsorption.

"Ductular bicarbonate secretion rate" was calculated as - (total bicarbonate secretion rate - [0.39 x bile salt secretion rate]). This correction of bicarbonate secretion rate was necessary to assure independence of the second independent variable (bicarbonate secretion) from the first (bile salt secretion), and could be applied since it had been shown that 0.39 mEq bicarbonate were secreted per mmole bile salt.

The results of the multivariable regression analysis showed that the model accounted for greater than 90% of the fluctuation in the dependent variable, i.e. the data fit the model very well. k_1 was 11.3 ml/mmole and k_2 9.8 ml/mEq. Both k_1 and k_2 were highly significant. The analysis demonstrated that the independent variable having the inconsistent effect on bile flow, in the fasting primate, is, or is related to, the "ductular bicarbonate secretion rate". k_1 was virtually identical to the slope of the linear regression line for bile flow and bile salt secretion rate in group 3 (11.7). This was a valuable external check on the model. Knowing k_1 and k_2 allows estimation of the four components of flow.

Canalicular bile salt dependent flow	= Bile salt secretion x 11.3
Canalicular bile salt independent flow	= ^{14}C erythritol clearance - Canalicular bile salt dependent flow
Ductular flow	= "ductular" bicarbonate secretion rate x 9.8
Ductular reabsorption	= Total canalicular flow (^{14}C erythritol clearance) + Ductular flow - Bile flow

Measurement of the four components of bile flow in a pathological state, by the method described above involves the following requirements:

1) The relationships between bile flow and bile salt secretion, and bile flow and "ductular bicarbonate secretion rate" must remain unchanged.

2) ^{14}C erythritol clearance and canalicular flow must continue to be quantitatively equal. If these conditions are met, then this method can be utilized to measure the four components of bile flow in different types of cholestasis.

SUMMARY

Certain of these studies provide an explanation for the differences in previously reported studies of bile flow. Factors affecting bile flow (other than bile salt secretion) must be considered when studying the relationship between bile flow and the bile salt secretion rate. The necessity to control food intake during control and experimental periods of studies of bile flow has been stressed.

Other studies have allowed the development of a model for describing the components of bile flow. The model was tested by multivariate linear regression analysis and found to fit the data well. This presents the possibility of characterizing various forms of cholestasis by their effects on the four components of normal bile flow.

ACKNOWLEDGEMENTS

Supported by the Medical Research Council of Canada, the J.P. Bickell Foundation, and the Toronto Western Hospital Research Foundation. Dr. Strasberg is a recipient of a Medical Research Council of Canada Scholarship 1973-1978.

REFERENCES

1. WHEELER HO, RAMOS OL: Determinants of the flow and composition of bile in the anesthetized dog during constant infusions of sodium taurocholate. J Clin Invest 39: 161-170, 1960.

2. PREISIG R, COOPER HL, WHEELER HO: The relationship between taurocholate secretion rate and bile production in the unanesthetized dog during cholinergic blockade and during secretin administration. J Clin Invest 41: 1152-1162, 1962.

3. DOWLING RH, MACK E, PICOTT J et al: Experimental model for the study of the enterohepatic circulation of bile in Rhesus monkeys. J Lab Clin Med 72: 169-176, 1968.

4. NAHRWOLD DL, GROSSMAN MI: Secretion of bile in response to food with and without bile in the intestine. Gastroenterology 53: 11-17, 1967.

5. STRASBERG SM, SIMINOVITCH KA, ILSON RG: Bile production in fasted and fed primates. Ann Surg 180: 356-363, 1974.

6. STRASBERG SM, SIMINOVITCH KA, ILSON RG: An analysis of the components of bile flow (F) in the rhesus monkey by multivariate linear regression. Gastroenterology 66: 895, 1974 (abstract).

7. STRASBERG SM, ILSON RG, SIMINOVITCH KA et al: Analysis of the components of bile flow in the rhesus monkey. Am J Physiol (in press)

8. BARBER-RILEY G: Measurement of capacity of biliary tree in rats. Am J Physiol 205: 1122-1126, 1963.

9. WHEELER HO, ROSS ED, BRADLEY SE: Canalicular bile production in dogs. Am J Physiol 214: 866-874, 1968.

10. FORKER EL: Two sites of bile formation as determined by mannitol and erythritol clearance in the guinea pig. J Clin Invest 46: 1189-1195, 1967.

CANALICULAR ANION TRANSPORT, PATHOGENETIC MECHANISMS AND A STEADY STATE DISTRIBUTED MODEL FOR MEASURING KINETICS

E. L. Forker

University of Iowa

Iowa City, Iowa

The purposes of this review are two-fold: 1) to present a brief overview of organic anion transport at the canalicular boundary of liver cells, emphasizing the kinds of mechanisms which might be important in the pathogenesis of defective anion transport. 2) To point out the importance of standing intralobular concentration profiles to the measurement of transport kinetics at this locus and to present a distributed model which takes this difficulty into account.

What little we know about the general physiology of canalicular anion transport rests almost exclusively on observations of the rate and concentration at which these materials appear in common duct bile, the complex anatomy of the canalicular network and the small dimensions of individual channels (diameter about 1μ)having thus far precluded sampling of the secretion at its source. Moreover, transport across the canalicular boundary is perforce preceded by uptake at the opposite face of the liver cell, often by metabolism of the anion to one or more polar conjugates, and usually by more or less extensive binding to cytoplasmic proteins. All of these factors add substantially to the difficulty of studying canalicular transport as a discrete phenomenon and largely account for the fact that we have only the barest outline of its physiology.

Nevertheless, the broad principles are reasonably clear. Several facts in particular can be accepted as well established. First, the canalicular membrane is capable of maintaining large concentration gradients. For example, concentration differences of the order of 100-fold are commonly observed for typical anions such as BSP and conjugated bilirubin. Since more or less extensive binding of these materials to cytoplasmic proteins is characteristic, the real or effective difference in concentration between intracellular fluid and bile is undoubtedly even more impressive. Second, like concentrative transport systems elsewhere in tbe body, the canalicular system displays saturation kinetics, reasonably well defined transport maxima having been described for conjugated bilirubin and several bile acids as well as a variety of dyes and cholecystographic agents. A third generalization is that the canalicular step has usually been found to be rate limiting for the overall movement of organic anions from blood to bile.

The only reasonably secure inferences one can draw from this limited information are first, that the transport is probably mediated by some sort of membrane carrier, and second, that the process is active in the sense that secreted anions probably move against a steep electrochemical gradient. The inferential nature of these conclusions should be clearly recognized, however. No carrier has been identified and the electrical potential difference across the canalicular membrane has never been measured. Moreover, it is possible that the secreted anions aggregate as polymolecular complexes either with themselves or in association with mixed bile salt micelles, so that the effective luminal concentration could be substantially less than that inferred from measurements made chemically or with radioisotopes. Nevertheless, the apparent difference between the concentration of free (dialyzable) anions in liver homogenate and the total concentration in bile is, in general, so large that it is difficult to believe that some sort of active anion pump is not involved.

The general picture which has emerged, therefore, is of an active transport system capable of sustaining high concentrations in bile relative to those in plasma or intracellular fluid, but operating with an intrinsically lower capacity than either uptake or conjugation. Of the many important details which remain to be clarified, two stand out as particularly important. First, it is not clear whether there is a single carrier, which serves to concentrate a variety of structurally unrelated anions or whether there are multiple systems which may interact with each other. Second, it is still not completely certain whether the transport system provides for bidirectional exchange of materials between cytoplasm and bile or whether for practical purposes organic anion excretion should be considered as irreversible.

The usual clinical manifestations of cholestasis are largely attributable to the retention of organic anions for which bile is normally the only excretory route. While the pathogenesis of this syndrome may ultimately be understood in terms of some more fundamental defect, it is practical to consider the kinds of mechanisms which could lead to failure of the final concentrative step which presumably occurs at the canalicular membrane.

One or more of the hypothetical carriers could be absent or defective on a genetic basis. For example this is a reasonable explanation for the jaundice and BSP retention that occur in mutant Corriedale sheep and patients with the Dubin-Johnson syndrome. It is of interest that the mutant sheep (1) and one patient who has been studied (2) showed no discernible defect in taurocholate excretion so that in this instance at least, the canalicular transport of bilirubin and BSP appears to be functionally distinct from the transport system for bile salts. These observations stand in contrast to a recent study in normal rats (3) in which taurocholate increased both the Tm and the apparent Km for BSP. The kinetic data for rats are consistent with a model for allosteric interaction between two separate carriers and raise the possibility that efficient transport of BSP and perhaps other organic anions may depend on the simultaneous transport of bile salts, not because of secondary effects in the canalicular lumen (*vide infra*), but because of some critical interaction within the canalicular membrane itself. Two other studies (4,5) of the interaction between pairs of anions have also revealed effects that are not readily explained by either simple competition or changes in bile flow. These findings are not necessarily in conflict with the earlier studies of mutant Corriedale sheep in which the effect of BSP on taurocholate excretion was not examined, but they do serve to emphasize the need for more refined methods with which to assess the actual kinetics of canalicular transport.

Under the general heading of pharmacological toxicity, one can visualize a variety of inhibitory or competitive phenomena by which drugs or their metabolites might interfere with anion transport. In very general terms a list of possible mechanisms would include poisoning of some critical enzyme within the membrane, competitive inhibition of one or more anion carriers, and diversion to other uses of the supply of energy required for active anion transport. At our present level of understanding, however, the distinction between these is probably somewhat artificial, because none of the factors at risk has been identified.

A third possible mechanism, which is at least conceptually distinct, is an increase in the passive permeability of the canalicular membrane which might allow solutes concentrated in bile to leak back into the cell or across the tight junctions between cells. This speculation is encouraged by the finding that canaliculi normally show a surprisingly high permeability to relatively large neutral solutes, which are thought to enter bile by simple diffusion and convection (6,7). For example, mannitol, which is virtually excluded from most other cells in the body, rapidly equilibrates in liver cell water and appears promptly in bile at concentrations very similar to those in plasma. Striking changes in canalicular permeability to sucrose do in fact occur in experimental estrogen cholestasis (8). Unfortunately it is not clear whether this effect is primary and of real functional importance or merely incidental to some more fundamental problem.

A fourth consideration is whether the rate of bile flow might be an important determinant of anion excretion. Obviously if there is no flow, there can be no solute excretion. But the important question from the point of view of trying to understand the normal physiology of organic anion transport is whether changes in bile flow are normally an important determinant of net solute flux. Reduced to its fundamentals, this issue centers around the question of whether anion excretion is normally bidirectional or whether it is effectively irreversible.

In principle, one can visualize the determinant of the transport maximum in two ways depending on whether the factor which limits the excretion rate is the maximum concentration that can be sustained in the lumen or the maximum carrying capacity of the membrane. In the first instance, the system is postulated to operate with a high flux ratio, the limitation in net flux occurring when the luminal concentration is sufficiently high that further increments in the forward flux are offset by equivalent increments in the opposite direction. Such a system will be sensitive to changes in the luminal concentration and accordingly will respond to changes in bile flow, or for that matter, to any factor which influences the rate at which the transported solute can be removed from the biliary face of the membrane. In the second instance, the limitation in net flux is imposed by the intrinsic capacity of the membrane itself - presumably by a limited number of carrier sites. At normal or high rates of bile flow, solute excretion by such a system should be nearly independent of luminal concentration.

The importance of this distinction is illustrated by the finding that taurocholate choleresis can increase the Tm for BSP (3,9,10,11, 12) and a variety of other anions, including iopanoic acid (13), indocyanine green (5) and conjugated bilirubin (14). The central question is whether a certain minimal bile salt flux is required for normal anion excretion and if so whether this requirement reflects critical interactions at the level of the membrane transport step itself or whether bile salts simply provide a necessary sink in the canalicular lumen. For BSP (3,15,16) and iopanoic acid (13), it is clear from experiments with several bile salt independent choleretics that the rate of bile flow *per se* is not an important determinant of the Tm. To this extent present evidence strongly favors the view that anion transport is for practical purposes irreversible.

The important question of whether mixed bile salt micelles bind polar anions or in some other way reduce the luminal activity of these solutes remains to be clarified in physical-chemical terms. Preliminary evidence from an examination of bile and bile salt solutions does suggest that some association with bile salts occurs with both BSP (17) and bilirubin (18,19). What is not clear is whether this phenomenon is quantitatively important in providing a sink for secreted anions or whether indeed any sink is needed for normal anion transport over and above the obvious requirement for some minimal rate of bile flow such as might be provided by the bile salt independent fraction of canalicular fluid production.

It is probable that new insights into at least some of the questions raised above might be achieved from steady state kinetic studies designed to isolate the parameters for canalicular transport from the much more complicated process of transport across the whole liver cell. The model to be presented here illustrates the importance of standing intralobular concentration profiles to this objective and provides an estimate of the errors that may be involved if these gradients are ignored. The model is based on the assumptions that excretion is irreversible and can be described by a simple hyperbolic relation between flux rate and substrate concentration, both of which are consistent with the data for BSP excretion in rats (3).

The lumped model in Fig. 1 is the familiar one in which plasma and intracellular fluid are considered to be single well stirred compartments. In effect, the lumped model replaces the whole liver by an equivalent liver cell. The coefficients, k_1 and k_2, are the conventional first order rate constants for uptake and efflux across the sinusoidal face of the cell, but the transfer coefficient for excretion at the canalicular face is a function of the intracellular concentration, C, and two kinetic parameters, V and K, which represent the maximum transport rate and the apparent Km respectively. The equation for steady state excretion rate in this case is $J = CV/(K+C)$ from which one could readily determine the values of V and K in the usual way by fitting observed values of J and C to a rectangular

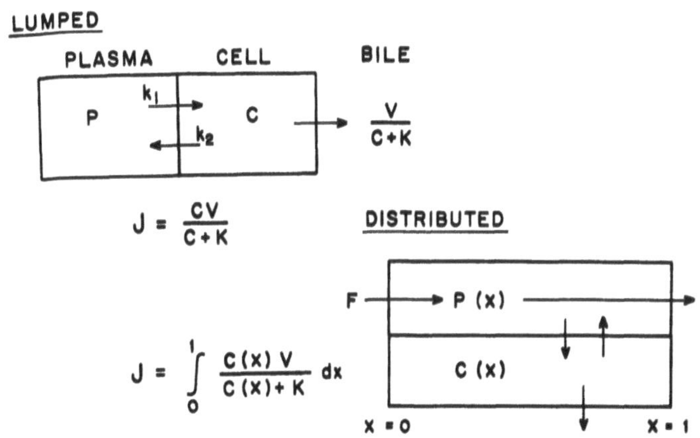

Fig. 1. Steady state models for canalicular anion transport.

hyperbola. The lumped model undoubtedly oversimplifies a number of details, but one of the potentially most important is that it ignores the structural organization of the liver lobule. In particular it assumes that each liver cell operates at the same substrate concentration, whereas in fact, if the solute in question is being progressively removed as it flows through the sinusoid, each cell along the way will be exposed to a lower concentration than its neighbor upstream. The distributed model in Fig. 1 takes this problem into account by treating the concentrations in plasma and intracellular fluid as functions of location along the sinusoid. In effect, the distributed model replaces the whole liver by an equivalent lobule.

Assuming that plasma and interstitial fluid are in diffusion equilibrium with respect to the transported solute, the starting equations for the distributed model are:

$$- F\frac{dP}{dx} = \frac{Cv}{K+C}$$

$$Pk_1 = Ck_2 + \frac{Cv}{K+C} \qquad (1)$$

in which F is the rate of plasma flow, x is the distance along the sinusoid, k_1 and k_2 are transfer rates per unit of concentration per unit length, and v is the maximum excretion rate per unit length. It is convenient to cast the variables in dimensionless form by setting $P' = P/K$, $C' = C/K$, and $x' = x/L$ where L is the length of an equivalent sinusoid. Equations (1) then become:

$$- F\frac{dP'}{dx'} = k'_3\, C'/(1+C')$$

$$P'k'_1 = C'k'_2 + k'_3\, C'/(1+C') \qquad (2)$$

in which $k'_1 = k_1L$, $k'_2 = k_2L$, and $k'_3 = vL/K = V/K$.

The new transfer coefficients (designated with primes) have the same units as F (volume per time) and V represents the maximum excretion rate for the whole liver. The solution to equations (2) is:

$$C' = C'(o) + \ln\frac{C'(o)}{C'} + \frac{k'_3}{k'_2}\ln\frac{C'(o)[1+C']}{C'[1+C'(o)]} - \frac{k'_1k'_3x'}{Fk'_2} \qquad (3)$$

Total excretion is the sum of the rates at each location, so that:

$$J' = \int_o^1 \frac{C'}{1+C'}\,dx' \qquad (4)$$

where $J' = J/V$ and C' is given by equation (3).

An important practical consequence of equation (4) is that by contrast with the lumped model, steady state excretion by the distributed model depends not only upon K and V, but upon k_1 and k_2 as well. Using the lumped model to interpret experimental data to which the distributed model actually applies therefore entails the risk of confusing changes in uptake with changes in excretion and vice versa.

To examine the errors that may be involved, it is useful to rewrite equation (3) by introducing a new parameter which can be determined experimentally. We call this new constant the extraction fraction, E, and define it to be the maximum value of $[P'(0)-P'(1)]/P'(0)$. E is thus the fraction of the solute removed from plasma in a single passage through the liver when the system is operating far below saturation. Taking the limit of equation (3) as $C'(0) \rightarrow 0$ and noting that for $C' \ll 1$, C' is proportional to P', we obtain:

$$\ln \frac{C'}{C'(0)} = \ln \frac{P'}{P'(0)} = \frac{k'_1 k'_3 x'}{F(k'_2 + k'_3)}$$

and for the whole liver, i.e., for $x' = 1$:

$$\ln \frac{P'(1)}{P'(0)} = \ln(1-E) = \frac{k'_1 k'_2}{F(k'_2 + k'_3)} \qquad (5)$$

If k'_3 is now eliminated between equations (3) and (5) we obtain:

$$C' = C'(0) = \ln \frac{C'(0)}{C'} - \left[\frac{\ln(1-E)}{k'_1/F+\ln(1-E)}\right] \ln \frac{C'(0)[1+C']}{C'[1+C'(0)]}$$

$$+ \frac{k'_1}{F}\left[\frac{\ln(1-E)}{k'_1/F+\ln(1-E)}\right] x' \qquad (6)$$

Moreover since $\ln(1-E)$ must be negative for positive values of k'_1, k'_2, k'_3, it follows from equation (5) that:

$$\frac{k'_1}{F} > [\ln(1-E)] \qquad (7)$$

A digital computer was used to construct the family of parametric curves relating the excretion rate defined by equations (4) and (6) to the mean intracellular concentration defined by

$$\overline{C}' = \int_0^1 C' \, dx' \qquad (8)$$

Representative curves for various values of the extraction fraction appear in Fig. 2. Operationally the mean intracellular concentration is defined by the total hepatic content of the solute corrected by the content of extracellular fluid, so that the plotted variables are those which should be accessible to direct measurement in an experiment.* The solid curve is a rectangular hyperbola representing the limiting case as E approaches zero. The broken lines show the progressive distortion that occurs as the extraction fraction increases. In each case the curve depicted in Fig. 2 is the one defined by setting $k'_1/F = 1.01 \ln(1-E)$ which is the smallest practical value consistent with inequality(7). This procedure has been adopted for purposes of illustration, because it was found that for any given value of E the displacement of the kinetic curve away from the ideal hyperbola diminished as k'_1/F increased. The parametric curves in Fig. 2 therefore illustrate the worst cases in the sense that for a particular value of E, any larger choice of k'_1/F would have yielded a curve closer to the one for E = 0.

Two features of practical importance that can be appreciated from Fig. 2 and readily verified directly from the equations are that the initial slope determined at low concetration and the final asymptote at high concentration are independent of E and k'_1/F. Since the initial slope is V/K and the final asymptote is V; in principle the desired kinetic parameters can always be extracted from a single experiment conducted at a tracer concentration of the solute, together with an independent measurement of Tm.

Since this approach may not be feasible or desirable in some instances, it is useful to have quantitative estimates of the error involved in determining K and V by more conventional means such as a Lineweaver-Burk plot. This information has been obtained with a sub-routine in the computer program which inverted the values for excretion rate and mean intracellular concentration and determined the least squares fit of the transformed variables to a straight line. Values of V and K were then determined in the usual way from the slope and the intercept of the regression line. The errors in estimating V and K by this procedure are virtually the same because, for values of J' less than .75 the method gives an accurate estimate

* For solutes such as BSP which accumulate inside the cell, the correction for sinusoidal plasma volume and the Disse space will have little effect on the estimate of intracellular concentration. Correction for the content of the intrahepatic biliary tree, however, may not be trivial. Estimates of biliary volume from which this correction can be made are available for the rat (20,21). The final value of $\overline{C}$ should also be corrected for protein binding, for example by dialysis (3) or gel filtration (22).

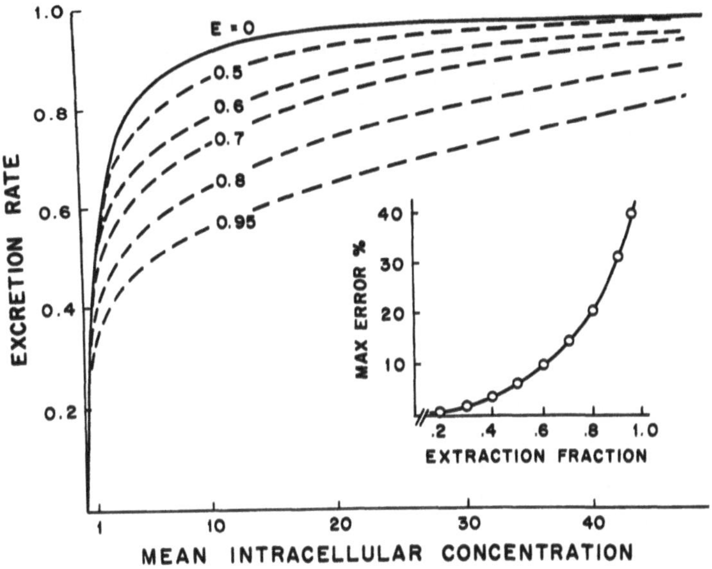

Fig. 2. Kinetic curves for canalicular anion transport for various values of the extraction fraction, E. The insert shows the maximum percentage error in determining either V or K from a double reciprocal plot of excretion rate vs mean intracellular concentration for various values of E.

of V/K, but a variable error in V. The graph at the bottom of Fig. 2 shows the percentage error in either V or K determined from 10 points equally spaced between $J' = .0005$ and $J' = .75$. It should be emphasized that the graph shows the maximum error that could occur in the absence of any information about the value of k'_1/F. In practice estimates of this quantity may be available to refine the analysis. For example, Goresky (23) has estimated the initial uptake rate of BSP by the dog from an analysis of multiple indicator dilution curves.

The distributed model obviously still contains a number of simplifications, probably the most important of which is the required assumption that the ratio, V/K, is not itself a function of location within the liver lobule. Moreover the coefficients, k_1 and k_2 are assumed to be first order rate constants whereas in fact transport at the sinusoidal face of the cell is probably saturable. While the assumption of first order kinetics for this step seems reasonable in view of the fact that saturation of the uptake process probably occurs at plasma concentrations much higher than those required to saturate canalicular transport, the error involved has not been evaluated. Final resolution of these difficulties will evidently require some way to measure the intralobular concentration profiles directly -- an experimental objective which seems remote, however, by any of the techniques presently available. In the interim the distributed model in its present form should serve as the best available approximation.

SUMMARY

The clinical manifestations of cholestasis largely reflect the retention of organic anions such as bilirubin and bile acids for which bile is normally the sole excretory route. The root cause or causes are unknown, but a final common defect is failure of concentrative transport at the canalicular border of the liver cell. A brief review in general terms of the kinds of pathogenetic mechanisms that might be important at this locus emphasizes the need for more detailed information about the kinetics of canalicular transport. Unfortunately the saturation kinetics which this step characteristically displays together with the presence of a non-linear standing concentration profile along the radius of the liver lobule make this a difficult experimental objective. A distributed model has been examined which takes these problems into account and provides quantitative estimates of the errors that may be involved. In principle the apparent affinity of canalicular transport for a given anion can be determined from measurements of Tm and the steady state hepatic content of the material when it is present at tracer concentration.

REFERENCES

1. ALPERT S, MOSHER M, SHANSKE A et al: Multiplicity of hepatic excretory mechanisms for organic anions. J Gen Physiol 53: 238-247, 1969.

2. GUTSTEIN S, ALPERT S, ARIAS IM: Studies of hepatic excretory function. IV. Biliary excretion of sulfobromophthalein sodium in a patient with the Dubin-Johnson syndrome and a biliary fistula. Israel J Med Sci 4: 36, 1968.

3. FORKER EL, GIBSON G: Interaction between sulfobromophthalein (BSP) and taurocholate, in The Liver. Quantitative Aspects of Structure and Function. Proc First International Gstaad Symposium, edited by PAUMGARTNER G, PREISIG R, S Karger, Basel, 1973, pp.326-336.

4. CLARENBERG R, KAO C-C: Shared and separate pathways for biliary excretion of bilirubin and BSP in rats. Amer J Physiol 225: 192-200, 1973.

5. VONK RJ, VEEN H, PROP G et al: The influence of taurocholate and dehydrocholate choleresis on plasma disappearance and biliary excretion of indocyanine green in the rat. Naunin Schmiededergs Arch Pharmacol 282: 401-410, 1974.

6. FORKER EL: Two sites of bile formation as determined by mannitol and erythritol clearance in the guinea pig. J Clin Invest 46: 1189-1195, 1967.

7. WHEELER HO, ROSS ED, BRADLEY SE: Canalicular bile production in dogs. Amer J Physiol 214: 866-874, 1968.

8. FORKER EL: The effect of estrogen on bile formation in the rat. J Clin Invest 48: 654-663, 1969.

9. O'MAILLE ERL, RICHARDS TG, SHORT AH: Factors determining the maximal rate of organic anion secretion by the liver and further evidence on the hepatic site of action of the hormone secretin. J Physiol 186: 424-438, 1966.

10. BOYER JL, SCHEIG RL, KLATSKIN G: The effect of sodium taurocholate on the hepatic metabolism of sulfobromophthalein sodium. The role of bile flow. J Clin Invest 49: 206-215, 1970.

11. GRONWALL R, CORNELIUS CE: Maximal biliary excretion of sulfobromophthalein sodium in sheep. Comp Gastroenterology (New Series) 15: 36-46, 1970.

12. GIBSON GE, FORKER EL: Canalicular bile flow and BSP Tm: The effect of a bile salt independent choleretic, SC-2644. Gastroenterology 66: 1046-1053, 1974.

13. BERK RN, LOEB PM, GOLDBERGER LE et al: Oral cholecystography with Iopanoic acid. New Eng J Med 290: 204-210, 1974.

14. GORESKY CA, HADDAD HH, KLUGER WS et al: The enhancement of maximal bilirubin excretion with taurocholate-induced increments in bile flow. Can J Physiol Pharmacol 52: 389-408,1974.

15. ERLINGER S, DUMONT M: Influence of canalicular bile flow on sulfobromophthalein transport maximum in bile in the dog. in The Liver. Quantitative Aspects of Structure and Function. Proc First International Gstaad Symposium, edited by PAUMGARTNER G, PREISIG R, S Karger, Basel, 1973, pp. 306-314.

16. BARNHART J, RITT D, WARE A et al: A comparison of the effects of taurocholate and theophylline on BSP excretion in dogs, in The Liver. Quantitative Aspects of Structure and Function, edited by PAUMGARTNER G, PREISIG R, S Karger, Basel, 1973, pp.315-325.

17. WARE A, HARDT M, BARNHART J et al: The interaction of bromsulphthalein sodium (BSP) molecules with themselves and with sodium taurocholate (TCA). Clin Res 21: 260, 1973 (abstract).

18. VERSCHURE JCM, MIJNLIEFF PF: The dominating macromolecular complex of human gallbladder bile. Clin Chim Acta 1: 154-166, 1956.

19. JUNIPER K: Physico-chemical characteristics of bile and their relation to gallstone formation. Amer J Med 39: 98-107, 1965.

20. FORKER EL: Hepatocellular uptake of inulin, sucrose and mannitol in rats. Amer J Physiol 219: 1568-1573, 1970.

21. HÄCKI W, PAUMGARTNER G: Assessment of bile salt independent bile formation by injection of taurocholate, in The Liver. Quantitative Aspects of Structure and Function. Proc First International Gstaad Symposium, edited by PAUMGARTNER G, PREISIG R, S Karger, Basel, 1973, pp. 360-367.

22. GIBSON JD, ROBERTS RJ: Effect of phenobarbital and the hepatotoxin alpha-naphthylisothiocyanate (ANIT) on the disposition and binding of sulfobromophthalein (BSP) to hepatic cytosol anion binding proteins under conditions of continuous sub-threshold BSP infusion. In press, J Clin Invest.

23. GORESKY CA: Initial distribution and rate of uptake of sulfobromophthalein in the liver. Amer J Physiol 206: 13-26, 1964.

DISCUSSION OF PAPERS ON BILIARY SECRETION

CHAIRMAN: A. SASS-KORTSAK

FORKER: Would Dr. Wheeler expand on how he obtained the data on bile osmolality? Are these figures from freezing point depressions and if so do they take into account the Krafft point or the critical temperature for micelle formation? Or does that tend to influence the kind of answers one would get from a freezing point determination?

WHEELER: Most of my figures have been derived from freezing point depressions. But they have subsequently been verified by vapor pressure measurements at 37°C and actually the agreement is quite good.

FORKER: Does the vapor pressure depend on surface tension?

WHEELER: No, I don't believe it does.

FORKER: Well, some kinds of vapor pressure determinations do, if they involve a drop of fluid. I raised the question simply because the bile salts, of course, influence the surface tension as well.

WHEELER: I can't rule this out. I am not sure how the two correlate. In other words if there were perfect agreement between the freezing point and the vapor pressure, is it conceivable that differing types of error lead to the same answer. If so, where would we go then?

FORKER: I am inclined to think that the effect must be minor.

ARIAS: Would Dr. Wheeler comment about the thesis that R.T. Williams and his colleagues have presented regarding the relationship between molecular weight of a substance and its appearance in the bile? Do you have any explanation for these seemingly clear-cut phenomena?

WHEELER: No, I am afraid I don't. The phenomenon is very interesting. Some mention has been made today, for example, about differences in protein binding and I think it is quite clear that this isn't a factor. But as far as molecular weight is concerned, I have no idea about possible mechanisms.

I would like to ask a question concerning another phenomenon. Bile salt independent secretion of a solution of inorganic electrolytes seems to be a rather constant component of bile even in Dr. Strasberg's comparison between feeding and fasting. What does he assume to be the canalicular bicarbonate component of this and how does he feel about the fact that the bicarbonate must be one of the components reabsorbed when there is ductular reabsorption?

STRASBERG: This study does not show that there is no canalicular bicarbonate secretion accompanying the bile salt independent canalicular flow. All it shows is that in the animals with the gastrointestinal tract excised there is no net bicarbonate secretion independent of bile salt secretion any more than there is any water secretion independent of bile salt secretion. There is water secretion but it is not net water secretion. There probably is bicarbonate secretion. In fact one might speculate that the trigger for reabsorption is bicarbonate or some other ion that isn't appearing in the net mass flow of ions or the net volume flow of bile.

GORESKY: Could you produce a stable preparation without taking out all the gut? If you infused bicarbonate into the duodenum will your conditions of bile flow become stable and will a lot of your scatter disappear?

STRASBERG: We tried this and so has Dr. Wheeler. All I can say is that it doesn't result in any consistent effect.

FORKER: What happens to portal blood flow in this eviscerated preparation? Might changes in portal blood flow be influencing your data?

STRASBERG: We do a Whipple procedure and remove the whole gut. We have not measured portal blood flow. All I can say is that the bile output for the amount of bile salts that we were infusing was in accord with that found in animals with an intact circulation. So bile salts appear to be getting to the liver.

GORESKY: One of the logical extensions of what Dr. Forker showed us would be to consider that bile flows in a countercurrent direction. This renders the situation much more complex. I would appreciate his comments on this.

FORKER: I was careful to make the final transport system unidirectional and I think there is good circumstantial evidence for this based on the failure of bile salts actually to increase the transport of a number of solutes. But some question remains and if one is forced to make the canalicular step bidirectional, the flow profile in the canaliculus becomes an important consideration and the arithmetic becomes very much more difficult.

HEMOLYSIS, JAUNDICE AND LIVER DISEASE

Michael C. Brain

McMaster University

Hamilton, Ontario L8S 4J9

INTRODUCTION

Jaundice due to elevation of serum unconjugated bilirubin only becomes evident when hemolytic anemia causes a two to three-fold or greater increase in hemoglobin catabolism. Even in rapid hemolysis, in which the production of bilirubin from hemoglobin reaches the maximum that can be handled of about six times the normal rate in an adult of 7.5 grams of hemoglobin per day, the serum level of unconjugated bilirubin rarely rises above 3 to 5 milligrams per 100 ml (Powell, 1972).

The level of conjugated bilirubin in the serum may rise in hemolytic anemia but this usually indicates underlying liver disease, especially when the conjugate fraction is greater than 15% of the total bilirubin (Tisdale et al, 1969). The capability of the normal liver to handle a massive increase in bilirubin load is demonstrated by a recent example of fulminating acquired Coombs-negative hemolytic anemia in a boy of 14 recently studied by my colleagues Drs. Derghazarian, Ali and Pineo (personal communication). This boy received 41 units of blood in 10 days in order to maintain his hemoglobin level above 7.0 g per 100 ml despite the absence of blood loss. The patient's unconjugated bilirubin reached a maximum of 12.8 mg% but the direct bilirubin never exceeded 1.0 mg%, although the destruction of the transfused red cells, not allowing for hemolysis of the patient's red cells, corresponded to a hemoglobin load in excess of 2,000 g over 10 days. The level of unconjugated bilirubin in patients with chronic hemolytic anemia is influenced by the rate at which the liver can take up the unconjugated bilirubin. Perona and co-workers (1973) have shown that the level of unconjugated bilirubin can be lowered by the administration of phenobarbitone and suggested that this effect was due to an enhanced rate of hepatic clearance of bilirubin.

The quantitative measurement of the excretion of bilirubin degradation products, urobilinogen and urobilin in the urine and feces, was first used to estimate the magnitude of hemolysis in hemolytic anemia. However, the problems encountered in collection and analysis of the products of bilirubin excretion limited the value of this approach. More accurate methods for the measurement of hemoglobin catabolism have been introduced and do permit the rate of hemolysis to be assessed. The rate of excretion of endogenous carbon monoxide (Coltman and Dudley, 1969, Landaw, 1974), and the rate of clearance of labelled bilirubin from the plasma (Berk et al, 1972, Berk, 1974) have been shown to correlate closely with the direct measurement of red cell survival. However, allowance has to be made for the 10 to 20% contribution to bilirubin formation and carbon monoxide excretion of the catabolism of non-hemoglobin heme proteins, and the breakdown of hemoglobin within the bone marrow due to ineffective erythropoiesis. Both methods require the accurate estimation of red cell volumes, in the determination of the total hemoglobin in the circulation.

The introduction of ^{51}Chromium provided a relatively simple and reliable method for measurement of red cell survival, and through the use of both the patient's and compatible donor cells and of surface counting, has enabled the mechanism of a hemolytic process to be explored and the sites of red cell destruction to be determined.

The application of biochemical and immunological techniques to the study of red cells in vitro has enabled both congenital and acquired causes of hemolytic anemia to be recognized as being due to disorders of a) the structure and function of the red cell membrane, b) red cell metabolism and its related enzymes, and c) the structure and stability of the hemoglobin molecule.

Although hemolytic anemia is a well recognized cause of jaundice it rarely gives rise to liver disease, except when both red cell survival and hepatic function are influenced by a common etiological agent, or when the pigmented biliary calculi resulting from excessive bilirubin excretion in chronic hemolytic anemia cause obstruction of the common bile duct.

Of greater interest to the hematologist, especially one interested in hemolytic anemia, are the disorders of the liver which can produce alterations in red cell morphology and, when liver disease is severe, an associated hemolytic anemia.

This association of hemolytic anemia with liver disease presents practical problems in both diagnosis and management. Furthermore, it is possible that the detailed studies of the disorders of red cell structure and function which accompany hemolysis in liver disease may throw light on more generalized disorders of cell function which may affect other cells in the body, including those of the liver itself.

Liver Disease and Hemolysis

Overt hemolytic anemia is uncommon in acute hepatitis, whether of viral or toxic etiology. Although measurement of red cell survival may demonstrate a shortening of erythrocyte life span, the hemolysis is usually brief in duration and well compensated. Hemolytic anemia in chronic hepatitis may be associated with a positive Coombs test. Of greater interest is the Coombs negative hemolytic anemia which not infrequently develops in patients with cirrhosis, especially alcoholic cirrhosis (Jandl, 1955), and which becomes more evident following heavy alcohol ingestion (Zieve, 1958). In both alcoholic cirrhosis and in severe obstructive jaundice changes in red cell morphology with the presence of target cells, in the absence of overt hemolysis, and "spur" cells with frank hemolysis, are associated with abnormalities in serum and red cell lipids. Hemolysis has also been described in association with the disorder of copper metabolism in Wilson's disease, and as a consequence of splenomegaly resulting from portal hypertenison.

Target Cells and Liver Disease

The presence of target cells in stained blood smears is associated with an increase in the surface area of the red cell membrane in relationship to the cell volume, and is accompanied by an increase in resistance to lysis by hypotonic saline in an osmotic fragility test. Reduced osmotic fragility may be present despite the absence of target cells in patients with obstructive jaundice or chronic liver disease. The increase in membrane area is acquired by normal red cells after transfusion into a jaundiced patient, and after incubation in vitro in the serum of patients with target cells (Cooper and Jandl, 1968). The increase in red cell membrane surface area is associated with an increase in red cell membrane cholesterol (Cooper and Jandl, 1968), and by a less marked rise in membrane phospholipid due to an increase in lecithin (Cooper et al, 1972). Target cells have a normal degree of deformability as shown by red cell filtration, which may account for their normal survival and absence of splenic sequestration (Cooper and Jandl, 1968).

The mechanism for cholesterol accumulation in target cells will be discussed later.

Spur Cells and Liver Disease

More marked changes in red cell morphology may be seen in patients with severe hepatocellular disease due to the late stages of alcoholic cirrhosis, and are associated with an episode of prolonged alcohol ingestion. Examination of the stained blood film in such patients reveals the presence of smaller red cells with an irregular outline. Such patients have an overt hemolytic anemia with a moderate to marked shortening of red cell life span and evidence of splenic sequestration of the labelled cells. The transfusion of normal donor cells into such patients is followed by an initial reduction in osmotic fragility after twenty-four hours, but thereafter the fragility of the transfused donor cells increases, a proportion of the cells being osmotically more fragile than normal (Cooper, 1969). Analysis of the red cell membrane lipids of patients with spur cell anemia has shown that whereas the phospholipid composition is relatively normal red cell cholesterol is greatly increased (Fig. 1), (Cooper, 1969, Cooper et al, 1972). Incubation of normal red cells in the serum of patients with spur cell anemia was shown to be accompanied by a dramatic increase in cholesterol uptake, whereas the red cells of the patient when incubated in normal serum lose cholesterol despite heating the serum to inhibit lecithin-cholesterol acyl transferase (LCAT), (Cooper, 1969, Cooper et al, 1972).

Mechanism of Target and Spur Cell Formation

The free cholesterol of the red cell membrane equilibrates rapidly and nearly completely with free cholesterol in the serum. The concentration of free cholesterol in the serum is governed by the concentration of low density lipoproteins with which it is associated and by the activity of LCAT which converts free cholesterol to esterified cholesterol. The fall in free cholesterol which takes place when red cells are incubated in unheated normal serum is predominantly due to the action of LCAT (Murphy, 1962). Bile salts are known to inhibit LCAT and this mechanism was initially thought to be responsible for the formation of cholesterol loading in target cells (Cooper and Jandl, 1968). More recently it has been shown that in patients with both target cells and spur cells the red cell free cholesterol correlates poorly with LCAT activity (Cooper et at, 1972). However, in both groups of patients the red cell membrane free cholesterol: phospholipid ratio correlates most closely with the free cholesterol: protein ratio in low density lipoproteins (Fig. 2),

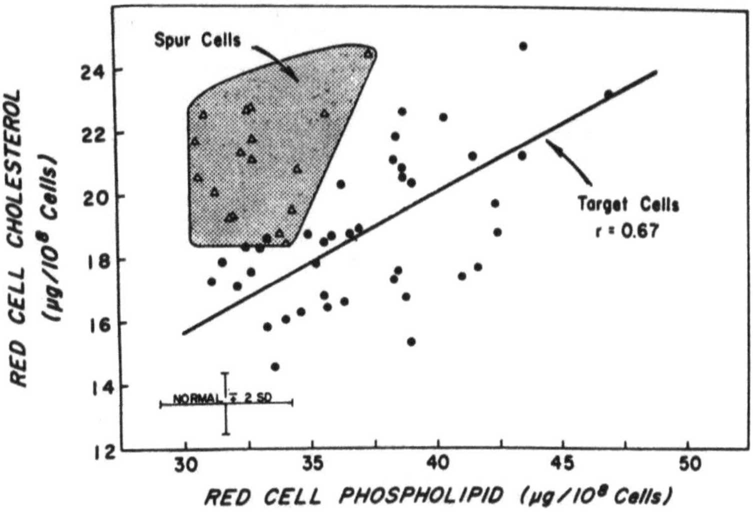

Fig. 1 The cholesterol and phospholipid content of target and spur cells from 17 patients with spur cells and 40 patients with target cells. The regression analysis calculated for target cells ($y = 2.5 + 0.44x$) was significant ($P < 0.01$).

Reproduced from Cooper et al (1972) with permission of the authors, and the editors of the Journal of Clinical Investigation.

(Cooper et al, 1972). It thus appears that the primary determinant of the raised cholesterol of both target cells and spur cells is due to an absolute reduction in low density lipoproteins, and a relative increase in the proportion of free cholesterol bound to this lipoprotein fraction in the patient's serum. This conclusion is supported by the demonstration that cholesterol loading and spur cells can be induced in monkeys by feeding them with lithocholic acid, a change which takes place in association with the reduction in low density lipoproteins with a consequent increase in the free cholesterol : phospholipid ratio in this fraction, (Cooper, Garcia and Trey, 1972), and by the observation that an increase in low density lipoproteins by the infusion of lecithin is associated with a reduction in free cholesterol in the serum and cholesterol depletion of the red cells (Robins and Miller, 1974).

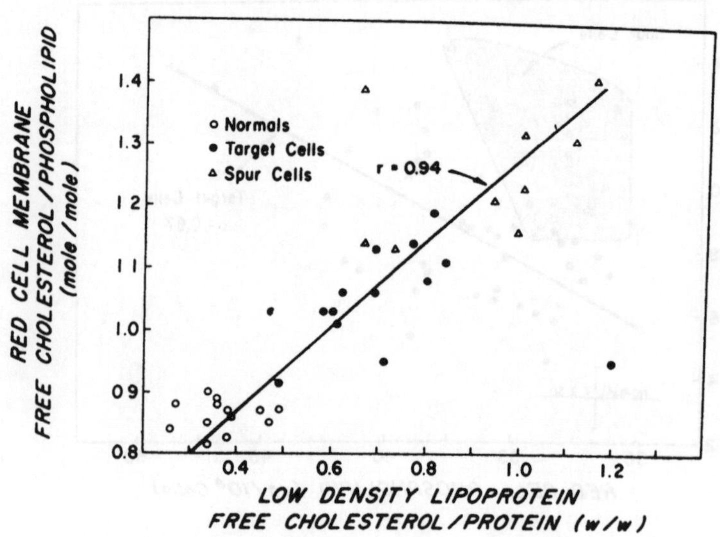

Fig. 2 Relationship between free cholesterol to protein weight ratio of low density lipoproteins and the free cholesterol to phospholipid mole ratio of red cell membranes. The two points distant from the curve were greater than 2 SD from the remainder of the data and were excluded from the regression analysis.

Reproduced from Cooper et al (1972) with permission of the authors, and editors of the Journal of Clinical Investigation.

Cooper and co-workers (1974) have recently demonstrated that the degree of morphological change of the spur cell, and the increased osmotic fragility and shortened red cell survival are probably due to the influence of the spleen on the cholesterol loaded cell. They have suggested that spur cell formation involves both excess membrane lipid and the loss of cell membrane, with formation of osmotically more fragile and distorted red cells, as a result of sequestration in the spleen. They base this conclusion on the change in morphology and the reduction in osmotic fragility which followed splenectomy in one patient despite the persistence of the abnormality of cholesterol: phospholipid ratio in the red cells.

Hemolysis in Obstructive Jaundice

Target cell formation and reduced osmotic fragility are not uncommon in obstructive jaundice. Overt hemolytic anemia due to obstructive jaundice is uncommon. Nevertheless, my colleagues and I have recently had the opportunity to study a 43 year old woman in whom the initial attempt to repair a biliary fistula which developed after cholecystectomy resulted in complete extra hepatic biliary obstruction (Fig. 3). The total serum bilirubin rose to 58 mg% and was associated with the presence of both target cells and spur cells in the peripheral blood and a reticulocytosis of 10 to 16 percent. The T1/2 ^{51}Cr survival of donor cells was 9.5 days. The cholesterol and phospholipid content of the red cells was markedly elevated at 35 mg and 33 mg per 10^8 cells. The hemolytic anemia and morphological changes in the red cells disappeared following surgical correction of the biliary obstruction.

Effects of Bile Acids and Bilirubin on Red Cells

The direct influence of bile acids and bilirubin on red cell shape and lipid composition is uncertain. In vitro bile acids at a concentration ten to twenty-fold of that found in disease can bring about an increase in red cell cholesterol content, probably through inhibition of LCAT activity (Cooper and Jandl, 1958). In vitro free unconjugated bilirubin at a concentration of greater than 20 milligrams percent induces both changes in membrane shape, loss of potassium ions and inhibition of metabolism (Cheung, Sanitsky, and Isenberg, 1966). However, it seems very unlikely that in disease states the concentrations of free, non-albumin bound, unconjugated bilirubin could rise to levels necessary to produce the effects observed in vitro.

Hemolysis in Wilson's Disease

Episodes of acute hemolytic anemia may precede the development of the more classical features of hepatic and neurological disease which characterize Wilson's disease (Walshe, 1962, Carr-Saunders and Laurance, 1965, McIntyre et al, 1967, Deiss, Lee and Cartwright, 1970). The mechanism of hemolysis in Wilson's disease appears to be related to transient elevation in serum copper concentration, exceeding the concentration of serum ceruloplasmin. Although toxic concentrations of copper sulphate induce hemolytic anemia with Heinz body formation, the concentrations of copper which cause similar effects in vitro exceed those reported in Wilson's disease. Boulard and co-workers (1972) have found that the main rate limiting enzymes of the red cell glycolytic pathway, hexokinase, phosphofructokinase, and pyruvate kinase, are

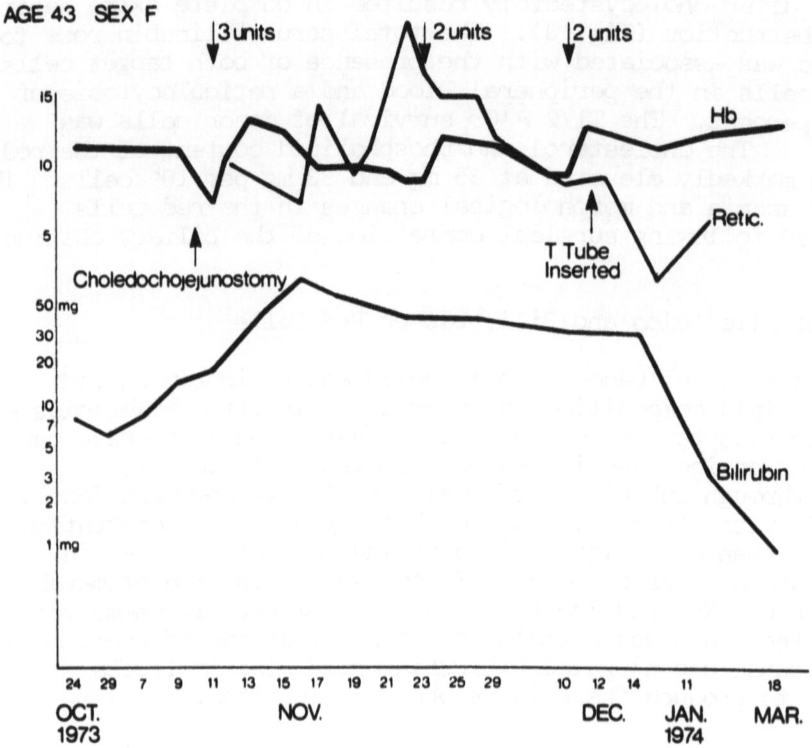

Fig. 3 Hemoglobin (g per 100 ml) and reticulocyte count (%) and total serum bilirubin (mg per 100 ml) in a patient with post-operative obstruction to the common bile duct. In mid-November the patient's blood contained both target cells and spur cells and T½ ^{51}Cr survival of compatible donor cells was 9 days.

completely or nearly completely inhibited at concentrations of copper of 15 μM which may be encountered episodically in Wilson's disease.

Hemolysis and Splenomegaly

Massive enlargement of the spleen however caused, including the congestive splenomegaly of portal hypertension, can give rise to hemolytic anemia due to the preferential destruction of red cells sequestered within the splenic sinuses. The hemolytic anemia is usually compensated and improves following surgical treatment of portal hypertension.

SUMMARY

The nature and causes of jaundice due to hemolytic anemia have been briefly reviewed. The associated morphological changes of the red cells (target cells and spur cells) have been discussed in relation to the alterations in red cell lipid and serum phospholipids. The mechanism of hemolytic anemia in Wilson's disease due to elevation of serum copper has been reviewed.

ACKNOWLEDGEMENTS

I am grateful to Drs. C.B. Derghazarian, M.A.M. Ali and G.F. Pineo for permission to quote findings in their patient with hemolytic anemia, and to Dr. J.F. Lind for data on his patient with obstructive jaundice. Dr. J.B. Somer kindly performed red cell lipid analysis in the latter patient. I am grateful to Dr. R.A. Cooper and his colleagues, and to the Editors of the Journal of Clinical Investigation for permission to reproduce Figs. 1 and 2.

REFERENCES

1. BERK PD, BLOOMER JR, HOWE RB, et al: Bilirubin production as a measure of red cell life span. J Lab Clin Med 79: 364-378, 1972.

2. BERK PD: Total body handling of bilirubin. In Jaundice, edited by C.A. Goresky and M.M. Fisher, New York, Plenum Press, 1975.

3. BOULARD M, BLUME KG, BEUTLER E: The effect of copper on red cell enzyme activities. J Clin Invest 51: 459-461, 1972.

4. CARR-SAUNDERS E, LAURANCE BM: Wilson's disease presenting as an acute hemolytic anemia. Proc Roy Soc Med 58: 614-615, 1965

5. CHEUNG WH, SANITSKY A, ISENBERG HD: The effect of bilirubin on the mammalian erythrocyte. Transfusion 6: 475-486, 1966

6. COLTMAN CA JR, DUDLEY GM III: The relationship between endogenous carbon monoxide production and total heme mass in normal and abnormal subjects. Am J Med Sci 258: 374-385, 1969

7. COOPER RA, JANDL JH: Bile salts and cholesterol in the pathogenesis of target cells in obstructive jaundice. J Clin Invest 47: 809-822, 1968

8. COOPER RA: Anemia with spur cells: A red cell defect acquired in serum and modified in the circulation. J Clin Invest 48: 1820-1831, 1969

9. COOPER RA, DILOY-PURAY M, LANDO P, et al: An analysis of lipoproteins, bile acids and red cell membranes associated with target cells and spur cells in patients with liver disease. J Clin Invest 51: 3182-3192, 1972.

10. COOPER RA, GARCIA FA, TREY C: The effect of lithocholic acid on red cell membranes in vivo. J Lab Clin Med 79: 7-18, 1972

11. COOPER RA, KIMBAL DB, DUROCHER JR: Role of the spleen in membrane conditioning and hemolysis of spur cells in liver disease. New Eng J Med 290: 1279-1284, 1974

12. DEISS A, LEE GR, CARTWRIGHT GE: Hemolytic anemia in Wilson's disease. Ann Intern Med 73: 413-418, 1970

13. ENGSTEDT L: Endogenous formation of carbon monoxide in hemolytic disease. Acta Med Scand Suppl 159: (332) 1-63, 1957

14. JANDL JH: Anemia of liver disease: Observation on its mechanism. J Clin Invest 34: 390-404, 1955

15. LANDAW SA: Carbon monoxide production as a measurement of heme catabolism. In Jaundice, edited by C.A. Goresky and M.M. Fisher, New York, Plenum Press, 1975.

16. MCINTYRE N, CLINK HM, LEVI AJ, et al: Hemolytic anemia in Wilson's disease. New Eng J Med 276: 439-444, 1967

17. MURPHY JR: Erythrocyte Metabolism III. Relationship of energy metabolism and serum factors to the osmotic fragility following incubation. J Lab Clin Med 60: 86-109, 1962

18. PERONA C, CORROCHER R, FREZZA M, et al: Phenobarbitone sensitivity of jaundice in haemolytic patients. Brit J Haemat 25: 723-736, 1973

19. POWELL LW: Clinical aspects of unconjugated hyperbilirubinemia. Seminars Hemat 9: 91-105, 1972

20. ROBINS SJ, MILLER A: Red cell cholesterol depletion and the formation of spiculated cells in vivo. J Lab Clin Med 38: 436-450, 1974

21. TISDALE WA, KLATSKIN G, KINSELLA ED: The significance of the direct fraction of serum bilirubin in hemolytic jaundice. Am J Med 26: 214-227, 1959

22. WALSHE JM: Wilson's disease. The presenting symptoms. Arch Dis Childh 37: 253-256, 1962

23. ZIEVE L: Jaundice hyperlipemia and hemolytic anemia. A heretofore unrecognized syndrome associated with alcohol fatty liver and cirrhosis. Ann Int Med 48: 471-496, 1958

THE FUNCTIONAL BASIS OF PHYSIOLOGIC JAUNDICE OF THE NEWBORN

Lawrence M. Gartner

Albert Einstein College of Medicine

Bronx, New York, 10461

INTRODUCTION

Jaundice in the newborn infant is a clinical sign which may lead both the clinician and investigator into vast areas of physiology and disease. Included within these areas of concern may be such widely disparate problems as infantile Gaucher's Disease, ABO hemolytic disease, neonatal hepatitis, prematurity, biliary atresia and kernicterus (1). The list is legion, but what these situations have in common is the retention of bile pigment in the tissues of the body and in the circulating plasma. In the neonate, as in the older child and adult, hyperbilirubinemia may be classified into those disorders in which conjugated bilirubin (direct-reacting) accumulates (i.e. neonatal hepatitis, biliary atresia and certain metabolic disorders) and those in which unconjugated bilirubin (indirect-reacting) accumulates. Physiologic hyperbilirubinemia of the newborn is of the unconjugated type.

By adult standards every newborn infant has some degree of unconjugated hyperbilirubinemia and, indeed, 50 percent of all infants will be visibly jaundiced at some time during the first five days of life, and will be diagnosed as having "physiologic jaundice". A far smaller proportion will have sufficient increase in their serum bilirubin concentration to be considered atypical or unusual and will require more extensive studies in an attempt to find a basis for the exaggerated hyperbilirubinemia. In some the cause will be found, but in many it will not and these infants will be considered to have an unknown disorder or to represent the extreme position on the normal distribution of physiologic jaundice. In all cases, however, regularly occurring functional abnormalities, resulting in "physiologic jaundice", are basic to the development of all unconconjugated hyperbilirubinemias in the newborn period. All more severe unconjugated hyperbilirubinemias are either exaggerations of one or more of the regularly occurring developmental disabilities or additional disorders superimposed on these developmental disabilities. In order to gain a better understanding of the transient physiologic limitations in the newborn, we undertook a series of detailed studies of bilirubin metabolism and transport in the newborn rhesus monkey.

Monkey Studies

The newborn rhesus monkey and probably newborns of all primate species develop a pattern of unconjugated hyperbilirubinemia comparable to that of the human neonate (2,3). The pattern of this hyperbilirubinemia in the full-term newborn monkey is characterized by a rapid rise from a value of less than 1 mg% at birth to a maximum of 4.5 mg% by 20 to 24 hours of age, (Fig.1). An equally rapid decline to 1 mg% occurs during the second 24 hour period of life. The full-term human newborn pattern is quite similar but has a time period approximately three times greater

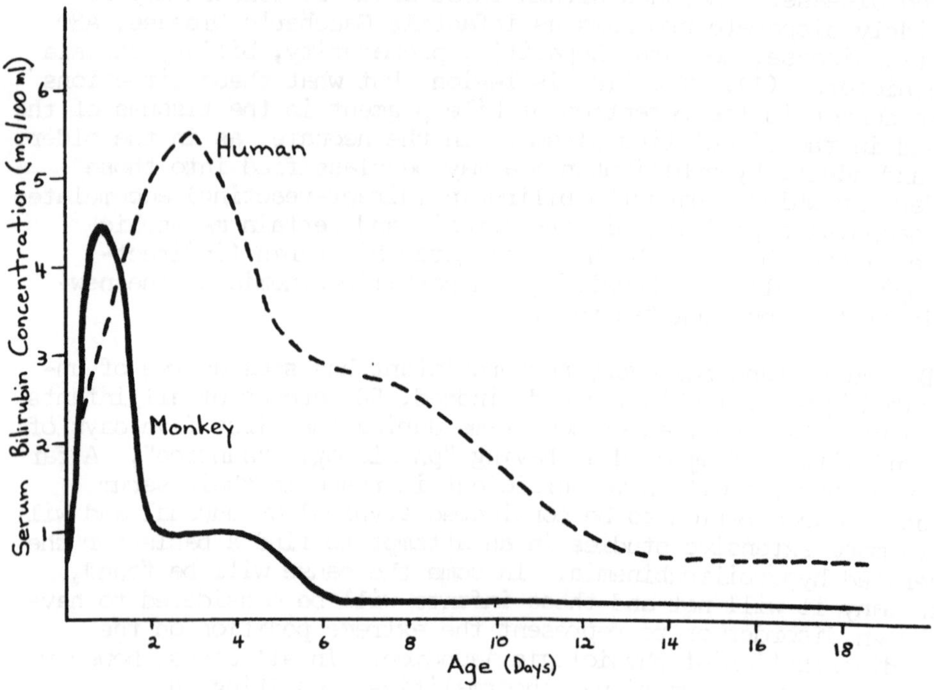

Fig.1. Mean serum bilirubin concentration (mg/100 ml) during the first 18 days of life in the newborn rhesus monkey (solid line) and in the full-term human newborn (dashed line).

than that of the monkey. In both the monkey and the human there is a period of approximately 3 to 4 days during which the serum bilirubin concentration remains fairly stable but elevated in comparison with adult values. This plateau period we have designated as Phase II physiologic jaundice, while the early peak we have called Phase I. Normal serum bilirubin concentrations in adult monkeys are 0.1 to 0.2 mg% while in the adult human they range from 0.5 to 1.0 mg%. Thus, in the full-term human neonate, normal serum bilirubin concentrations may not be found until near the end of the second week of life, although the more marked early rise, Phase I, will have disappeared by approximately day 5.

In order to examine the mechanisms responsible for physiologic jaundice we surgically prepared newborn rhesus monkeys at various ages during the first month of life for collection of bile, blood, urine and liver biopsies, and for constant infusion of saline or bilirubin intravenously (4). Without detailing the methodology used, let me define the parameters determined and the possible mechanisms which could explain the accumulation of unconjugated bilirubin in the newborn.

The five major compartments of bilirubin transport and metabolism are represented diagramatically in Fig. 2. Abnormalities in function of four of these five compartments could result in the accumulation of unconjugated bilirubin. Increased bilirubin synthesis whether from shortened erythrocyte life-span (5), increased

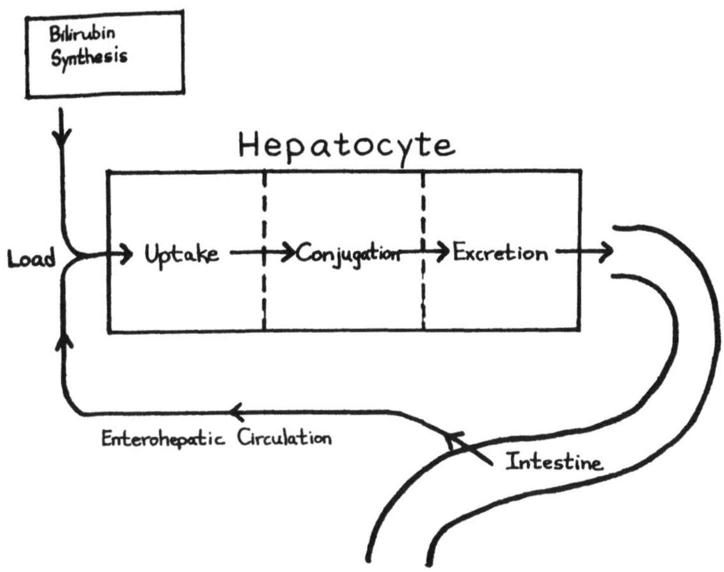

Fig. 2. Hepatic bilirubin pathways in the transport of bilirubin from blood into the intestinal tract.

cytochrome or other nonhemoglobin heme-protein turnover (6), or from resorption of immature or pre-circulating erythrocytes in erythropoietic tissue could and probably does increase bilirubin synthesis significantly in the newborn. Defective hepatic cell uptake of bilirubin, as suggested by our previous studies in the newborn guinea pig (7) and by studies in the newborn monkey (8) could also produce significant hyperbilirubinemia. Defective uptake could result either from deficiency of "Y" protein (ligandin), the cytoplasmic bilirubin binding protein of the liver, as indicated by the work of Arias (8), or from disordered liver cell membrane function.

Defective conjugation of bilirubin with glucuronic acid or other substances (glucose, xylose, etc.) to convert the water insoluble unconjugated bilirubin into the water soluble compound which can be excreted by the liver into bile would also result in retention of unconjugated bilirubin. It has generally been accepted that deficiency of the conjugating enzyme, glucuronyl transferase, is responsible for the development of physiologic jaundice (9). Direct evidence that this metabolic transformation is the rate-limiting step in the transfer of bilirubin from blood to bile in the newborn with physiologic jaundice is lacking, however. It should also be pointed out that deficiency of enzyme synthesis is not the only possible explanation for deficient conjugation of bilirubin. Thus, enzyme inhibition and/or insufficient substrate (UDPGA) would also account for deficient conjugation.

Deficient hepatic excretion of conjugated bilirubin would not directly result in conjugated hyperbilirubinemia since the pigment retained if this step were rate-limiting would be conjugated or direct-reacting bilirubin. However, deficient hepatic excretion of substances which are inhibitors of hepatic uptake mechanisms, or of the conjugating enzyme glucuronyl transferase could indirectly result in unconjugated hyperbilirubinemia.

The fifth step in the movement of bilirubin takes place in the intestinal tract, where conjugated bilirubin undergoes both conversion to urobilinogens and hydrolysis back to unconjugated bilirubin. Unconjugated bilirubin can be reabsorbed by the intestinal mucosa to return to the liver for reprocessing and excretion once more. In the newborn the reabsorption of bilirubin in the intestinal tract may well be increased in comparison with the adult (10,11). The newborn lacks the intestinal bacteria for conversion of bilirubin to urobilinogen, therefore leaving a greater proportion of the unconjugated bilirubin unconverted and available for reabsorption. In the newborn the surface to volume ratio of the bowel is greater than in the adult giving a large surface for reabsorption. Intestinal motility may also be slow during the first few days of life, further enhancing reabsorption.

Finally, meconium contains a very large quantity of unconjugated bilirubin which is a potential contributor to the total bilirubin pool. The combination of de novo synthesis of bilirubin and intestinally reabsorbed bilirubin is the quantity of bilirubin presented to the liver for disposal, and designated as load.

Hepatic Bilirubin Load

The bilirubin load presented to the liver was determined by the rate of endogenous excretion of bilirubin into bile during the first 21 days of life in the newborn monkey as compared with adult animals (Fig. 3). During the first 24 hours of life the load appears to be increasing. However, during this early period of time of restricted plasma clearance of bilirubin this increasing excretion reflects the increasing capacity of the liver to excrete the accumulated load of bilirubin. From 24 hours of life through the second day of life, there is further increase in endogenous excretion reflecting disposal of additional previously retained

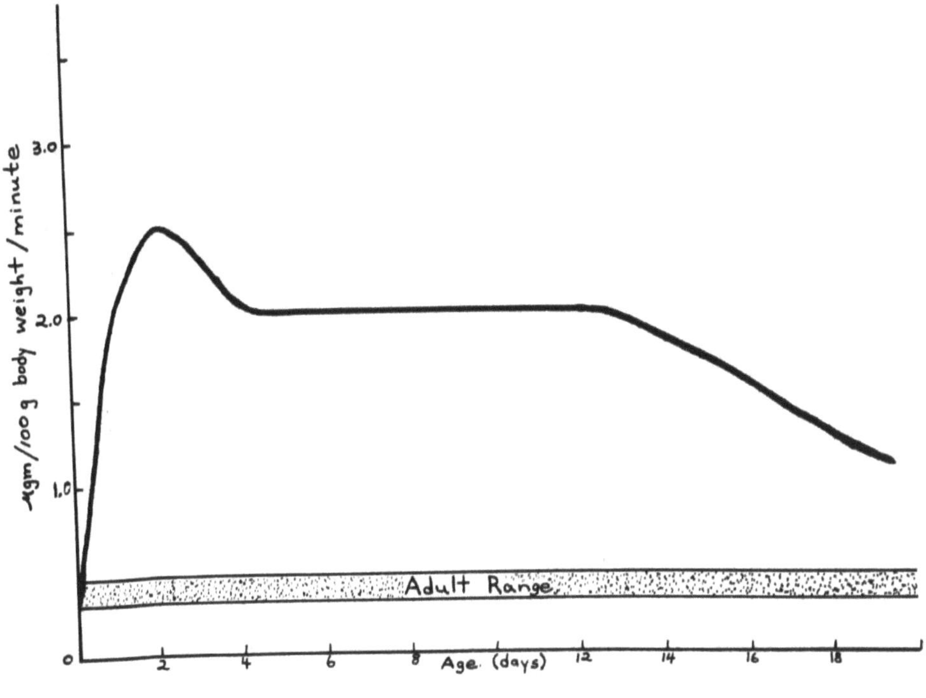

Fig. 3. Mean endogenous excretion of bilirubin in bile in the full-term newborn rhesus monkey during the first 18 days of life expressed as μg/100 grams body weight/minute (solid line) as compared with adult rhesus monkey range of normal endogenous excretion (dotted bar).

bilirubin. After the end of the 2nd day of life, endogenous bilirubin excretion declines somewhat to approximately 2.0 μg/100 g body weight/minute, a rate of excretion 7 times greater than in adult monkeys. Only during the third week of life does the load or endogenous excretion rate begin to fall toward that of the adult. Whether this increased load of bilirubin presented to the liver in the newborn is the result of increased *de novo* synthesis of bilirubin or from reabsorbed enteric bilirubin has not yet been determined. Other published evidence (5,6,10,11) suggests that both factors contribute, though the relative contribution of each is not known.

Hepatic Bilirubin Uptake

Deficiency of maximal cumulative hepatic bilirubin uptake or absolute uptake capacity during the first 24 hours of life has been observed, followed by rapid maturation of uptake capacity to normal by 48 hours of life (Fig. 4). This suggests that uptake may be the rate-limiting step during the first 24 hours of life in the passage of bilirubin from blood to bile. However, other evidence indicates that although uptake is low in capacity it is not the limiting function during this first day. Uptake is a process of facilitated diffusion and the rate of entry of bilirubin into a cell is determined, in part, by the serum bilirubin concentration. With the techniques used in this study serum bilirubin concentrations were extremely high and the uptake rates indicated on this slide are maximal; that is, further increase in the serum bilirubin concentration will not enhance uptake. In more recent studies, hepatic bilirubin uptake has been examined in relation to lower serum and liver unconjugated bilirubin concentrations. Preliminary results from these new studies suggest that *relative* hepatic uptake deficiency extends beyond the second day of life and probably explains Phase II Physiologic Jaundice and correlates temporally with maturation of "Y" protein. Thus, in order to clear a 7 fold increased load of bilirubin during the newborn period, it is necessary that the serum bilirubin concentrations be elevated. As uptake mechanisms mature further the rate of uptake at any bilirubin concentration increases, resulting in a reduction in serum bilirubin concentration to normal and thus the termination of Phase II.

Hepatic Bilirubin Conjugation

Hepatic glucuronyl transferase activity was estimated *in vitro* under optimal conditions using bilirubin as substrate.

During the first 24 hours of life, glucuronyl transferase activity is very close to zero but rises rapidly beginning at 24 hours, coincident with the decline of the serum bilirubin (Fig.5).

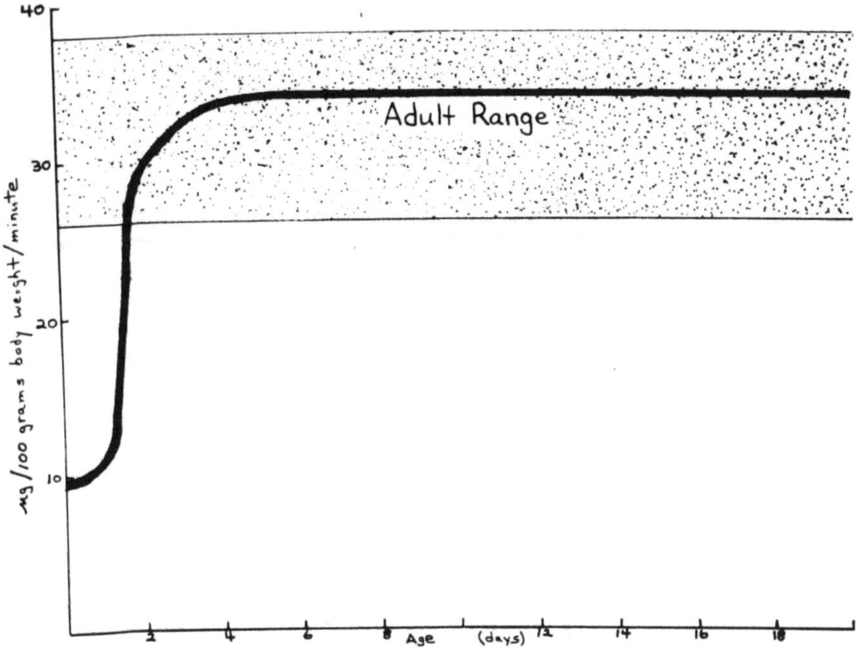

Fig. 4. Mean cumulative uptake of bilirubin in the full-term newborn rhesus monkey during the first 18 days of life expressed as μg/100 grams body weight/minute (solid line) as compared with adult rhesus monkey range of normal cumulative hepatic uptake (dotted bar).

By the third day of life enzyme activity has nearly approximated adult levels of activity. By a series of calculations we have estimated that the conjugating capacity of the liver during the first 24 hours of life is less than the load of bilirubin presented to the liver. If the load of bilirubin were not 7 times normal, then this very reduced conjugating capacity would have been sufficient to prevent accumulation of bilirubin. Thus, from these data we have drawn the conclusion that Phase I Physiologic Jaundice results from a combination of increased bilirubin load and markedly reduced conjugating capacity. We also believe that relative hepatic uptake deficiency contributes to Phase I and although not the critical rate-limiting step during Phase I does prevent accumulation of bilirubin in the liver.

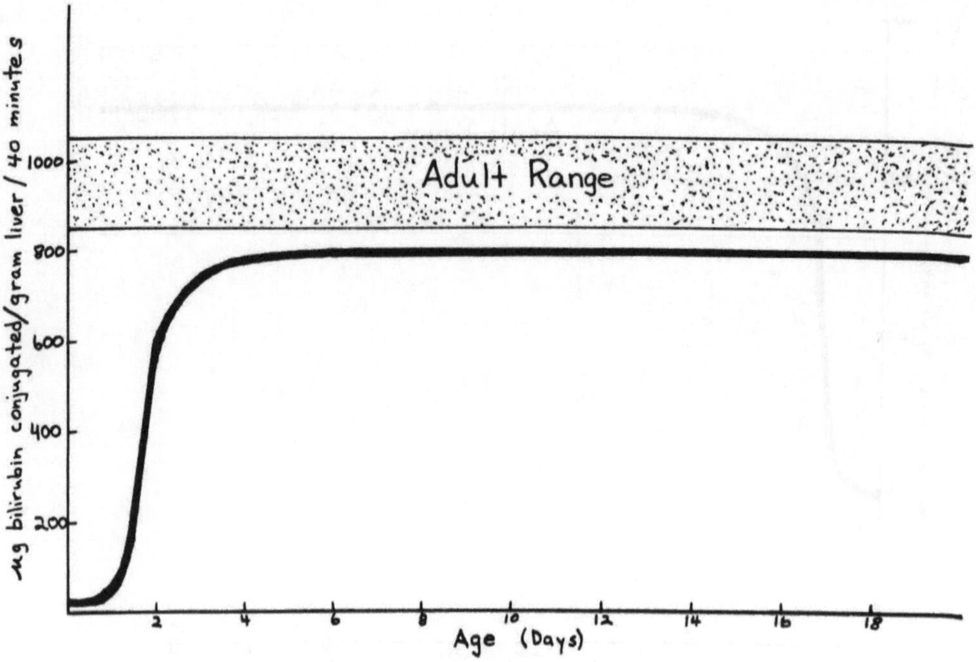

Fig. 5. Mean hepatic glucuronyl transferase activity in the full-term newborn rhesus monkey during the first 18 days of life expressed as μg bilirubin conjugated/gram liver wet weight/40 minutes (solid line) as compared with adult rhesus monkey normal range of enzyme activity (dotted bar).

SUMMARY

The concepts of the mechanisms of physiologic jaundice of the newborn developed from the rhesus monkey studies are summarized in Fig. 6. During Phase I, a large load of bilirubin coupled with a marked reduction in conjugation results in retention of unconjugated bilirubin, with the conjugation step being rate-limiting and the actual output of bilirubin reflecting conjugating capacity. During Phase II conjugation is no longer rate-limiting but at moderately increased loads of bilirubin, as seen in the newborn, uptake is the rate-limiting step. Should the load of bilirubin increase markedly, with a resultant sharp rise in the serum bilirubin concentration, then the rate of uptake will increase significantly so that excretory capacity is exceeded, and excretion will then become the rate-limiting step. During Phase II output is the same as load but this is only achieved at the expense of a slightly increased serum bilirubin concentration.

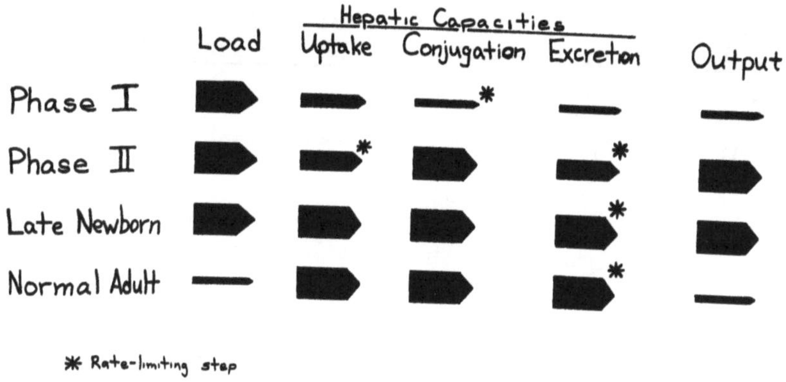

Fig. 6. Diagrammatic representation of hepatic bilirubin load, hepatic capacities for uptake, conjugation and excretion of bilirubin by the liver and output of bilirubin in bile during Phase I and Phase II of physiologic hyperbilirubinemia, the late newborn period and in the normal adult rhesus monkey.

During the late newborn period hepatic capacities for uptake, conjugation and excretion are normal and serum bilirubin concentrations are normal, but load is still increased, as reflected in increased output. In this period of life and during the adult period, excretion is the potential rate-limiting step as would become apparent if the bilirubin load were increased very markedly, resulting in conjugated hyperbilirubinemia.

On the skeletal outline of bilirubin transport in the newborn can be placed the various clinical situations which alter hepatic bilirubin load, uptake, conjugation and excretion to result in exaggerations of the regularly occurring physiologic status of the newborn.

REFERENCES

1. GARTNER LM, HOLLANDER M: Disorders of bilirubin metabolism. In Pathophysiology of Gestation, Vol. III, edited by Assali N, New York, Academic Press, 1972, p. 455-503.

2. LUCEY JF, BEHRMAN RE, WARSHAW AL: Physiologic jaundice in newborn rhesus monkey. Am J Dis Child 106: 350-355, 1963.

3. GARTNER LM, LANE DL: The physiology of physiologic hyperbilirubinemia of the newborn. In Medical Primatology 1972, Part I, Basel, Karger, 1972, p. 237-247.

4. GARTNER LM, LANE DL, CORNELIUS CE: Bilirubin transport by liver in adult Macaca mulatta. Amer J Physiol 220: 1528-1535, 1971.

5. PEARSON HA: Life-span of the fetal red blood cell. J Pediat 70: 166-171, 1967.

6. ROBINSON SH, LESTER R, CRIGLER JF, TSONG M: The early labeled peak of bile pigment in man: studies with glycine-C^{14} and delta-aminolevulinic acid-H^{3}. New Eng J Med 277: 1323, 1969.

7. GARTNER LM, ARIAS IM: The transfer of bilirubin from blood to bile in the neonatal guinea pig. Pediat Res 3: 171-180, 1969.

8. LEVI AJ, GATMAITAN Z, ARIAS IM: Deficiency of hepatic organic anion-binding protein, impaired organic anion uptake by liver and "physiologic" jaundice in newborn monkeys. New Eng J Med 283: 1136-1139, 1970.

9. BROWN AK, ZUELZER WW: Studies on the neonatal development of the glucuronide conjugating system. J Clin Invest 37: 332-340, 1948.

10. ULSTROM RA, EISENKLAM E: The enterohepatic shunting of bilirubin in the newborn infant. I. Use of oral activated charcoal to reduce normal serum bilirubin values. J Pediat 65: 27, 1964.

11. POLAND RD, ODELL GB: Physiologic jaundice: the enterohepatic circulation of bilirubin. New Eng J Med 284: 291, 1971.

PHOTOPHARMACOLOGY AND BILIRUBIN

Jerold F. Lucey and Jean Hewitt

University of Vermont College of Medicine

Burlington, Vermont 05401

I will confine my remarks to the effect of light on the hyperbilirubinemia of newborn infants for three reasons:

1) It is important and new.

2) This effect has been largely ignored by internists until recently.

3) It is controversial, which in turn should make it interesting.

A great deal of research has gone into defining the optimal microenvironment of the newborn infant with respect to oxygen, humidity, temperature and bacterial flora. Very little attention has been paid to the infant's light environment. I suggest that the reasons for this are largely emotional. We have in our medical training been taught very little about the effects of this potent energy source in our environment. No serious consideration before 1958 was given to the effect of light upon serum concentration of bilirubin(1). Light therapy was introduced into the U.S.A. in 1968(2). The only specialists interested in its effects have been dermatologists. They have largely confined their interests to the effects of the ultraviolet portion of the radiation spectrum upon skin. The effects of light I am discussing today occur due to light energy in 400 - 500 nm range, or blue visible light, and can occur when human infants or adults are exposed to bright fluorescent light.

TABLE I

PROVEN EFFECTS OF SUPPLEMENTAL LIGHT ON NEONATAL INFANTS

LOWER LEVELS OF SERUM BILIRUBIN DUE TO PHOTODEGRADATION IN TISSUES
INCREASED EXCRETION OF UNCONJUGATED BILIRUBIN IN BILE AND STOOL
INCREASED URINE PIGMENT EXCRETION
INCREASED SKIN BLOOD FLOW
DECREASED GASTROINTESTINAL TRANSIT TIME
INCREASED INSENSIBLE WATER LOSS
TRANSIENT SKIN RASHES AND PIGMENTATION
INCREASED BILE ACID TURNOVER (ADULTS)

Table 1 summarizes what I consider to be the proven effects of this light. It is a fairly impressive list. I suggest it is but the beginning as research in this field has only recently become respectable. We, as pediatricians, have been priviledged to observe these effects because our prematurely born patients are not usually clothed and they remain jaundiced and in incubators for days. They are, in effect, nude prisoners in our artificially designed adult oriented light environment called a nursery!

The recent demonstrations by Ostrow(3), Lund(4) and Thaler(5) that in jaundiced animals and human adults and infants one can increase the excretion of unconjugated bilirubin is, I believe, going to be of major significance. At the least, it will require a re-thinking of the present dogma that conjugation is a necessary step before excretion of bilirubin. In this regard I would like to digress a moment to suggest an interesting, neglected animal model for study. Adult frogs were shown by Lester et al(6) to have UDP glucuronyl transferase in their livers but to excrete unconjugated bilirubin. Biliary excretion of bile pigment as a glucuronide did not occur. Levine et al(7) have demonstrated that this species has Y and Z protein (ligandin) in the liver cell. This species has no measurable circulating bilirubin in the serum. We exposed some adult frogs whose "bile" duct was cannulated to alternate five hour periods of darkness and intense light. Bile flow rates

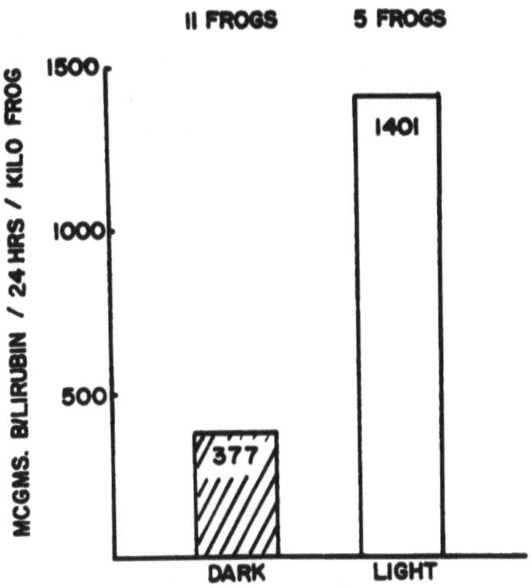

Fig. 1 Average Bilirubin Excretion in the Frog

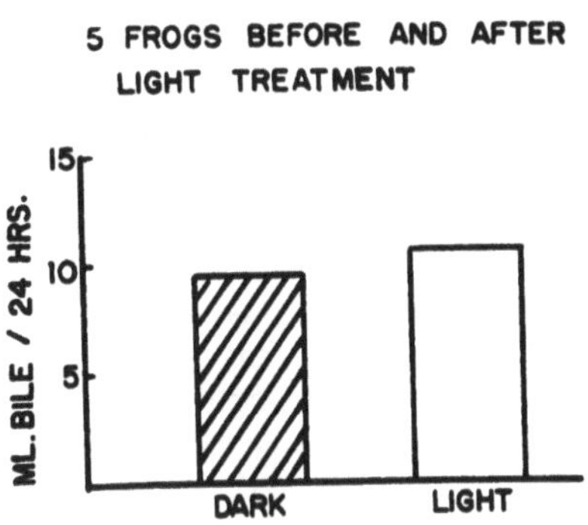

Fig. 2 Effect of Light Upon Hepatic Bile Flow in Frogs

(cc/kg of body Wt.) did not change during these contrasting periods. There was, however, a four fold increase in the excretion of unconjugated bilirubin (diazo positive material) during the light exposure period(Fig 1 & 2). We interpret this to indicate that peripheral photodegradation products are not involved in whatever the mechanism is by which unconjugated bilirubin is excreted by the liver. If light can have this profound, unexpected effect in man and animals on bilirubin metabolism, it seems to me highly likely that a number of other compounds metabolized in the liver will also be effected. A new area of research probably called photopharmacology seems likely to emerge in the near future.

One of the first very promising studies in this field has been recently reported by Ballowitz(8). She has found that the well known toxicity of bilirubin in infant Gunn rats which is potentiated by sulfonamide therapy can be nearly completely reversed or prevented if the animals are treated with light at the time of the sulfonamide administration (Fig. 3). One possible explanation for this protective effect of light is that in this situation light destroys in the periphery the unbound bilirubin displaced by the sulfonamide, thereby, allowing this animal to survive. This neuroprotective effect of light in this experimental situation obviously has profound implications for possible clinical use in humans. A similar photoprotective effect of light has been noted when gentamycin was being tested for its toxicity in jaundiced neonatal Gunn rats(8). (Fig.4).

The present lighting conditions in our hospitals were not selected with any great care. It was assumed that if adequate light existed for adult personnel to see, then this would be a satisfactory environment for infants. Later some consideration was given to lighting that would enable physicians to visually assay jaundice and cyanosis. Little attention is still paid to the cyclical variation of light during the day and night. In many intensive care nurseries windows have been eliminated, continuous artificial light is used and small premature infants may not experience any natural sunlight for several weeks after birth. How do we know that this is correct? The answer, of course, is that we do not. It is assumed, by some workers, that our present lighting conditions are optimal and, therefore,

	CONTROLS	SULFA	LIGHT & SULFA
NUMBER	86	44	40
SURVIVAL	77%	25%	80%

(600 - 1000 MG / KG)

Fig. 3 Effect of Light upon Sulfonamide Mortality in Infant Gunn Rats. Ballowitz (8).

	GENTAMYCIN	LIGHT + GENTAMYCIN
NUMBER	24	25
SURVIVAL	4%	70%

(100 - 200 MG / KG)

Fig. 4 Effect of Light upon Gentamycin Mortality in Infant Gunn Rats. Ballowitz 1974

deviations from present practice might be fraught with disaster. It is also assumed that "light therapy" is exposing infants to vastly increased amounts of radiant energy exposure. This is not always true. A good deal of misunderstanding exists on this point. Let's examine what we do know about our present light conditions. MacLeod and Stern(9) have documented the well known fact that great variations in light intensity of from 15 F.C's to 2500 F.C's can occur. It has also been documented that a general level of 90 F.C.'s in a nursery is effective in decreasing the incidence of hyperbilirubinemia(10). The majority of "phototherapy" studies have been done using 200-400 F.C.'s of broad spectrum light -- an amount arbitrarily selected in 1958 by Creemer(1).

A number of factors listed on Table II are very important in assessing the present normal light environment. The infant lives in a rapidly changing sea of radiant energy of very variable intensities. We initially assumed when we carried out our study in 1966(2) of the effects of light on serum bilirubin in premature infants that we had two groups -- "normal controls" and a "light treated" group. I would now challenge this assumption made by us and many others as gross oversimplification of a difficult problem.

We have carried out careful studies over a 24-hour period in our nursery using a number of different spectroradiometers. These devices are more appropriate to use than light meters because they measure the amount of radiation energy in selected wavelengths -- the irradiance in micro watts/sq.cm. -- instead of supplying an expression of the sensation of brightness as do light meters.

TABLE II

FACTORS IMPORTANT IN ASSESSING NURSERY LIGHT ENVIRONMENT

SUN AND CLOUD FORMATION
WINDOW LOCATION
SEASON
CLOTHING
TYPE OF INCUBATOR
FEEDING
ENVIRONMENTAL LIGHT
EQUIPMENT ON INCUBATOR
SKIN LOTIONS
EXPOSURE ANGLE - REFLECTING SURFACES

Figure 5 represents a schematic version of the type of radiant energy exposure expressed as microwatts per square centimeter between 440-470 nanometers an infant receives in our nursery in a day if the incubator was near a window with an eastern exposure. One sees that this infant receives a high amount of total light exposure for a short period of the day as compared to the infant receiving lower but fairly continuous amounts of light exposure under conventional phototherapy. At different seasons this exposure would obviously vary. This highly variable but potent source of light exposure has in the past been neglected, as no studies I am aware of have measured it in the control group.

Another way of expressing these data is to compare the 24 hour theoretical exposures received expressed either as irradiance, (Fig. 6) or as dosage (joules) (Fig 7). Whether expressed as irradiance or as dosage, it is obvious that at least in some nurseries the natural light exposure of an infant is an important variable.

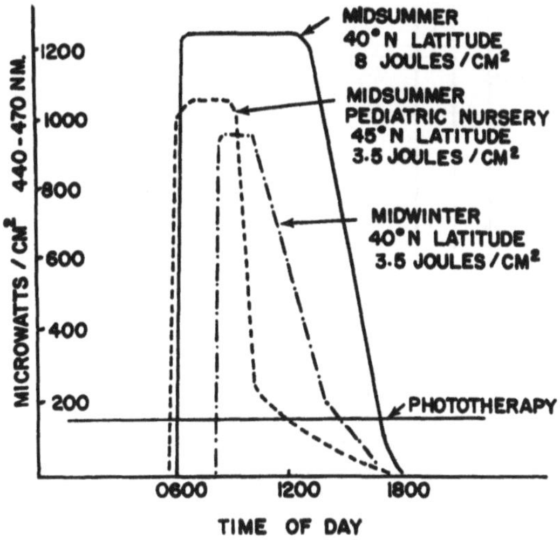

Fig. 5 A Flux Day in Life of a Premature Infant in Nursery with Windows

We are suggesting that in the future one should perhaps compare the radiant energy exposure of these infants on the basis of a total 24-hour exposure period. The term flux day, at various specific wavelengths, could then be used. This would allow more meaningful comparisons of light dosage than now exist. Looked at in this fashion one sees that the infant near a window in Vermont for 6 hours can actually receive more radiant energy exposure in the 440-470 nanometer range than does the infant under conventional phototherapy with daylight bulbs for 24 hours. I appreciate that few infants are exposed to direct sunlight via a window but in this comparison we have actually used levels of natural light intensity that are commonly achieved in some nurseries with windows.

The point we wish to make is that intermittent phototherapy has been going on in nurseries for years under uncontrolled conditions. This important point has been ignored. The value of studies where the light conditions of the controls have not been precisely defined must now be questioned. The repeated concerns expressed by some that so-called light therapy might be dangerous or highly experimental should be tempered by this consideration. There is no evidence available -- other than tradition -- which establishes the present conditions as optimal. In fact, a good

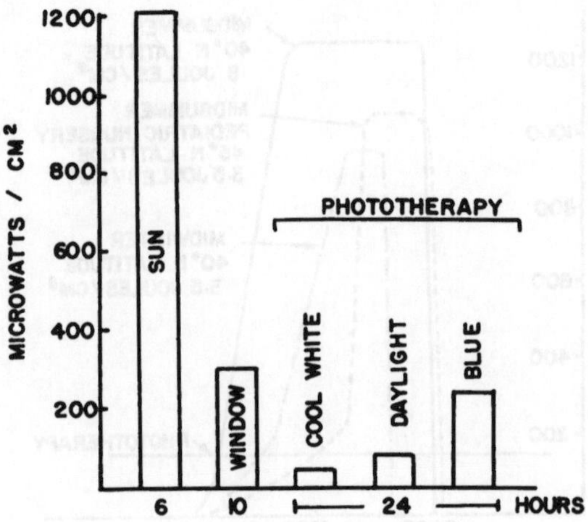

Fig. 6 Light irradiance in the Newborn Nursery 440-470 nm

case can be made for the hypothesis that a component of neonatal jaundice is due to light deprivation! It would be but another example of our inability to correctly select, from adult standards, the best environment for the infant.

It will not be easy to select the correct amount of radiant energy exposure an infant should receive. As with all radiation, the least amount of exposure that will accomplish the desired effect seems to be the best goal. On the basis of animal studies in the Gunn rat(11) we estimate that to be effective in lowering serum bilirubin, a light must supply at least 100 microwatts/sq.cm. at 440-470 nanometers. Present phototherapy units usually supply much more than this.

A number of important variables keep us from applying this figure to humans. The skin is one such variable. Its thickness obviously varies with gestational age and area of the body.

The amount of light that will penetrate in these areas is obviously different. No studies of this important point have been carried out.

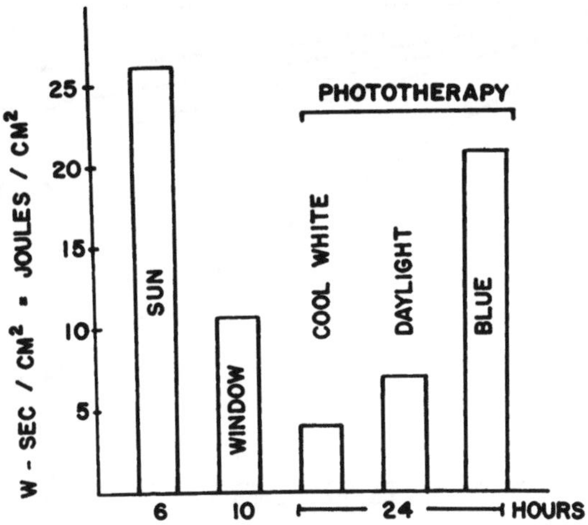

Fig. 7 Light Dosage in the Newborn Nursery 440-470 nm

The exact site of action of light is still not known. In the future calculations of light dosage, the area exposed, skin thickness and penetration will all have to be considered.

If an important site of action is intravascular, another factor which may be important is the hematocrit. This has been suggested by Blackburn and Orsalezi(12). In an in vitro study (Fig. 8) we compared the effects on a solution of bilirubin in serum in which the only variable was the hematocrit. All samples were agitated constantly during the 24-hour light exposure. The blood with a high hematocrit had less of a fall in bilirubin concentration than the low hematocrit blood. In a clinical situation this may be a contributing factor to the differences in response of serum bilirubin to light which one observes in different infants.

We have carried out a few postmortem studies on the relative penetration of light through the newborn scalp and skull bones. Simple proof that light penetrates the skull is supplied by the well known use of light for transillumination of infants' heads in the nursery.

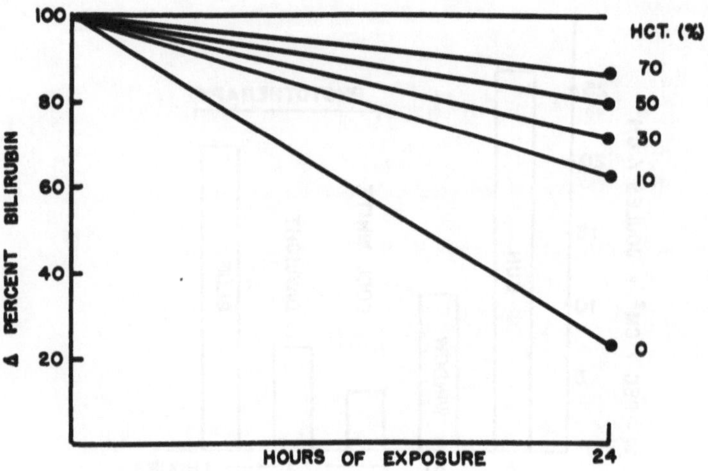

Fig. 8 In Vitro Effect of Hematocrit on Photodegradation of Bilirubin

In this study shown in Figure 9 an I.S.C.O. spectroradiometer cosine corrected probe was placed within the empty cranium of two prematurely born infants at postmortem examination. The light source tested was a standard Air Shields phototherapy unit equipped with 6 daylight fluorescent tubes. In each study a small percentage of the incident light at wavelengths 490-520 nanometers penetrated the skull. It is important to note that wavelengths commonly used for heating had great penetration. No studies of the effects of this common widespread use of radiant energy have been carried out.

We have recently reviewed our clinical experience with the use of phototherapy (supplemental light) in low birth weight infants for "physiologic jaundice of prematurity", and mild A.B.O. or Rh blood group incompatibility, in the pre-supplemental light era (1960-66) of our nursery and in the (1967-73) period when we have been using "more light" in the nursery environment.

In 1960-66 we had 949 low birth weight (less than 2500 gms B.W.) infants admitted to our unit. We performed serum bilirubins

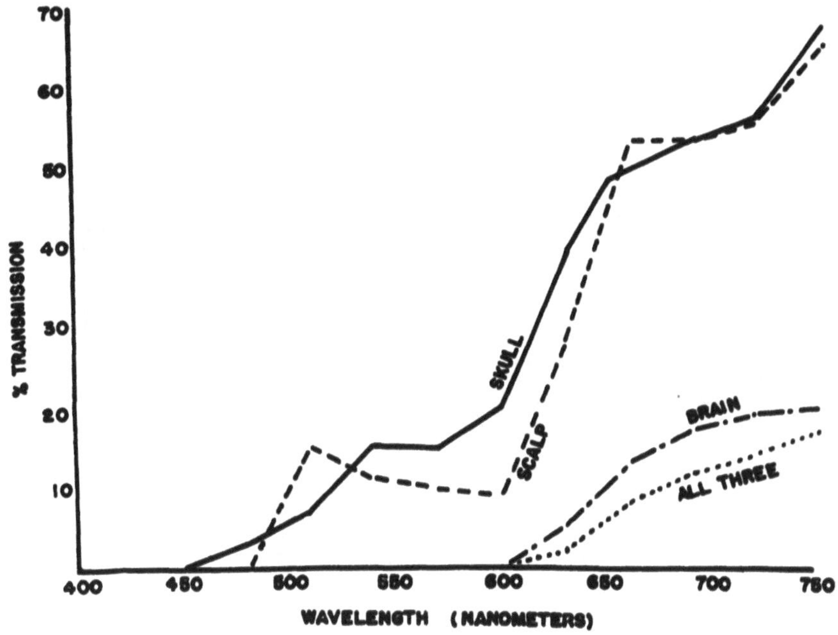

Fig. 9 Light Penetration Skull of 1500 Gram Infant

on 60% of these infants and 14% were found to have serum bilirubin concentrations of over 15 mg%.

During the next six year period 1967-73 we had 870 infants admitted. During this era we were using increased amount of environmental lighting in a variety of ways. We treated 47% of these infants with light. We did serum bilirubin studies on 60% of the total infants admitted. We found that 4% developed serum concentrations of over 15 mg%. (See Table III).

An analysis of our recent experience indicates that we tend to be using light on a higher % of infants in 1972-73 and doing more serum bilirubins, but that the incidence of hyperbilirubinemia, defined as a serum bilirubin of greater than 15 mg%, hasn't changed appreciably. The significance, if any, of this is difficult to interpret because since 1972 we have experienced an increased

TABLE III

PHOTOTHERAPY EXPERIENCE

LOW BIRTH WEIGHT INFANTS

University of Vermont 1967-73

YEAR	NO. OF INFANTS	% LIGHT THERAPY	% BILIRUBINS DONE	% SERUM BILIRUBINS <10	10-15	>15
1967-8	156	33	54	69	25	5
1968-9	135	47	47	73	20	6
1969-70	192	44	52	63	33	4
1970-1	140	47	65	45	52	3
1971-2	130	47	58	61	35	4
1972-3	117	71	84	43	53	3
TOTAL	870	AVR 47%	59%	59%	36%	4%

number of infants being transferred from other hospitals with severe respiratory distress and other illnesses. These are factors which would tend to increase the incidence of hyperbilirubinemia.

The only conclusion we draw from looking back at this experience is that one can significantly decrease, but not eliminate, hyperbilirubinemia in such a population of infants by the use of phototherapy of "supplemental light" in approximately one-half of the infants. We have not had a low birth weight infant with a serum bilirubin of over 20 mg% in the last seven years. We have not had any cases of kernicterus at postmortem examination nor clinically observed during the last 12 years. We make no claim that our experience can answer the important question of whether the incidence of "low bilirubin kernicterus" can be changed by phototherapy. Our experience combined with others is, however, most reassuring in that there is no evidence that neurologic damage is occurring in treated infants. If a "kernicterus like" picture were going to show up due to a change in say bilirubin binding capacity of serum albumin, as has been hypothesized, it would be apparent by now as the clinical experience in the U.S.A. and world is now of 15 years duration and involves thousands of

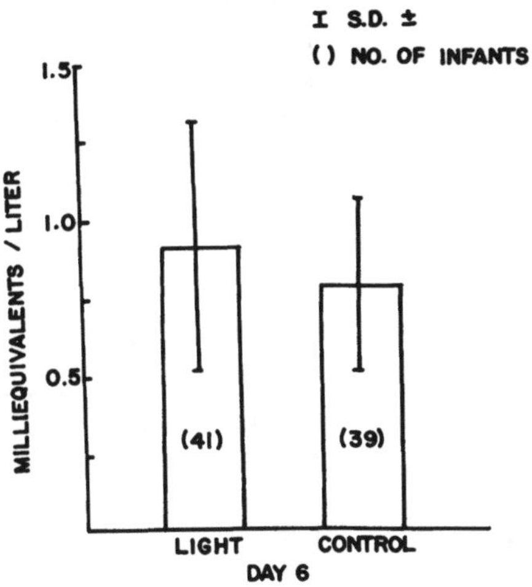

Fig. 10 Serum Free Fatty Acid Values: Phototherapy and Control Infants

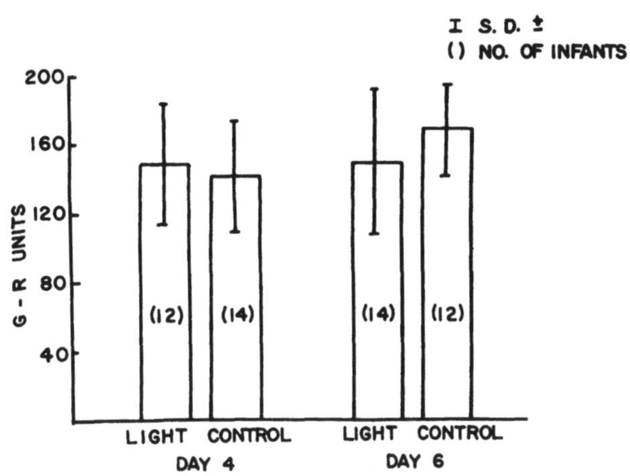

Fig. 11 Serum Leucine Amino Peptidase Values: Phototherapy and Control Infants

TABLE IV

RESULTS OF A SIX YEAR FOLLOW-UP IN 1972-3
OF A CONTROLLED STUDY OF 99 LOW BIRTH
WEIGHT INFANTS TREATED WITH PHOTOTHERAPY
IN 1966

NUMBER OF INFANTS		AVERAGE WGT.	HEAD CIRCUMFERENCE		PSYCHOMETRIC		HEARING		NEUROLOGIC	
			NL.	SM.	NL.	ABNL.	NL.	ABNL	NL.	ABNL.
CONTROL	44	2134 gms	43	1	30	10	40	8	34	2
LIGHT	55	2072 gms	48	5	22	9	31	6	46	3

infants. No research workers I am aware of have observed any unusual increase in the incidence of neurologic damage thought to be due to bilirubin. In fact, a decreased incidence of kernicterus at postmortem examination has been reported by Ploussard(13), and Petrich(14).

We have carefully followed up 99 infants (55 controls and 44 light treated) of our original study carried out in 1966(15). These infants have been seen by a pediatric neurologist. They have had psychometric evaluation and speech and hearing evaluation, all carried out by examiners who did not know the status of the child at the time of the study.

We failed to detect any significant differences in these two groups in I.Q., speech and hearing, neurologic status, or head circumference. (Table IV).

The whole question of an effect, if any, upon head circumference and I.Q. of phototherapy is going to be an exceedingly difficult one on which to do a control study. The basic reason for this is that we of course do not know, nor can we control, the important factors (genetic, environmental - both pre and postnatal, calories, and viral infections) which are known to have very profound effects upon these parameters.

A question has also been raised as to the possible effect of light upon serum free fatty acid concentrations. Figure 10 summarizes our experience on this point. We were unable to detect any difference on the second, fourth or sixth day of life when the light group was compared to controls. These were the infants in our original study(9). We have not published these observations previously. We were also not able to detect any difference in serum leucine amino peptidase values (Fig.11). This was reassuring to us, as this test is a sensitive index of biliary tract damage.

SUMMARY

We have called attention to the profound effects light may have upon bilirubin metabolism in the neonatal infant. A new field, photopharmacology, has appeared and shows great promise of being clinically important. It is suggested that a useful model for exploring the mechanism by which light increases the excretion of unconjugated bilirubin is the frog, who naturally excretes unconjugated bilirubin. In light this animal can increase its excretion of unconjugated bilirubin fourfold. The mechanism remains unknown.

Very little is known about the light environment of the newborn infant. We challenge the assumption that the present lighting conditions are either optimal or inviolate. If one accepts our concept of a flux day, normal infants in many nurseries can receive more radiant energy exposure than is being received by infants under phototherapy.

Controlled clinical studies of the long term effects of light will be very difficult to carry out and interpret unless the light conditions of both groups are carefully monitored.

ACKNOWLEDGEMENTS

The authors acknowledge the invaluable consultation and help given in these studies by Dr. Richard Klein, Department of Botany, University of Vermont. Mr. Tom Wolk and Mr. James Bottiggi carried out the light measurement under Dr. Klein's direction. The work was aided by grants from N.I.C.U.D. (PUS R01 05561-02) and United Cerebral Palsy (R-242-73).

REFERENCES

1. CREMER RJ, PERRYMAN PW, RICHARDS DH: Influence of light on the hyperbilirubinemia of infants. Lancet 1: 1094-1097, 1958.

2. LUCEY J, HEWITT J: Prevention of hyperbilirubinemia of prematurity by phototherapy. Pediat 41: 1047-1054, 1968.

3. OSTROW J, BERRY C: Excretion of exogenous and endogenous bile pigments after intravenous administration of bilirubin photoderivatives to Gunn rats. Gastroenterology 64: 152, 1973 (Abstract).

4. LUND H, JACOBSEN J: Influence of phototherapy on unconjugated bilirubin in duodenal bile of newborn infants. Acta Pediat Scand 61: 693-696, 1972.

5. THALER M, DAWBER N, KRASNER J, YAFFE S, MOSOVICH L: Effects of phototherapy on bilirubin metabolism and sulfobromophthalein excretion in unconjugated hyperbilirubinemia. Pediat Res 7: 106, 1973 (Abstract).

6. LESTER R, SCHMID R: Bile pigment excretion in amphibia. Nature 190: 452, 1961.

7. LEVINE R et al: Phylogenetic study of organic anion transfer from plasma into the liver. Nature New Biology 231: 277-279, 1971.

8. BALLOWITZ L, HANEFIELD F: Phototherapy of infant Gunn rats under the influence of different drugs. Symposia on Bilirubin Metabolism, edited by H. Blondheim. Original Article Series, National Foundation, N.Y.C. 1974 (in press).

9. MACLEOD P, STERN L: Natural variations in environmental illumination in a newborn nursery. Pediat 50: 131-133, 1972.

10. GIUNTA F: Phototherapy and neonatal hyperbilirubinemia. Hosp Pract 7: 87-92, 1972.

11. HEWITT J, KLEIN R, LUCEY J: Photodegradation of serum bilirubin in the Gunn rat. Biol Neonate 21: 112-119, 1972.

12. BLACKBURN M, ORZALESI M: Personal communication.

13. PLOUSSARD JP: Growth retardation - a reversible side effect of phototherapy. Phototherapy of Hyperbilirubinemia of Prematurity - A Symposium. N.I.H., Bethesda, Md. April 1974 (in press).

14. PETRICH C: Idiopathic hyperbilirubinemia and phototherapy. Pediat 54: 654-655, 1974.

15. LUCEY J, HEWITT J, EMERY E, GOLDSTEIN S, COLLINS S: A controlled follow-up study of low birth weight at 4-6 years of age treated with phototherapy. Pediat Res 7: 169, 1973 (Abstract).

DISCUSSION OF PAPERS ON BILIRUBIN METABOLISM

CHAIRMAN: L.G. ISRAELS

LESTER: Your results concerning the excretion of the increased bilirubin load by the newborn Rhesus monkey were expressed in terms of body weight. I wonder if they might not be expressed as legitimately in terms of body surface and if this might not considerably lower the apparent load. Small animal to large animal comparisons are difficult, but in trying to compare neonatal bile salt secretion to adult bile salt secretion we found that the match-up between liver weight and one or two other things was better when the data were expressed in terms of body surface.

GARTNER: We chose body weight because it yielded fairly consistent values in different species which varied widely in size and because it relates to liver size as well. I have not calculated the results in terms of surface area.

LESTER: The cell plates of the adult liver are one cell thick and are perfused on two sides with blood. In contrast the liver cell plates of the fetus and newborn are two or more cells thick and one would think that liver cell perfusion might be a great deal less efficient than in the adult. Do you think that the diminished uptake of bile pigment by the liver of the newborn might in part be caused by this relatively diminished perfusion of the liver cells?

GARTNER: Yes. The whole question of blood flow in the newborn liver has not been looked at carefully enough.

LESTER: The subject was discussed in 1961 during a meeting held at the New York Academy of Sciences. Radiographs of the fetal liver show big blunted blood vessels which appear to shunt blood away from functional liver tissue.

ZIMMON: The neonatal liver really has a functioning portacaval shunt. During the first few days after birth this shunt is closing as the hepatic circulation changes from arterial to portal venous. It seems to me that there must be a tremendous variation in hepatic blood flow as well as microscopic anatomy during this time and that this would exert a considerable influence on the phenomena which you have been discussing.

ROY: Conjugated bilirubin can be deconjugated in the newborn gut and I wonder if you have looked at the enterohepatic circulation of bilirubin and considered how this might influence your findings.

GARTNER: We have not looked at the rate of hydrolysis in vivo or at the rate of bilirubin reabsorption in the monkeys. This is something we are beginning to do.

SCHMID: You made the statement that the rate-limiting step in bilirubin secretion is that of canalicular secretion. Now this is something which we all preach but it does not really correlate with the observations that, if you give a load of bilirubin, you get an unconjugated and not a conjugated hyperbilirubinemia. How do you deal with this discrepancy?

GARTNER: When infusing unconjugated bilirubin into adult mammals there is a progressive accumulation in conjugated bilirubin in the liver and plasma but not until you exceed the Tm. Bilirubin excretion has an absolute maximum and not until you get enough bilirubin into the liver cell to exceed the rate of excretion will you get conjugated bilirubin accumulating within the liver. In a sense it is a matter of terminology and it depends upon how much bilirubin. I talk about it being the rate-limiting step. I am really talking about saturation down the line when we are giving enough bilirubin to saturate both uptake and conjugation.

SCHMID: I am sure that that is the real answer. Some years ago we looked at this problem in rats and found that although unconjugated bilirubin increases as you increase the load, the fraction of direct reacting bilirubin increases proportionately. If you give the rat a load of 5-10 mg of bilirubin for hours the unconjugated bilirubin will perhaps be 2 mg% and another 0.3 mg% will be conjugated. If you double the load the bilirubin goes up but the proportion between the conjugated and the unconjugated bilirubin remains the same. This really doesn't fit with any of the regular steps proposed.

GARTNER: That is not what we found in the adult monkey studies and I am sorry that I don't have the data here. In these studies the amount of conjugated bilirubin increased disproportionately as the canalicular secretory capacity was exceeded.

SCHMID: In your studies with the Rhesus monkey, how did you actually measure hepatic uptake?

GARTNER: The method is indirect. We calculated the amount of conjugated bilirubin excreted into the bile, the increasing concentration of total bilirubin in the liver cells, the amount of conjugated bilirubin excreted in the urine and the increase in the conjugated bilirubin in the plasma having measured plasma volume. From these we calculated the cumulative hepatic uptake or net increase over a finite period of time. In the monkeys this was done hourly for three consecutive hours.

LAMALA: I would like to ask Dr. Brain to comment about the increased osmotic fragility in spur cells in relation to their increased cholesterol content. Vandeenen and co-workers and also Breen increased the cholesterol content of normal erythrocytes using a liposome exchange technique and both groups reported a decrease in osmotic fragility.

BRAIN: With some of these alterations you get an actual loss of membrane from the cells, possibly by some fragmentation process, and they can go on to look like spherocytes. I think that there is a derangement of the membrane similar to that which takes place if you deplete the red cells of cholesterol and the alteration results in a loss of membrane from the cell.

SIMON: Although free cholesterol and lipoproteins exchange readily with red cell membrane cholesterol, there is clear evidence that this exchange is independent of the actual concentration of cholesterol in the serum. This appears instead to be related to the relative saturation of free cholesterol in lipoproteins. The lecithin-cholesterol acyl transferase reaction contributes to this exchange in that its deficiency is one of the factors that would lead to a relatively high free cholesterol in relation to the apoprotein and other lipids in patients with liver disease. It is this relative rather than absolute increase in lipoprotein free cholesterol that will enhance exchange with red cell membrane and lead to an increased free cholesterol in red cells.

THE FUTURE OF ENDOSCOPIC RETROGRADE CHOLANGIOPANCREATOGRAPHY (ERCP) AS A CLINICAL AND RESEARCH TOOL

David S. Zimmon

Veterans Administration Hospital

408 First Avenue, New York, New York, 10010

The initial reception of endoscopic retrograde cholangiopancreatography (ERCP), particularly in North America, was tinged with pessimism and skepticism (1,2). In the short span of two years, a spate of reports documenting experiences at centers throughout the world testifies to the rapid development of individual skill in the technique and to the value of ERCP in the clinical management of pancreatic and biliary tract diseases (3,4,5,6,7). Therefore, it seems appropriate to venture an estimate of the future clinical and research value of this tool so that individuals and institutions will be encouraged to invest the time and treasure necessary to master the technic. The opinion expressed here results from experience gained through more than 400 attempts at endoscopic retrograde cannulation of the papilla of Vater.

Endoscopy: Fiberoptic endoscopy is the best general method currently available for the diagnosis or exclusion of upper gastrointestinal tract pathology (8,9). Endoscopy has greater precision than barium contrast radiography in detecting lesions that deform the mucosa (peptic ulcer, submucosal tumors or mucosal malignancies). In addition, endoscopy allows the diagnosis of subtle alterations of the mucosal surface (esophagitis, esophagogastric varices, gastritis, duodenitis, and early carcinoma) that may escape radiography. Modern endoscopy yields mucosal biopsies and samples of gastrointestinal secretion. Although still infrequently used the potential for obtaining cytologic specimens has been emphasized by Japanese endoscopists.

In the current medical circumstance where the daily cost of hospitalization is high, endoscopy allows the examination of the upper tract before the traditional exclusion of colonic disease by barium enema in a patient where symptoms or signs may be the result of either upper or lower gastrointestinal tract disease. Since barium is not introduced, endoscopy may be followed immediately by cannulation of the papilla of Vater, angiography, laparoscopy, colonoscopy, barium enema, intravenous pyelography, or surgical intervention if necessary. For these reasons, upper gastrointestinal tract endoscopy has rapidly come to the forefront as a primary diagnostic procedure for patients suspected of having disease of the upper gastrointestinal tract, pancreas or biliary tract.

In jaundiced patients or patients suspected of having pancreatic disease, we combine endoscopy and endoscopic retrograde cholangiopancreatography as a primary diagnostic procedure. The endoscopy is performed with the Olympus JFB cannulating duodenoscope on the x-ray couch. If a diagnosis is not established by the endoscopic portion of the examination, the papilla of Vater is cannulated and pancreatography or cholangiography performed. In a consecutive series of 91 patients, this approach established a correct clinical diagnosis in 85% of patients (10). Since the procedure requires no preparation except fasting, it may be performed on an out-patient basis. It does not incur the risk of hemorrhage or bile peritonitis or the necessity for the hospitalization or immediate surgery of transhepatic cholangiography, transjugular cholangiography, or minilaparotomy.

Pancreatography: Since the pancreatic duct exits at right angles from the duodenal wall it is more easily cannulated than the biliary system. Endoscopic pancreatography allows the identification of pancreatic disease and the differentiation of pancreatitis, pancreatic pseudocyst or carcinoma. Although no comparative studies of angiography and pancreatography in the detection of pancreatic carcinoma have been published to date, the pancreatographic patterns observed in pancreatic carcinoma by a number of groups are manifestations of late disease and show gross obstruction or distortion of the pancreatic duct system. These findings suggest that pancreatography will ultimately be demonstrated to have greater precision than angiography in the diagnosis of pancreatic carcinoma and particularly in differentiating chronic pancreatitis from pancreatic carcinoma. The biochemical work up of a patient with suspected pancreatitis or pancreatic insufficiency including fecal fat quantitation, secretin test and the like, has given way to a rapidly performed pancreatogram that is capable of establishing the presence of chronic pancreatic disease (Fig. 1) and ruling in or out an operative lesion in the pancreatic duct system or obstruction suspicious of carcinoma.

We have performed more than 100 pancreatograms in patients with pancreatic inflammatory disease and find the technique extremely

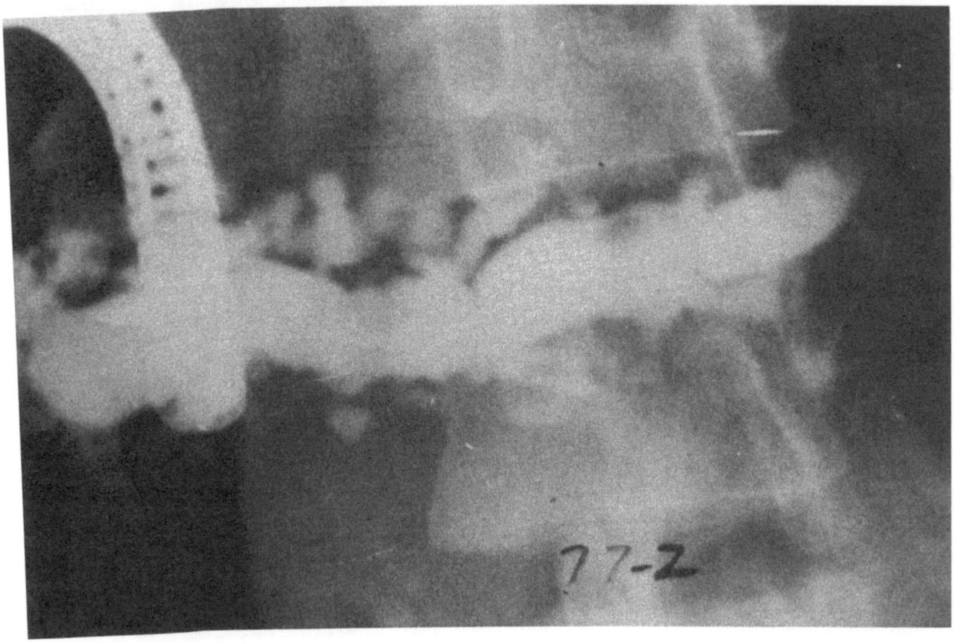

Fig. 1 Endoscopic pancreatogram in a patient without a previous history of abdominal pain or pancreatic calcification demonstrating markedly dilated pancreatic duct system with a reduction in overall length of the pancreas indicative of chronic pancreatitis with pancreatic exocrine insufficiency.

useful in classifying patients with pancreatitis and finding those with operable lesions (11). The preoperative pancreatogram allows the surgeon to plan his operation and his incision in advance (Fig. 2). He may approach a portion of the pancreas if necessary and need not enter the duodenum or perform an operative pancreatogram. If a sphincterotomy has been performed in the past, it can be examined endoscopically and its function ascertained. Similarly a distal pancreatic drainage operation (pancreaticojejunostomy) can be examined by retrograde pancreatography to determine if the anastomosis is patent and adequately drains the pancreas. These advantages of endoscopic pancreatography hopefully will initiate a new era in the treatment of pancreatic disease. Early precise classification of pancreatic inflammatory disease with the detection of strictures or duct blockage is now possible (Fig. 3). The appropriate surgical remedies undertaken to relieve these self-perpetuating obstructive lesions can now be evaluated by post-operative pancreatography. It should be possible to establish

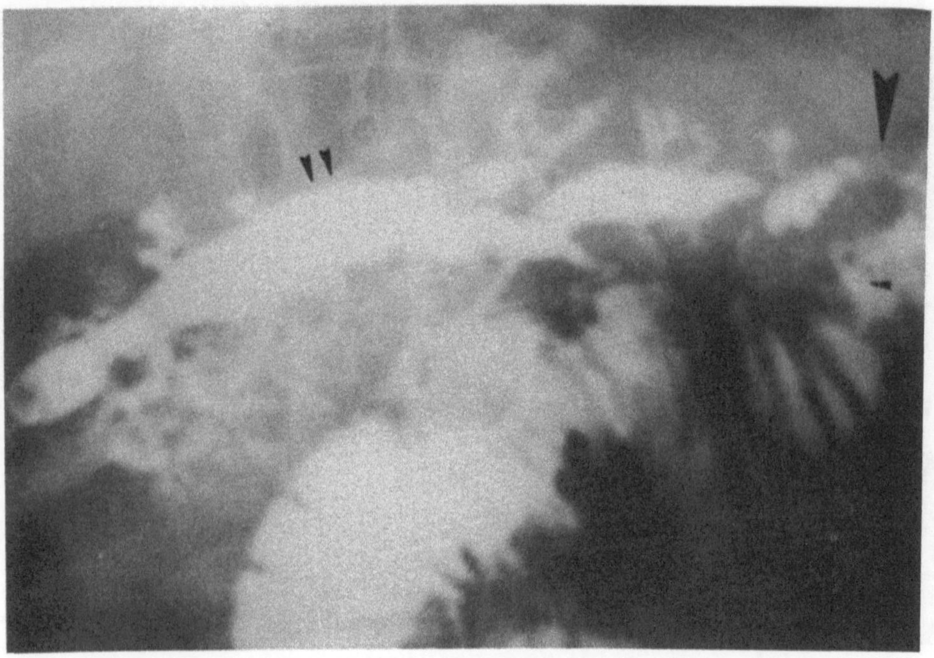

Fig. 2 Endoscopic pancreatogram demonstrating moderate dilatation of the pancreatic duct system with obstruction in the head of the pancreas indicating chronic pancreatitis (small arrow). Distal pancreatectomy and pancreaticojejunostomy have been performed and the dye injected through the stenosed head of the pancreas exits through pancreatico-jejunostomy demonstrating its patency (large arrow).

precise indications for pancreatic surgery and the efficacy of various surgical procedures. The picture for pancreatic carcinoma remains bleak since the majority of lesions are found late in their course when the opportunity for resection is past. This circumstance will only be reversed by the free use of pancreatography at an early time when symptoms are subtle.

The research value of pancreatography with its potential for sampling pancreatic secretion directly from the duct system and measuring pressure within the pancreatic duct system or across the papilla of Vater is already being explored. Nebel (12) has recently reported the normal transsphincter pressure in the pancreas to be 28 mm of mercury as measured at cannulation of the papilla of Vater and has documented the efficacy of atropine and glucagon in reducing sphincter pressure.

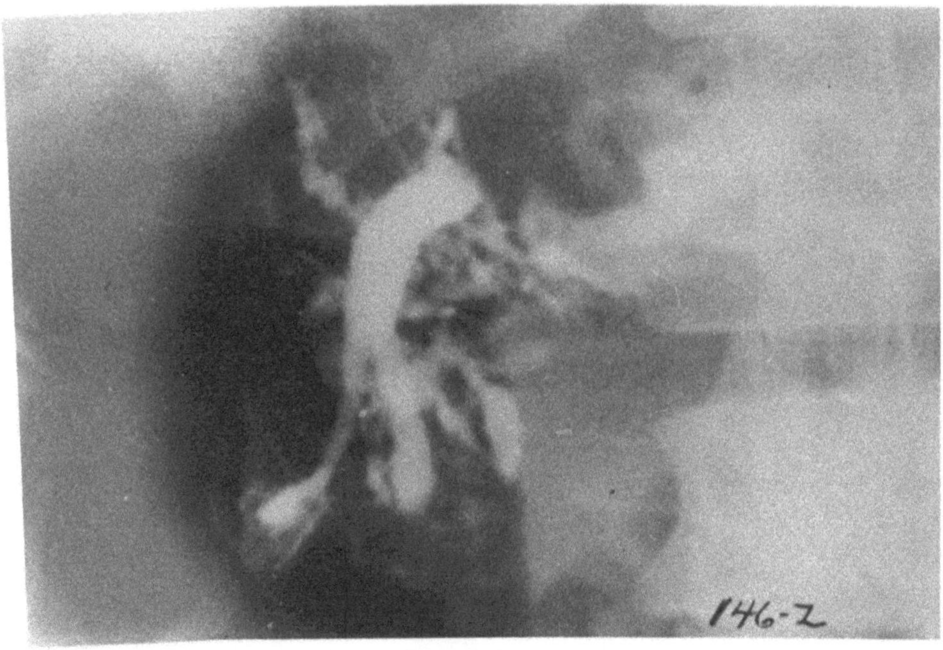

Fig. 3 Endoscopic pancreatogram demonstrating a short segment of pancreatic duct in the pancreatic head. The duct system in the pancreatic head is dilated indicating chronic pancreatitis. The acute obstruction of the duct system could be due to superimposed carcinoma of the pancreas or pancreatic pseudocyst. In this case a pancreatic pseudocyst was found at surgery and drained.

Cholangiography: Endoscopic retrograde cholangiography has made both simple and safe the visualization of the extrahepatic biliary tree, gallbladder and cystic duct in patients with jaundice, liver disease or non functioning gallbladder after oral cholecystography. The impact of this new technique for visualizing the biliary tract in individuals with jaundice need not be emphasized. Retrograde cholangiography excludes biliary tract obstruction (Fig. 4). The usefulness of this procedure in gallbladder disease is yet to be explored. When oral cholecystography fails and cholecystectomy is contemplated, retrograde cholangiography allows confirmation of gallbladder disease, demonstrates the anatomy of the biliary tract and allows exclusion of common duct stone prior to surgery. In particular, the intraoperative decision as to the advisability of exploring the common bile duct or the necessity to perform an operative cholangiogram is obviated by the preoperative retrograde cholangiography.

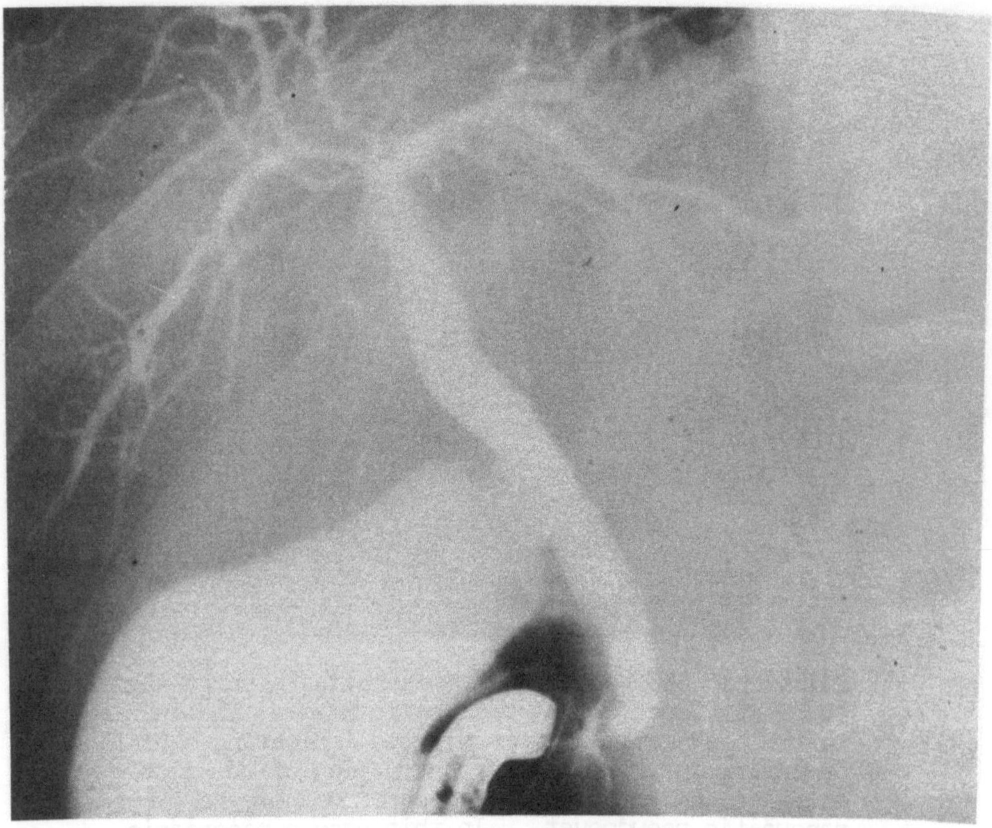

Fig. 4 Retrograde cholangiogram in a patient with known cirrhosis, a portacaval shunt performed three years earlier and presenting with jaundice. Cholangiography demonstrates a normal common bile duct without obstruction. The gall-bladder contains multiple radiolucent stones. The intrahepatic biliary tree is diffusely distorted and irregular compatible with cirrhosis.

In experienced hands retrograde cholangiography is successful in more than 90% of cases. By contrast, even when bilirubin levels are below 3 mg% intravenous cholangiography fails to visualize the common bile duct adequately in 30 to 40% of patients. When the surgeon relies on intraoperative examination to determine the need for common duct exploration, many common ducts are explored unnecessarily (range 28-73%) or common ducts are not explored when stones are present (4%) (13). Common duct exploration with the placement of a T-tube prolongs the patient's hospital course and adds a small but distinct risk of common duct injury. This should be avoided when not necessary. The retained common duct stone in

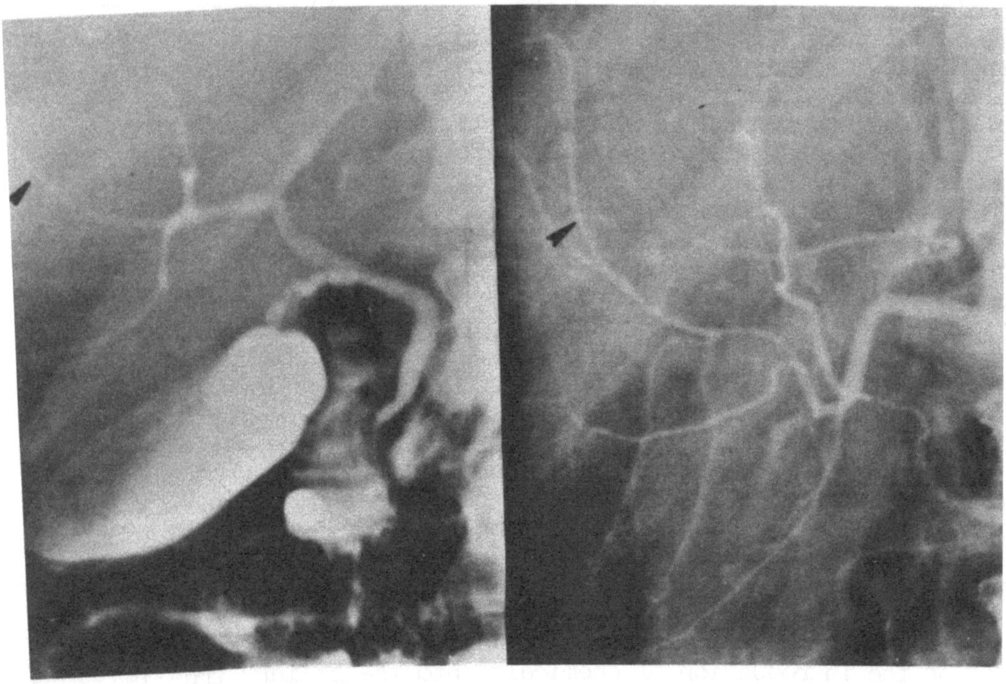

Fig. 5 Retrograde cholangiography on the left demonstrates widely splayed intrahepatic bile ducts displaced by a mass within the center of right hepatic lobe. Angiography in the right hand picture demonstrates an identical displacement of hepatic arterial branches. This 43 year old diabetic was admitted to hospital with fever and right upper quadrant pain. Cholecystitis was suspected. Retrograde cholangiography demonstrated a normal extrahepatic biliary tract and the presence of a hepatic abscess. Confirmatory arteriogram was then performed.

the absence of a T-tube is a serious problem that frequently leads to a second operative procedure. This cholecystectomy conundrum can be alleviated by the use of preoperative retrograde cholangiography.

Retrograde cholangiography provides a unique opportunity to visualize the intrahepatic biliary tree. It allows the diagnosis of specific diseases of the intrahepatic bile ducts (Caroli's disease) or the presence of intrahepatic ductal stones. Since the intrahepatic bile ducts lie within the portal triad, the same diagnostic potential exists for the intrahepatic cholangiogram as for visualization of the portal venous or the hepatic arterial systems. By visualizing the intrahepatic bile ducts, the presence of hepatic cirrhosis, hepatic infiltrative diseases (fatty liver, sarcoidosis, myelofibrosis), and the presence of hepatic mass lesions (abscess, tumor) may be appreciated (Fig. 5). In comparison with the noninvasive technique of scanning, intrahepatic cholangiography offers the accuracy of venography or arteriography. Umbilical vein venography requires a surgical procedure. The contrast between arteriography and intrahepatic cholangiography is important since these techniques should yield similar diagnostic results. As yet, there is no study comparing the risks or sensitivity of the two methods. Retrograde cholangiography does not require the expensive equipment necessary for selective angiography. Furthermore, in cholangiography no radio-opaque contrast is actually within the body and contraindications such as allergy to the contrast material or renal disease are not operative. In the elderly or those with advanced vascular disease in whom the risk of vascular complications is considerable, retrograde cholangiography might be preferred. Most importantly, the performance of an intrahepatic cholangiogram is simply an extension of a combined diagnostic procedure of endoscopy and endoscopic retrograde cholangiopancreatography. Intrahepatic cholangiography extends the diagnostic spectrum of endoscopic retrograde cholangiopancreatography to diseases within the hepatic parenchyma (14).

The potential for instrumental manipulation with the biliary tract or the introduction of chemicals into the biliary tree is only beginning to be explored. In cholecystitis or cholangitis with obstruction, antibiotics may be injected into the gallbladder or bile duct at cholangiography. We have attempted to extract common duct stones with a Dormia basket in a fashion similar to that used through an indwelling T-tube (Fig. 6) (15). We have also had some success in dislodging mud or small stones during the performance of retrograde cholangiography by forcefully injecting fluid or by passing a 3 mm balloon catheter into the bile duct through the impacted area. In collaboration with Dr. Victor Zakkay, we are developing a double lumen catheter for infusion and withdrawal of sodium cholate into the bile duct through the papilla of Vater. Individual reports of endoscopic electrosurgical sphincterotomy for the relief of impacted common duct stones (16) and endoscopic removal of obstructing material from the bile duct (17) have recently appeared. These early developments preview a field of operative endoscopic cholangiography which may permit the removal or dissolution of obstructing biliary lesions. Simultaneously, opportunities will arise for fruitful research in biliary tract physiology and hepatic excretory function in man.

Early estimates of ERCP suggested that this procedure could be delegated to a technician or that it might be so complex and difficult to be restricted to 10 or 20 major centers in the

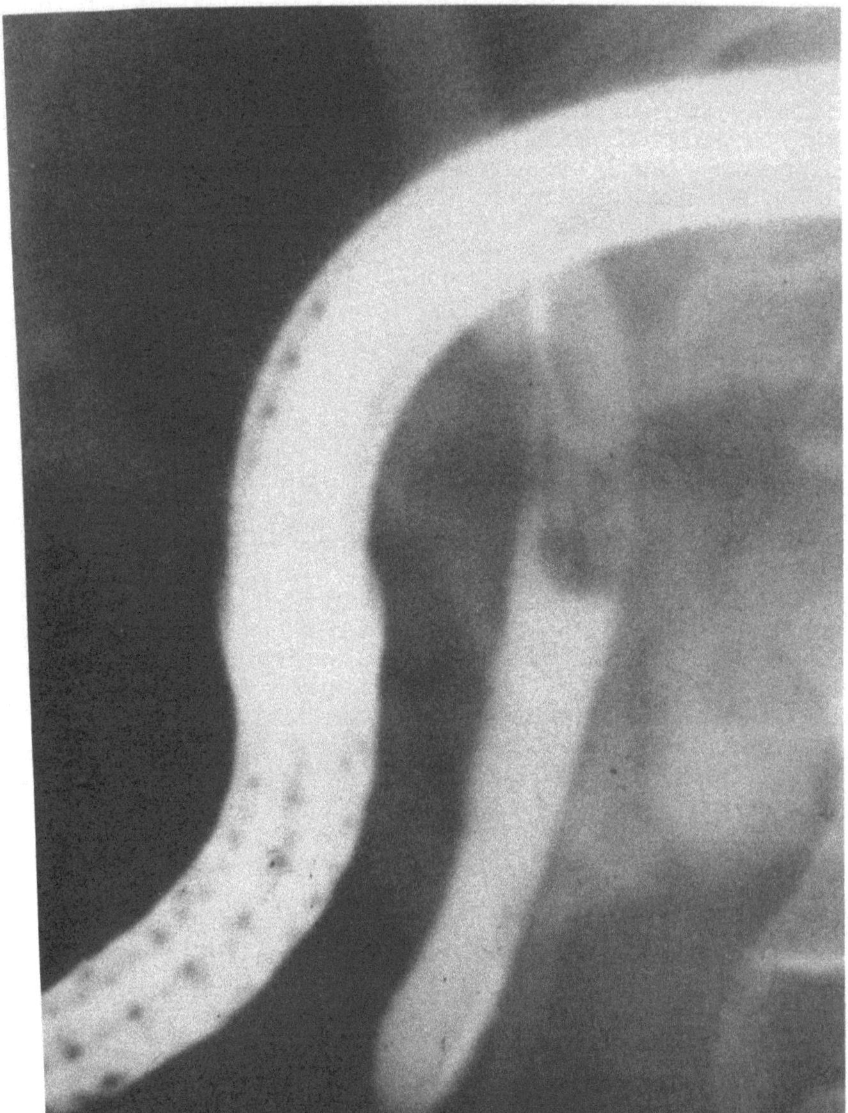

Fig. 6 Retrograde cholangiogram in a patient with a retained common duct stone two months after cholecystectomy for cholelithiasis. Dormia basket introduced through the papilla of Vater (15mm in diameter) has been opened within the common bile duct and grasps the stone. This large cholesterol stone (1.3 cm in diameter) could not be fractured by compressing the basket and was too large to remove through the papilla of Vater. It was removed surgically on the following day.

United States. The rapid development of individual skill in performing the technique and advances in its application for the diagnosis and management of biliary tract diseases, suggest a much broader role. ERCP is a valuable tool that can be at the disposal of any individual wishing to devote the time and effort to develop his personal skill and any institution that supports his development. The broad value of this technique for both the diagnosis and eventual treatment of disease in the pancreas and biliary tract suggests that it is a diagnostic maneuver essential to the armamentarium of those wishing to diagnose and manage disease of the pancreas, biliary tract and liver.

SUMMARY

The technique of endoscopic retrograde cholangiopancreatography (ERCP) is a combined endoscopic and radiographic procedure that has great diagnostic potential and relatively little hazard. The procedure combines endoscopic examination of the upper gastrointestinal tract with pancreatography for visualization of the pancreatic duct system and cholangiography for visualization of the biliary tree, gallbladder and intrahepatic biliary radicles. In addition to diagnosis this technique allows for instrumentation of both the pancreatic and biliary ducts. This rapidly evolving technique provides opportunities which have yet to be fully evaluated, but which hold promise for dramatically advancing diagnosis, treatment and research in the areas of pancreatic and biliary tract disease.

REFERENCES

1. MORRISSEY JF: To cannulate or not to cannulate. Gastroenterology 63: 351-352, 1972.

2. INGELFINGER FJ: Endoscopic pancreatocholangiography; progress and problem. New Eng J Med 287: 879-880, 1972.

3. CLASSEN M, KOCH H, DEMLING L: Diagnostische bedeutung der endoskopischen kontrastdarstellung des pankreasgangsystems. Leber Magen Darm 2: 79-81, 1972.

4. COTTON PB, SALMON PR, BLUMGART LH, et al: Cannulation of papilla of Vater via fiber-duodenoscope. Lancet 1: 53-58, 1972.

5. KASUGAI T, KUNO N, KOBAYASHI S, et al: Endoscopic pancreatocholangiography. I. The normal endoscopic pancreatocholangiogram. Gastroenterology 63: 217-226, 1972.

6. KASUGAI T, KUNO N, KIZU M, et al: Endoscopic pancreatocholangiography. II. The pathological endoscopic pancreatocholangiogram. Gastroenterology 63: 227-234, 1972.

7. VENNES JA, JACOBSON JR, SILVIS SE: Endoscopic cholangiography for biliary system diagnosis. Ann Int Med 80: 61-64, 1974.

8. COTTON PB, ROSENBERG MT, WALDRAM RPL, et al: Early endoscopy of oesophagus, stomach, and duodenal bulb in patients with haematemesis and melaena. Brit med J 378: 505-509, 1973.

9. NEBEL OT, FARRELL RL, KIRCHNER JP et al: Duodenoscopy in the evaluation of patients with upper gastrointestinal symptoms. Gastrointestinal Endoscopy 19: 142-143, 1973.

10. BRESLAW JS, KESSLER RE, ZIMMON DS: Diagnosis of pancreatic and biliary disease by endoscopy combined with retrograde cholangiography and pancreatography (abstract). Gastroenterology 64: 704, 1973.

11. ZIMMON DS, FALKENSTEIN DB, ABRAMS RM, et al: Endoscopic retrograde cholangiopancreatography in the diagnosis of pancreatic inflammatory disease . Radiology (in press).

12. NEBEL OT: Endoscopic manometry: A new technique for the physiologic study of the human sphincter of Oddi (abstract). Gastro Endo 20: 182, 1974.

13. WAY LW, ADMIRAND WH, DUNPHY JE: Management of choledocholithiasis. Ann Surg 176: 347-359, 1972.

14. FALKENSTEIN DB, RICCOBONO C, ABRAMS R et al: The endoscopic retrograde intrahepatic cholangiogram (abstract). Gastro Endo 20: 179, 1974.

15. BURHENNE HJ: Nonoperative retained biliary tract stone extraction: a new roentgenologic technique. Am J Roent, Radium Therapy & Nuclear Med 117: 388-399, 1973.

16. KAWAI K, AKASAKA Y, MORAKAMI K, et al: Endoscopic sphincterotomy of the ampulla of Vater. Gastro Endo 20: 148-151, 1974.

17. SHAPIRO HA, CARLSON R: "Succotash" cholangitis diagnosis by retrograde endoscopic cholangiography (abstract). Gastro Endo 20: 185, 1974.

5. [illegible] T, [illegible] M, et al: Endoscopic pancreato-cholangiography. III: The pathological endoscopic pancreatocholangiogram. Gastroenterology 53: 227-233, [illegible]

6. VENNES JA, JACOBSON JR, SILVIS SE: Endoscopic cholangiography for biliary system diagnosis. Ann Intern Med 81: 61-64, 1974

8. [illegible], [illegible] RL, et al: Early endoscopy of oesophagus, stomach, and duodenal bulb in patients with peptic ulcer and [illegible]. Brit Med J [illegible], 1973

9. [illegible] et al: Endoscopy in the evaluation of patients with upper gastrointestinal symptoms. Gastroenterology [illegible], 1972

10. [illegible], ZIMMON DS: Diagnosis of pancreatic and biliary disease by endoscopy combined with retrograde cholangiography and pancreatography. [illegible] Gastroenterology [illegible]

11. [illegible]

12. [illegible]

13. [illegible]

14. [illegible]

THE ADVANTAGES OF PRE-OPERATIVE UMBILICOPORTAL CATHETERIZATION AND VENOGRAPHY IN EXTRAHEPATIC BILIARY OBSTRUCTION

Pierre Lavoie, André Légaré, and André Viallet

Hôpital Saint-Luc, University of Montréal

1058 Rue Saint-Denis, Montréal 129, Québec

Some 350 patients with extrahepatic biliary obstruction have been investigated and operated at the "Hôpital Saint-Luc" of Montreal since 1964.

From this experience, three procedures have proved to be essential in the evaluation of these cases: (1) cholangiography; (2) portography; (3) arteriography.

Each one of these methods has its particular advantages and indications, and must be used accordingly. Even though our surgical team was probably the first to utilize, in 1965, the so-called "minilap" for the investigation of extrahepatic biliary obstruction (16), this complete procedure, including liver biopsy, transhepatic cholangiography, umbilical vein catheterization with portography and manometry, has been considered too often unnecessary to be performed routinely, as recently proposed by others (19, 23). As an example, there is absolutely no need of liver biopsy and portal catheterization in common calculous biliary tract obstruction.

For this reason, a sequential approach has been rather preferred in the investigation of icteric patients.

Since the differential diagnosis between hepato-cellular and obstructive jaundice is usually easy, the real problem resides in the distinction between intrahepatic and extrahepatic cholestasis. This situation will sometimes require pre-operative cholangiography (17), which can be performed in many ways: percutaneous transhepatic (5,20), trans-vesicular under laparoscopic control (1), trans-jugular (7), retrogradely at endoscopy (2), or even more simply, after a 3 cm laparotomy under local or general anesthesia (12,15,16,19,23).

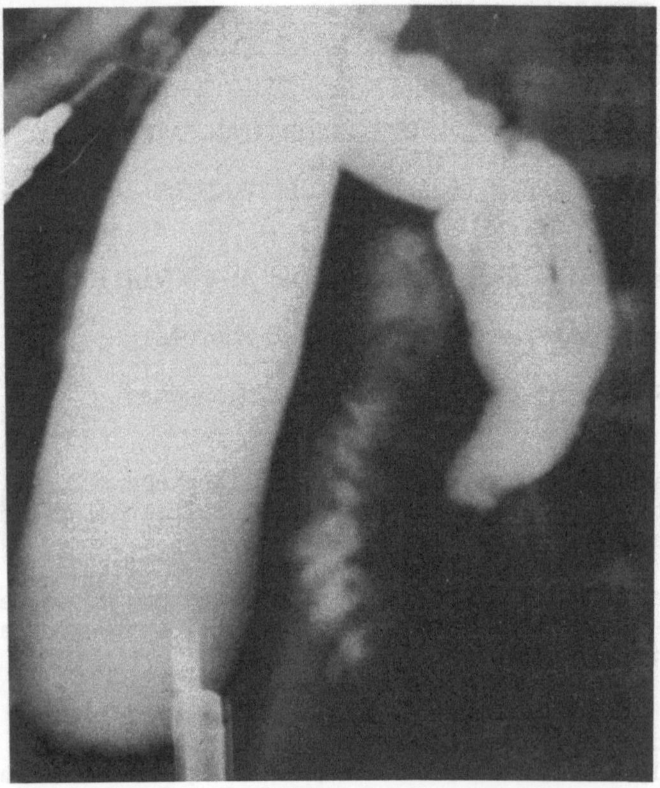

Fig. 1: Trans-vesicular cholangiography under laparoscopic control (as performed by Dr. André Viallet). Nearly complete obstruction of the common duct with Courvoisier's gallbladder, typical of a distal choledochal carcinoma.

When gallstones are the presumed cause of biliary tract obstruction, the patient can be brought to surgery and a cholangiogram obtained during the operation. Whenever there is suspicion of malignancy, the cholangiography must be performed preoperatively. If a diagnosis of calculous obstruction is in fact determined, appropriate surgery is accomplished without further investigation, possibly during the same anesthesia when the examination has been realized by "minilap". If gallstone cholestasis is ruled out, the level and the appearance of the obstruction generally permit the diagnosis of a benign lesion (stenosis of the sphincter of Oddi, pancreatitis) or a cancer (16). In this last eventuality, it is even possible to ascertain regularly a precise diagnosis of ampulloma, cancer of the distal common duct (Fig. 1), or cancer of the head of the pancreas (Fig. 2), each of these implying, of course, different prognoses and specific indications as regards the extent of the operation (6,16,18,20).

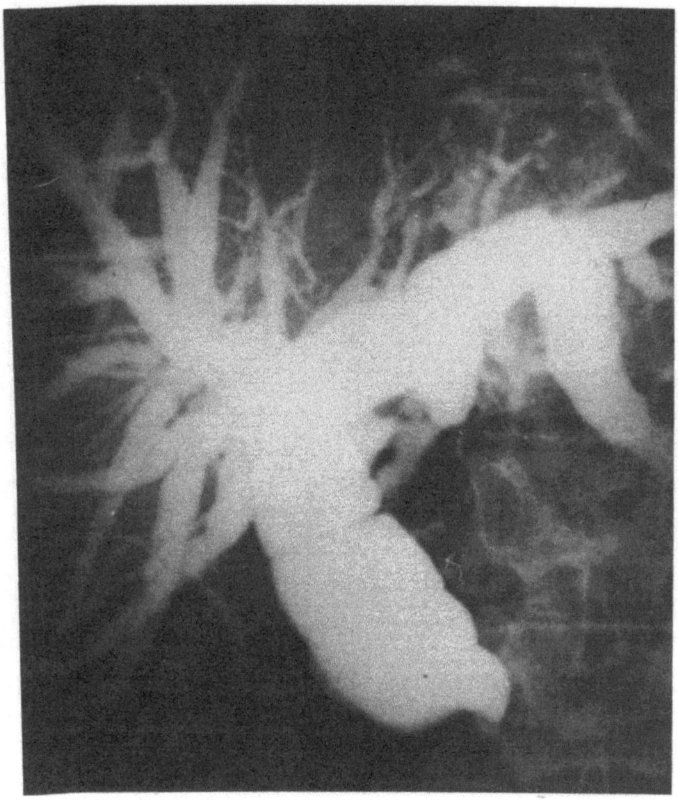

Fig. 2: Cancer of the head of the pancreas as revealed by total biliary tract obstruction with rat-tailing effect at the superior margin of the gland. The gallbladder had been removed anteriorly.

When a malignant lesion is recognized as the cause of biliary tract obstruction, complementary information is mandatory. It is best obtained by portal catheterization and venography (4,12,15, 16,18), which indicates whether or not there is invasion of the venous system and usually permits a sound appreciation of the liver parenchyma as regards the presence or absence of metastases.

Finally, if hepatic or pancreatic resection is contemplated, arteriography must be performed to rule out any anatomic anomaly, such as a right hepatic artery originating from the superior mesenteric artery, whose accidental ligation could obviously result in serious complications (3). Arteriography however should not be considered as very useful for the positive diagnosis of jaundice secondary to extrahepatic obstruction.

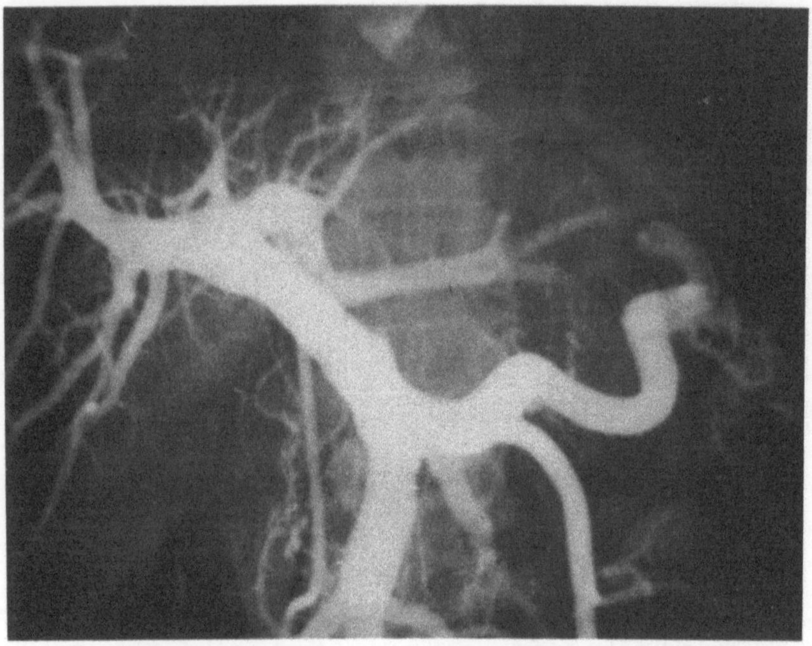

Fig. 3: Normal portogram after umbilicoportal catheterization. Precise delineation of the superior mesenteric and splenic veins. The absence of portal involvement allowed a Whipple procedure in this patient with cancer of the head of the pancreas.

Several authors have resorted to umbilicoportal catheterization following the initial report of Gonzalez (Carbalhaes). Our group has improved the original technique of simple catheterization of the left branch of the portal vein by positioning the catheter exactly into the portal and splenic veins, as desired, so permitting complete opacification of the whole splanchnic area and collateral circulation (Fig. 3). This technique of selective catheterization has been described elsewhere (12-15).

In our institution, more than 400 cases of portal catheterization via the round ligament of the liver have been performed during the past ten years, with no mortality and a very low morbidity. Most authors have reported a significant degree of failures with this procedure. In contrast, our last 150 consecutive cases have been successful in the exact positioning of the catheter within the portal vein, with a 90% rate of selective splenic catheterization provided this vein was still patent. These very good results can perhaps be explained by the fact that the technique has continuously been performed by the same team of surgeons.

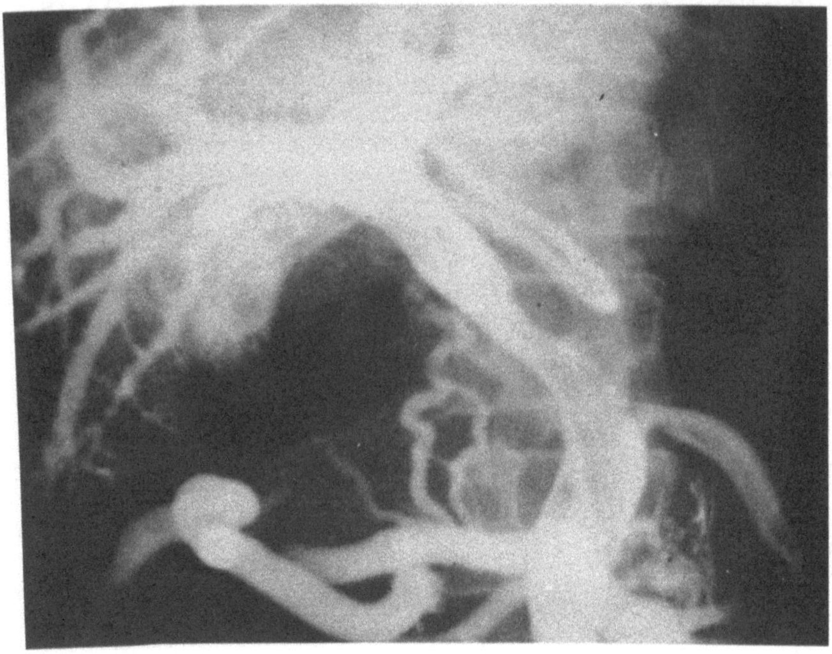

Fig. 4: Cancer of the pancreas with major invasion of the superior mesenteric vein and malignant amputation of the splenic vein. Portal obstruction resulting in segmental portal hypertension with hepatopetal and mesentericolumbar (Retzius) collaterals. Biliary diversion was the only possible procedure.

The most obvious indication of portal catheterization is the investigation of portal hypertension, usually secondary to cirrhosis of the liver, where a complete hemodynamic evaluation is compulsory when considering surgical therapy. In such circumstances, the insertion of a catheter into the portal system provides, among other advantages, more reliable portograms (12,15), precise assessment of the portal pressure and the level of obstruction (10,11,21, 22) and simultaneous estimation of hepatic and portal blood flows (9).

Another application of this approach has been in the evaluation of expanding lesions within the liver: abcesses, cysts, benign tumors, hepatomas, and metastases. The information thus obtained is absolutely necessary when considering surgery (12,15).

A last very important indication of this method is in the evaluation of biliary tract obstruction by a malignant tumor. Since venous invasion usually precedes arterial involvement (16,18), portography is certainly superior to arteriography in the assessment of operability.

First, a fine delineation of the mesentericoportal axis is possible (Fig. 3). This is an important point when one considers that pancreatoduodenal cancers invade primarily the superior mesenteric vein (Fig. 4), whose opacification cannot be obtained by any other pre-operative method including splenoportography (4). The venous phase of celiac and superior mesenteric arteriographies reveals gross invasion only.

Second, umbilicoportal catheterization with portography permits the detection of very small liver metastases which could escape even accurate surgical exploration, particularly when located within the parenchyma (12,15).

Every patient must then be considered as an individual case. An exact diagnosis of gallstones, pancreatitis, cancer of the ampulla of Vater, of the common duct or of the head of the pancreas, is to be recognized as the cause of biliary tract obstruction prior to surgery. One must also establish if a curative or palliative treatment is to be undertaken, and when a resection is contemplated, what should be its extent.

A curative resection for cancer of the head of the pancreas is indeed a radical procedure (Fig. 5). It implies a clean denudation of the hepatic artery, the mesentericoportal vein, and

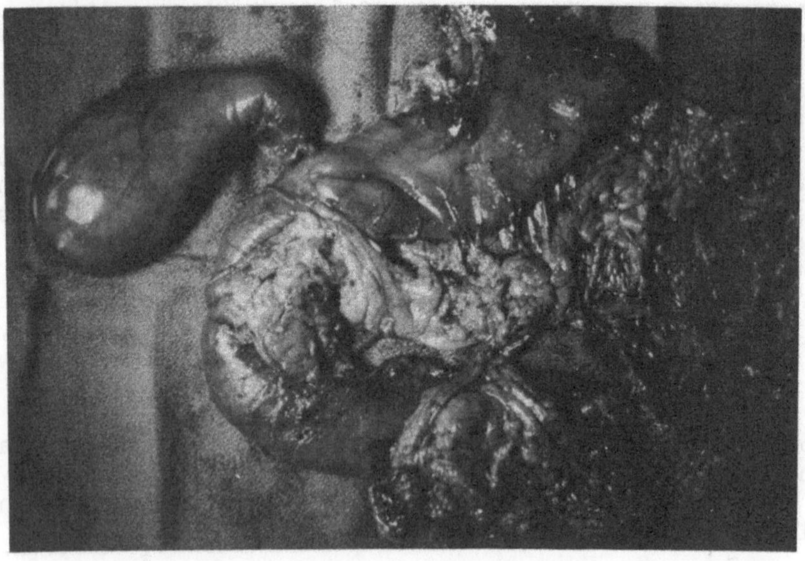

Fig. 5: Anatomic specimen after a radical Whipple procedure for cancer of the head of the pancreas without portal invasion, as shown in Figure 3.

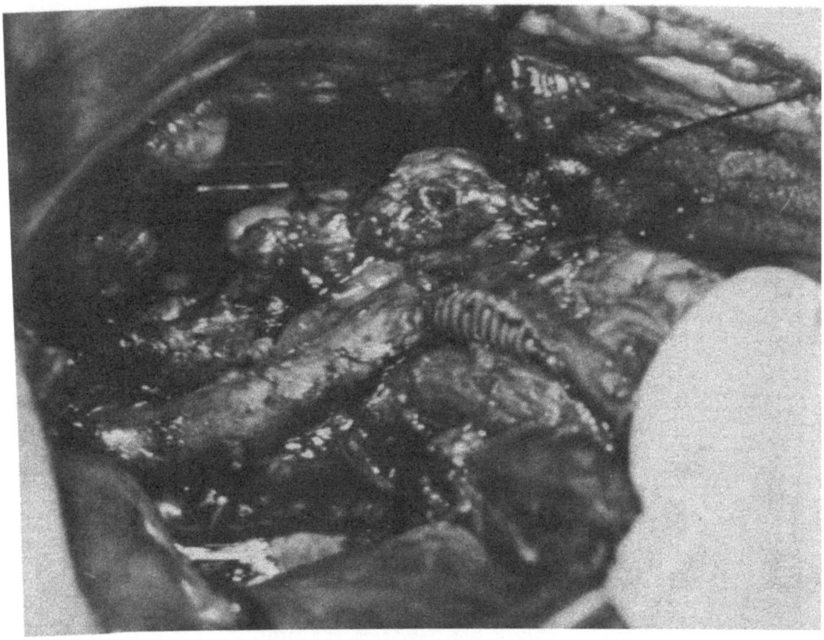

Fig. 6: Prosthetic roofing of the superior mesenteric vein after pancreatoduodenectomy with lateral excision of the vein for parietal involvement.

the inferior vena cava. A Whipple procedure effected for the treatment of an ampulloma does not need to be that extensive. This is also true of pancreatoduodenectomies done for palliation or for pancreatitis. Palliative Whipple resection is sometimes the soundest approach for well-circumscribed cancers. Such decisions necessitate information disclosed only by an appropriate investigation.

Moreover, surgeons generally reject resection of a cancer when there is any invasion of the portal vein (4). A more circumspect approach may prove to be very fruitful (8). A patient with cancer of the pancreas involving the superior mesenteric vein has been submitted to a Whipple procedure with parietal excision of the vein and a prosthetic roofing (Fig. 6). He is still doing well, with no sign of recurrence, more than two years after his operation. Another one had total pancreatoduodenectomy with segmental excision of the portal vein (Fig. 7), because she was very young and her tumor was still well localized in spite of gross portal involvement. She regrettably did not survive the operation, but the operation most likely to cure her had been tried. Such decisions cannot be taken too lightly, when hurried by the limitations imposed by the operating time. These delicate problems must be solved before

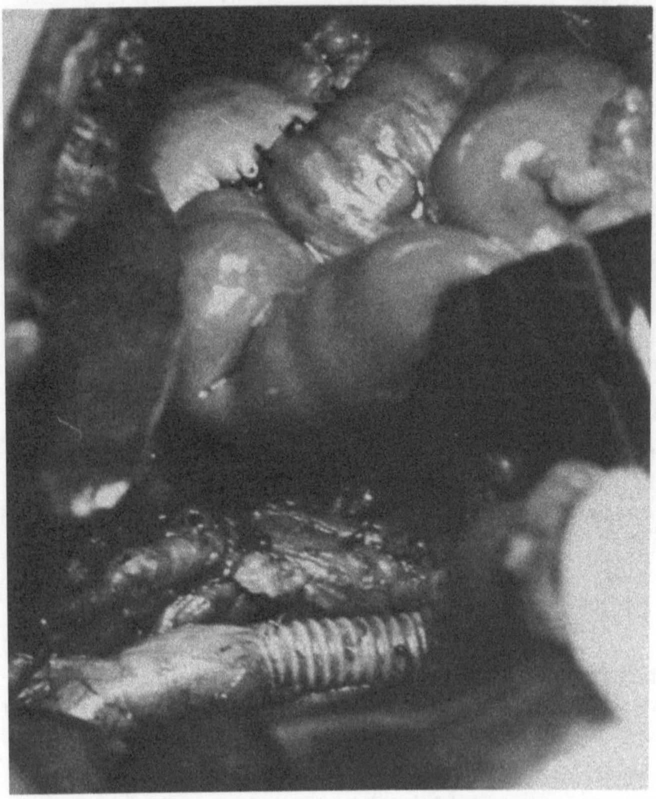

Fig. 7: Segmental excision of the portal vein with graft replacement. A pancreatoduodenectomy was carried out despite gross venous invasion because of the patient's young age and a particularly well circumscribed tumor.

surgery, so that both the patient and the surgeon can be adequately prepared.

It seems reasonable to think that many surgeons, when confronted with an unexpected cancer of the pancreatoduodenal region, will not consider a resection, even though feasible, since the problem is of such magnitude that one must be psychologically and technically ready to proceed.

In other cases, surgery is attempted, and after perhaps hours of tedious dissection, the surgeon realizes that the tumor cannot be sensibly removed because of invasion of essential vessels (4). At that time, the stomach, the common duct and the pancreas may have been transsected, and the final resection unavoidable. It is indeed always difficult, often impossible, to assess the resectability of a malignant tumor on operative findings only, not to mention the precious time spent in that manner. Currently, such an attitude is inappropriate since these trying situations, usually lethal, can be prevented by a simple, yet adequate, preoperative investigation.

In conclusion, it should be emphasized that rushed operations must be discouraged in dealing with surgical jaundice. In fact, we know of no biliary obstruction which commands emergency surgery, apart from purulent cholangitis with septicemic shock where the biliary tract must be quickly decompressed in order to prevent acute renal tubular necrosis.

It is naive to think that all the problems are solved at laparotomy. Pancreatoduodenal cancer is a severe and complex disease requiring vigorous and experienced surgery (4). Relying constantly upon the same team of physicians and surgeons for its treatment seems to be a most promising and beneficial approach.

SUMMARY

From a series of 350 patients with extrahepatic biliary obstruction observed in 10 years, three procedures of investigation are considered: cholangiography, portography, and arteriography.

Transhepatic cholangiography is the first choice method in the etiologic diagnosis of cholestasis. It is useful in intrahepatic and peremptory in extrahepatic obstruction. The anatomic aspect of the biliary block can even furnish a diagnosis of ampulloma, cancer of the common duct or the pancreas.

Surgery is readily undertaken in gallstone obstruction. Preoperative portography is imperative to assess resectability when malignancy is detected.

The disclosing of vascular anomalies is the main interest of arteriography whenever pancreatic or hepatic resection is anticipated.

Over 400 umbilicoportal catheterizations have been performed in 10 years with a 100% success rate in the last 150 cases. Most of them were done for the investigation of portal hypertension, others for expanding lesions of the liver, and at last, for the assessment of operability in malignant obstruction of the biliary tract.

The gravity of pancreatoduodenal cancers is emphasized and a preoperative specialized approach is urged for their investigation and adequate treatment.

REFERENCES

1. BERCI G, MORGENSTERN L, SHORE JM, et al: A direct approach to the differential diagnosis of jaundice. Laparoscopy with transhepatic cholecystocholangiography. Am J Surg 126: 372-378, 1973.

2. BLUMGART LH, SALMON P, COTTON PB, et al: Endoscopy and retrograde choledochopancreatography in the diagnosis of the jaundiced patient. Lancet 2: 1269-1273, 1972.

3. BRITTAIN RS, MARCHIORO TL, HERMANN G, et al: Accidental hepatic artery ligation in humans. Am J Surg 107: 822-832, 1964.

4. CHILD CG, FREY CF: Pancreaticoduodenectomy. Surg C N A 46: 1201-1213, 1966.

5. FLEMMA RJ, CAPP MP, SHINGLETON WW: Percutaneous transhepatic cholangiography. Arch Surg 90: 5-10, 1965.

6. GLENN F, THORBJARNARSON B: Carcinoma of the pancreas. Ann Surg 159: 945-958, 1964.

7. HANAFEE W, WEINER M: Transjugular percutaneous cholangiography. Radiology 88: 35-39, 1967.

8. HUBBARD TB Jr: Carcinoma of the head of the pancreas: Resection of the portal vein and portacaval shunt. Ann Surg 147: 935-944, 1958.

9. HUET M, LAVOIE P, VIALLET A: Simultaneous estimation of hepatic and portal blood flows by an indicator dilution technique. J Lab Clin Med 82: 836-846, 1973.

10. JOLY JG, BERNIER J, LAVOIE P, et al: Hemodynamic and radiological evaluation of patients with hepatic or pancreatic disease by combined umbilico-portal and systemic venous catheterization. Can Med Ass J 98: 16-24, 1968.

11. JOLY JG, MARLEAU D, LEGARE A, et al: Bleeding from esophageal varices in cirrhosis of the liver: Hemodynamic and radiological criteria for the selection of potential bleeders through hepatic and umbilicoportal catheterization studies. Can Med Ass J 104: 576-580, 1971.

12. LAVOIE P, JACOB M, LEDUC J, et al: The umbilicoportal approach for the study of splanchnic circulation: Technical, radiological and hemodynamic considerations. Can J Surg 9: 338-343, 1966.

13. LAVOIE P, FERREIRA V, LEGARE A, et al: Phlébographie sélective splénique, mésentérique ou portale par voie ombilicale. Presse Méd 74: 2607-2608, 1966.

14. LAVOIE P, VIALLET A: L'ombilicoportographie. Arch Franc Mal Appareil Digest 55: 915-918, 1966.

15. LAVOIE P, LEGARE A, VIALLET A: Portal catheterization via the round ligament of the liver. Amer J Surg 114: 822-830, 1967.

16. LAVOIE P: Les ictères chirurgicaux. Etude de 140 malades opérés. Union Med Canada 98: 1135-1147, 1969.

17. REDMAN HC, REUTER SR, JOSEPH RR: Roentgenographic evaluation of patients with suspected obstructive jaundice. Surg Gynec Obstet 131: 1100-1104, 1970.

18. SATO T, SAITOH Y, KOYAMA K, et al: Preoperative determination of operability in carcinomas of the pancreas and the periampullary region. Ann Surg 168: 876-886, 1968.

19. STRACK PR, NEWMAN HK, LERNER AG, et al: An integrated procedure for the rapid diagnosis of biliary obstruction, portal hypertension and liver disease of uncertain etiology. New Eng J Med 285: 1225-1231, 1971.

20. THORBJARNARSON B, MUJAHED Z, GLENN F: Percutaneous transhepatic cholangiography. Ann Surg 165: 33-40, 1967.

21. VIALLET A, LEGARE A, LAVOIE P: Hepatic and umbilicoportal catheterization in portal hypertension. Ann N Y Acad Sci 170: 177-192, 1970.

22. VIALLET A, JOLY JG, MARLEAU D, et al: Comparison of free portal venous pressure and wedged hepatic venous pressure in patients with cirrhosis of the liver. Gastroenterology 59: 372-375, 1970.

23. WEXLER MJ, McLEAN APH, SKINNER GB, et al: "Minilap": An accurate, rapid and safe approach to the diagnosis of liver disease and jaundice. Ann Surg 178: 736-744, 1973.

BILIARY EXCRETORY FUNCTION AND EXCRETORY PATTERNS IN INFANTILE CRYPTOGENIC CHOLESTASIS

M.M. Thaler

University of California

San Francisco, California 94143

INTRODUCTION

Cholestasis is the hallmark of all liver disease in infancy. Neonatal cholestatic jaundice occurs in conditions which differ widely in etiology and outcome, including heritable metabolic disorders (galactosemia, alpha-1-antitrypsin deficiency, cystic fibrosis, storage diseases) and intrauterine infections (cytomegalic inclusion disease, syphilis, toxoplasmosis). In a large majority of infants with cholestasis, however, the underlying liver disorder is not readily apparent.

Cryptogenic infantile cholestasis[1] may be classified into two broad categories of hepatobiliary pathology. Type I cholestasis is a manifestation of primary parenchymal dysfunction which may be of multiple origin and is usually misnamed "neonatal hepatitis". Type II cholestasis reflects structural malformations of the biliary system, mainly variants of intrahepatic and extrahepatic biliary atresia and choledochal cysts (1). Atresias of the major extrahepatic biliary passages account for nearly 90% of duct abnormalities in newborns. Most are inoperable and uniformly lethal.

Distinction between the two types of infantile cholestasis is relatively difficult, because physical findings and results of standard liver function tests lack specificity at this age. Many young infants with cryptogenic cholestasis are surgically explored

1 This term is preferable to "neonatal obstructive jaundice" which suggests a mechanical block.

in search of the rare duct malformations which can be repaired. This invasive diagnostic approach is potentially harmful to those with parenchymal liver disease (2). Non-surgical means of separating primary hepatocellular lesions from biliary abnormalities include measurement of ^{131}I-Rose Bengal quantitative fecal excretion (3,4), red cell peroxidation (5,6), lipoprotein X (7), and serum bile salts (8). These procedures reflect - directly in the case of ^{131}I-Rose Bengal, indirectly in the rest - the relative efficiency with which biliary components are excreted by the liver. It is apparent, therefore, that the clinical usefulness of available diagnostic aids depends on whether quantitative differences in biliary excretion exist between the two types of cryptogenic cholestasis.

The qualitative aspects of biliary function have received little attention, although bile formation and secretion are intermittent processes influenced by nutritional, hormonal (circadian?) and other factors (9). The periodicity in bile flow caused by these factors may be eliminated in patients in whom the major biliary passages are blocked or absent; in patients with severe liver disease bile flow may be greatly reduced but its irregularities preserved in the presence of intact extrahepatic bile ducts.

Studies were undertaken in infants with cryptogenic cholestasis to characterize the quantitative and qualitative aspects of biliary excretory function in the two major types of infantile liver disease.

STUDY PROTOCOL

Study subjects were selected among infants admitted to the University of California Medical Center, San Francisco, for investigation of liver disease in the first three months after birth. Known causes of infantile liver disease were excluded with appropriate metabolic studies and cultures. Infants with cryptogenic cholestasis who were unable to excrete more than 10% of radioactivity in feces during the 72-hour period following intravenous injection of a standard dose of ^{131}I-Rose Bengal were chosen for performance of the entire study protocol. Parental consent was obtained in all cases.

Standard 72-hour ^{131}I-Rose Bengal fecal excretion tests were performed as previously described (4). For kinetic studies, 3 uCi/Kg of the labeled dye was injected intravenously after administration of Lugol's iodine solution to minimize thyroid uptake. Individual stool specimens were placed in separate plastic containers, weighed, and mixed with preservative solution for storage. Urine was collected separately into plastic bags equipped with catheters and pooled as 12-hour aliquots. Blood (1ml) was obtained by venipuncture at specified intervals. Radioactivity in blood, urine and feces was measured in a Nuclear Chicago gamma counter and results analyzed as described elsewhere (4).

Red cell peroxidation tests were performed by the procedure of Lubin et al, (5), and serum bile salts were determined by methods employed in previous studies (10).

The entire protocol was repeated in each subject after one month, and again after complete recovery from Type I cholestasis. Infants with persistent severe biliary insufficiency for one month in whom percutaneous liver biopsies suggested Type II cholestasis were surgically explored. The protocol was repeated in infants with extrahepatic biliary atresia 1 to 3 months after surgery. Thus, all study subjects acted as their own controls.

RESULTS

Among 49 infants with cryptogenic cholestasis, 21 had Type I cholestasis ("neonatal hepatitis") and 28 had Type II cholestasis. Of the 28 with Type II cholestasis, 22 had extrahepatic biliary atresia and 6 had intrahepatic biliary atresia or hypoplasia. Quantitative ^{131}I-Rose Bengal fecal excretion tests performed on admission revealed that all 22 infants with extrahepatic biliary atresia and 5 of the 21 infants with Type I cholestasis excreted less than 10% of the total radioactivity (Fig. 1). The remaining 16 infants with Type I cholestasis and all 6 with intrahepatic biliary lesions excreted more than 10% of the radioactive label.

The investigations described in the study protocol were performed in 18 infants with cryptogenic cholestasis whose fecal ^{131}I-Rose Bengal excretion was below 10%. Of these, 8 were shown to have Type I cholestasis ("neonatal hepatitis"), and 10 had Type II cholestasis due to extrahepatic biliary atresia. The results of these tests, summarized in Table I, revealed no differences between infants with Type I cholestasis during the acute "shut-down" phase of hepatocellular dysfunction, and infants with Type II cholestasis. Furthermore, plasma clearance, half-time in plasma (T 1/2), and urinary excretion of ^{131}I-Rose Bengal during the shut-down phase of Type I cholestasis were in the range observed in Type II cholestasis (Table II). Thus, neither quantitative indices nor kinetic measurements differentiated the two types of cholestasis when parenchymal excretory function was severely depressed.

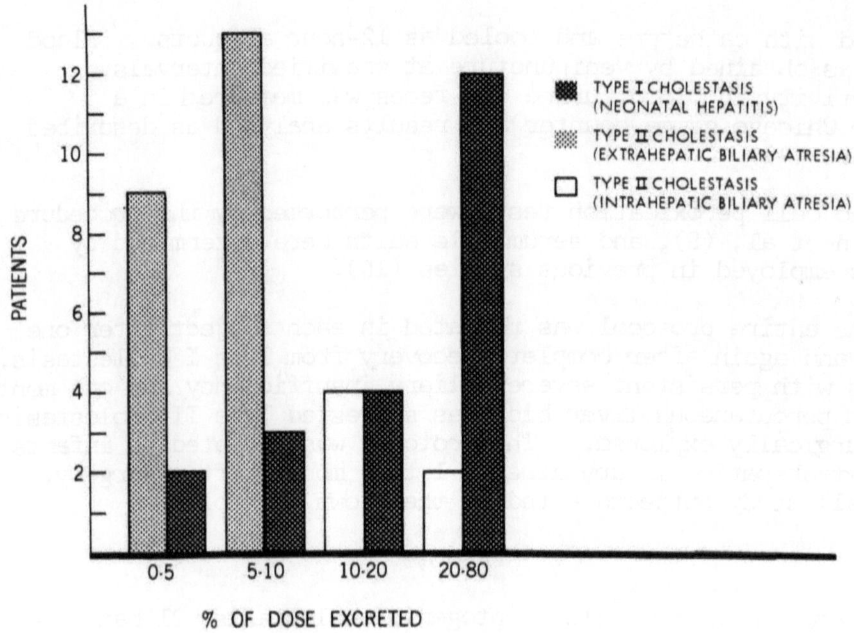

Fig. 1: Total 72-hour fecal excretion of ^{131}I-Rose Bengal in 49 infants with cryptogenic cholestasis.

Resolution of the parenchymal disease process in Type I cholestasis was reflected in increased excretion of radioactive Rose Bengal in feces, increased resistance of red cells to peroxidation, decreased total serum bile salt levels, and gradual reversal of the cholate to chenodeoxycholate ratio (Table I). In the course of recovery, plasma clearance of ^{131}I-Rose Bengal was accelerated, T 1/2 was shortened, and urinary excretion of label was markedly reduced (Table II). No changes in these indices were observed at any time in the course of extrahepatic biliary atresia.

Monitoring of fecal excretion of ^{131}I-Rose Bengal for 72 hours revealed obvious differences in excretory patterns in the two types of cholestasis. The label was excreted at relatively uniform rates in feces of infants with extrahepatic biliary atresia (Fig. 2A). Fecal radioactivity decreased very slowly, in parallel with its clearance from plasma. (Fig 2B). Urinary counts indicated that 7 to 30 times as much radiodye was eliminated by the kidneys compared with the intestine (Fig. 2C). Thus, in "steady state" conditions, i.e. when body compartments were uniformly labeled, plasma clearance reflected mainly renal excretion of Rose Bengal.

TABLE I

INDICES OF BILIARY EXCRETION IN INFANTILE CRYPTOGENIC CHOLESTASIS

TEST	TYPE I CHOLESTASIS			TYPE II CHOLESTASIS
	ACUTE	RESOLVING	RECOVERED	CHRONIC
Quantitative ^{131}I-Rose Bengal (% excreted in feces/72 hours)	<10	15-22	45-80	<10
Red cell peroxidation (%)	80-90	50-80	<10	80-95
Serum bile salt concentrations (ug/ml)				
Cholate	45-200	20-80	-	30-280
Chenodeoxycholate	32-120	15-30	-	45-300
Average cholate/chenodeoxycholate ratio	0.5	1.3	-	0.7

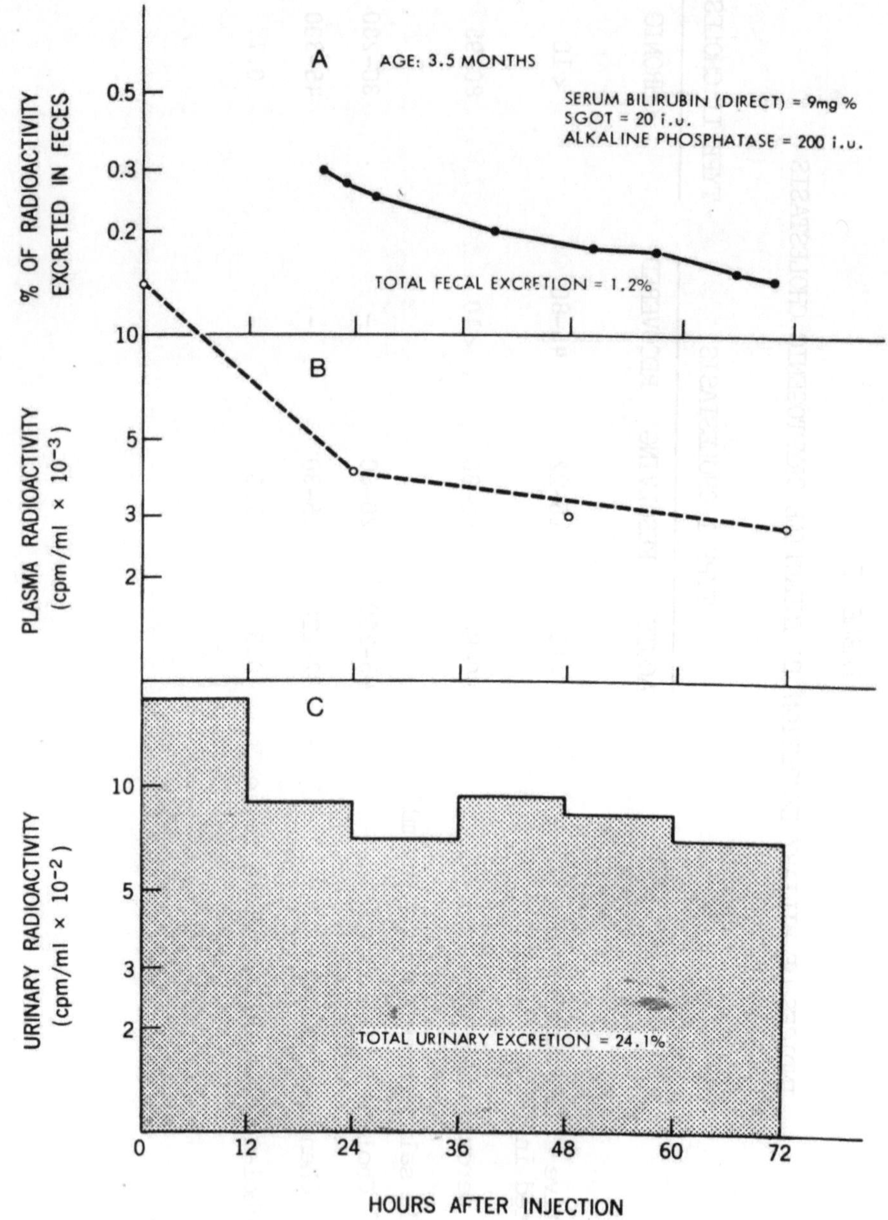
A
AGE: 3.5 MONTHS
SERUM BILIRUBIN (DIRECT) = 9mg %
SGOT = 20 i.u.
ALKALINE PHOSPHATASE = 200 i.u.
% OF RADIOACTIVITY EXCRETED IN FECES
0.5
0.3
0.2
TOTAL FECAL EXCRETION = 1.2%
B
PLASMA RADIOACTIVITY (cpm/ml × 10⁻³)
10
5
3
2
C
URINARY RADIOACTIVITY (cpm/ml × 10⁻²)
10
5
3
2
TOTAL URINARY EXCRETION = 24.1%
0
12
24
36
48
60
72
HOURS AFTER INJECTION

In contrast with Type II cholestasis, fecal excretion of ^{131}I-Rose Bengal in infants with parenchymal dysfunction and intact extrahepatic biliary passages revealed a remarkable periodicity (Fig. 3). This was discerned most clearly in cases with nearly complete biliary insufficiency, (total fecal excretion of radioactivity in the range associated with complete arrest of bile flow) because most of the label had not been eliminated and was readily measurable throughout the entire 72-hour test period (Fig. 3A). Radioactive dye was excreted into the intestinal lumen in pulses which occurred at approximately 24-hour intervals, and which did not relate to the exponential decline in plasma and urinary radioactivity. The beginning of the recovery phase was signalled in Type I cholestasis by an increase in total radioactivity in feces (Table I), and a shift of most of the label to the initial peak (Fig. 3B). However, periodicity continued to be apparent, and intervals of active biliary excretion alternated with periods when little or no radioactivity was detectable in feces. As resolution of the parenchymal disease process progressed, nearly all of the label in feces was excreted during the first day (Fig.3C). In fully recovered infants, up to 80% of the injected radioactive dye was eliminated as a single peak.

A positive relationship between patency of extrahepatic bile ducts and periodicity of fecal excretion of ^{131}I-Rose Bengal was also evident in Type II cholestasis due to intrahepatic biliary hypoplasia (Fig. 4).

DISCUSSION

Tests which determine the degree of biliary insufficiency in infants with cryptogenic liver disease indicated that bile flow may be nearly completely inhibited in the course of severe Type I cholestasis ("neonatal hepatitis"). During this acute "shut-down" phase of parenchymal disease, quantitative procedures could not discriminate between primary hepatocellular dysfunction and atresia of the extrahepatic bile ducts (Tables I and II).

Fig. 2: Typical excretory and plasma clearance patterns of ^{131}I-Rose Bengal in Type II cholestasis, exemplified by an infant with extrahepatic biliary atresia (total 72-hour fecal excretion = 1.2%).

A: Fecal radioactivity declines exponentially in line with plasma clearance, and urinary excretion curves.

B: Plasma radioactivity reaches equilibrium within 24 hours. Thereafter clearance proceeds slowly, with T 1/2 of 6.3 days.

C: Elimination of label is largely a function of urinary excretion, which is 20 times greater than fecal excretion. Bars represent 12-hour aliquots of urine.

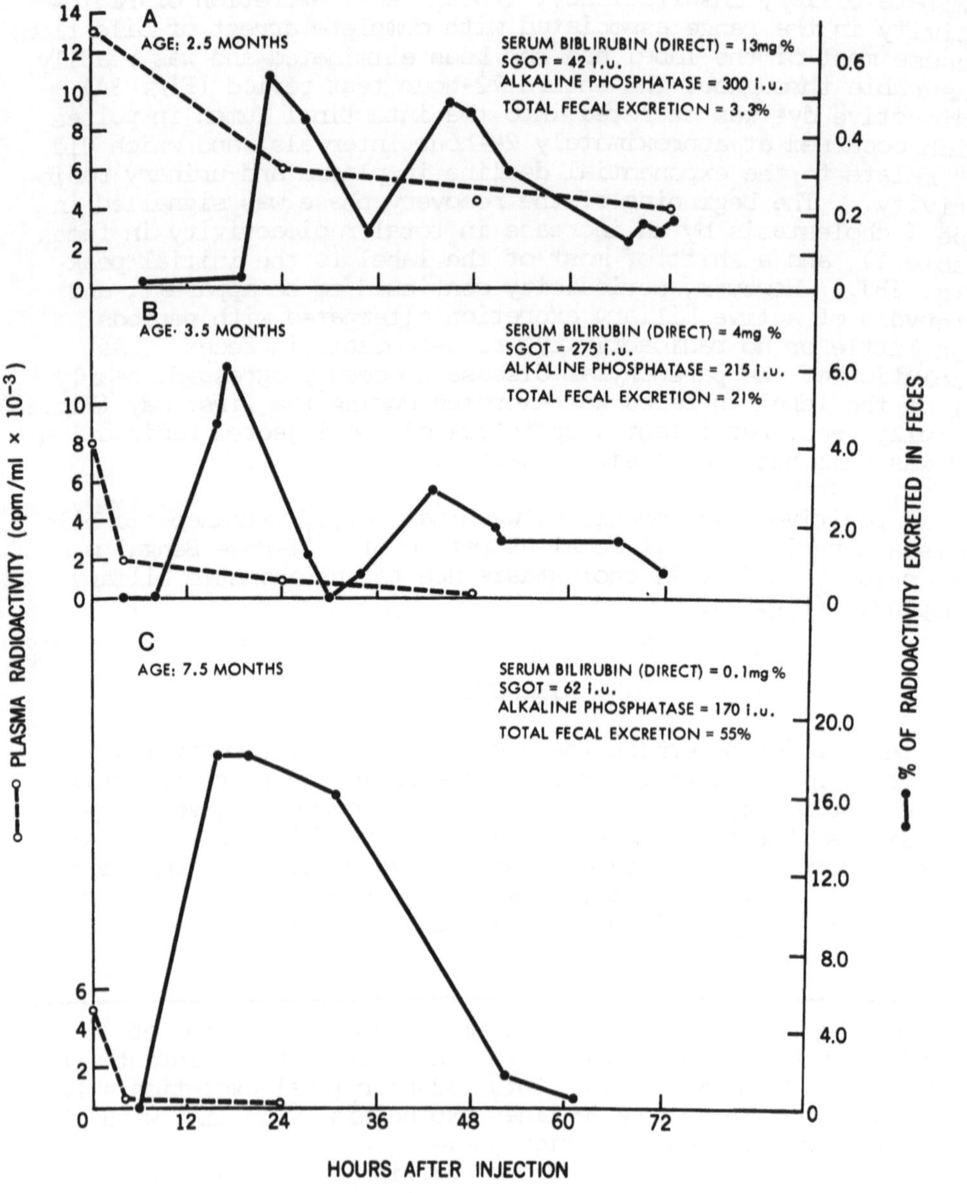
A
AGE: 2.5 MONTHS
SERUM BIBLIRUBIN (DIRECT) = 13mg %
SGOT = 42 i.u.
ALKALINE PHOSPHATASE = 300 i.u.
TOTAL FECAL EXCRETION = 3.3%
B
AGE· 3.5 MONTHS
SERUM BILIRUBIN (DIRECT) = 4mg %
SGOT = 275 i.u.
ALKALINE PHOSPHATASE = 215 i.u.
TOTAL FECAL EXCRETION = 21%
C
AGE: 7.5 MONTHS
SERUM BILIRUBIN (DIRECT) = 0.1mg %
SGOT = 62 i.u.
ALKALINE PHOSPHATASE = 170 i.u.
TOTAL FECAL EXCRETION = 55%
PLASMA RADIOACTIVITY (cpm/ml × 10⁻³)
% OF RADIOACTIVITY EXCRETED IN FECES
HOURS AFTER INJECTION
0
12
24
36
48
60
72

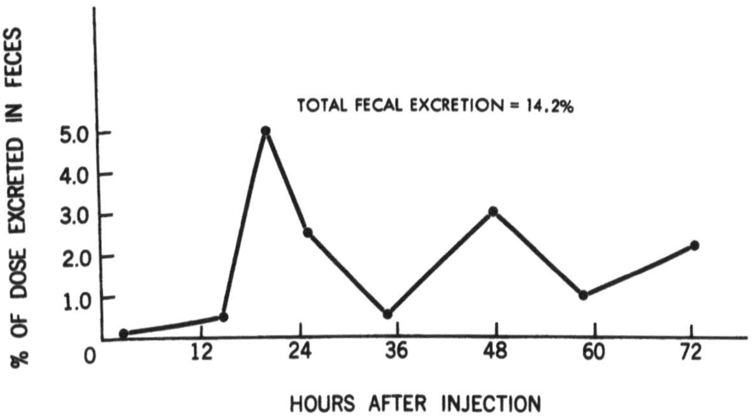

Fig. 4: Fecal excretion of radioactivity following ^{131}I-Rose Bengal administration in an infant with hypoplasia of intrahepatic bile ducts. Major bile ducts were visualized by operative cholangiography, and the diagnosis was established by percutaneous and surgical liver biopsy.

Fig. 3: Typical patterns of radioactivity in plasma and feces in Type I cholestasis following administration of ^{131}I-Rose Bengal. The entire course of illness in an infant with "neonatal hepatitis" is illustrated.

A: "Shut-down" phase. Severe biliary insufficiency consistent with nearly complete arrest of bile flow. (Total 72-hour fecal excretion = 3.3%). Diurnal periodicity of label in feces is unrelated to plasma radioactivity curve which declines at rates similar to rates observed in extrahepatic biliary atresia.

B: Resolution phase. Fecal diurnal pattern is still apparent, with larger proportion of label in the initial peak.

C: Recovery phase. Most of the label is excreted as a single broad peak. Note changes in scale of fecal radioactivity during the three stages of disease.

TABLE II

KINETICS OF ^{131}I-ROSE BENGAL IN INFANTILE CRYPTOGENIC CHOLESTASIS

	TYPE I CHOLESTASIS			TYPE II CHOLESTASIS
	ACUTE	RESOLVING	RECOVERED	CHRONIC
Activity remaining*: at 4 hours	15-20	7-10	3-4	18-25
at 24 hours	10-15	5-8	1-2	12-16
T 1/2 in plasma (hours)	90-140	35-60	18-22	120-160
Excretion (% in 72 hours):				
Urine	24-35	5-10	2-4	20-33
Feces	10	15-22	45-80	10

* Expressed as percent of plasma radioactivity 5 min after intravenous injection of ^{131}I-Rose Bengal (for details see ref. 4).

In infants with severe biliary deficiency of either type, plasma clearance and T 1/2 of ^{131}I-Rose Bengal were dependent upon urinary excretion of the dye. Thus, Rose Bengal may persist for several weeks in infants with depressed renal clearance mechanisms, and a relatively greater proportion of the radioactive label may leak into the intestine in such cases. However, in extrahepatic biliary atresia this intestinal fraction was never greater than 10% of the total dose administered, indicating that severe degrees of biliary insufficiency are reliably reflected by this procedure.

Bile appears to flow intermittently in infants with Type I cholestasis. Most of the biliary label recovered in feces of infants with this type of liver disease was concentrated in radioactivity peaks which were especially easy to detect when cholestasis was severe and the total amount of bile delivered to the intestine correspondingly small. It is of diagnostic interest that the presence of intact extrahepatic bile ducts was also reflected in periodic fecal radioactivity patterns in Type II cholestasis due to hypoplasia of the intrahepatic biliary system. Infants with Type II cholestasis of the extrahepatic ducts cannot transfer bile directly from the liver into the intestine. Radioactive label in the feces of such infants appears to be "filtered" through the intestinal wall at constant rates which reflect radioactivity levels in plasma and tissues.

These observations provide a means of distinguishing between infants with patent extrahepatic bile ducts and those with extrahepatic biliary atresia. Phenobarbital enhances fecal excretion of ^{131}I-Rose Bengal (4) and bile salts (11), and reduces serum bilirubin levels and pruritus (10,11) in jaundiced infants with intact bile ducts. Detection of intermittent fecal excretory patterns with ^{131}I-Rose Bengal should help identify those infants with severe cryptogenic cholestasis who do not require surgical repair of bile ducts, and who may be aided by drugs which stimulate bile flow.

ACKNOWLEDGEMENT

This work was supported by USPHS Grant HD-03148.

REFERENCES

1. THALER MM: Biliary disease in infancy and childhood. In Gastrointestinal Disease, edited by Sleisenger M and Fordtran J. Saunders, Philadelphia. 1973. Chapter 83, pp 1087-1097.

2. THALER MM and GELLIS SS: Studies in neonatal obstructive jaundice. II. Effect of diagnostic laparotomy on long-term prognosis of neonatal hepatitis. Amer J Dis Child 116: 262-270, 1968.

3. GHADIMI H and SASS-KORTSAK A: Evaluation of the radioactive rose-bengal test for the differential diagnosis of obstructive jaundice in infants. New Eng J Med 265: 351-358, 1961.

4. THALER MM: Effects of phenobarbital on hepatic transport and excretion of ^{131}I-Rose Bengal in children with cholestasis. Pediat Res 6: 100-110, 1972.

5. LUBIN BH, BAEHNER RL, SCHWARTZ E, et al: The red cell peroxide hemolysis test in the differential diagnosis of obstructive jaundice in the newborn period. Pediatrics 48: 562-565, 1971.

6. MELHORN DK, GROSS S, IZANT RJ Jr, et al: The red cell hydrogen peroxide hemolysis test and vitamin E absorption in the differential diagnosis of jaundice in infancy. J Pediat 81: 1082-1087, 1972.

7. POLEY JR, SMITH EI, BOON DJ, et al: Lipoprotein-X and the double ^{131}I-Rose Bengal test in the diagnosis of prolonged infantile jaundice. J Pediatr Surg 7: 660-669, 1972.

8. JAVITT NB, MORRISSEY KP, SIEGEL E, et al: Cholestatic syndromes in infancy: diagnostic value of serum bile acid pattern and cholestyramine administration. Pediatr Res 7: 119-125, 1973.

9. WHEELER HO: Secretion of bile. In Diseases of the Liver, edited by Schiff, L. Lipincott, Philadelphia. 1969. pp 84-96.

10. STIEHL A, THALER MM and ADMIRAND WH: The effects of phenobarbital on bile salts and bilirubin in patients with intrahepatic and extrahepatic cholestasis. New Eng J Med 286: 858-861, 1972.

11. STIEHL A, THALER MM and ADMIRAND WH: Effect of phenobarbital on the kinetics of bile salts in cholestasis due to intrahepatic biliary atresia. Pediatrics 51: 992-997, 1973.

DISCUSSION OF PAPERS ON EXTRAHEPATIC BILIARY OBSTRUCTION

CHAIRMAN: N.B. JAVITT

JABBARI: Is pancreatitis a contraindication to retrograde cholangiopancreatography?

ZIMMON: Not at all, if there is something to be gained from doing a cholangiogram. But you must be careful, and even in the best hands there is a 1-2% incidence of clinically insignificant pancreatitis. I am aware of only one case of serious pancreatitis. In order to avoid this relatively rare but important problem we do not do a pancreatogram unless there are clinical benefits to be derived from the procedure.

JABBARI: Is Trasylol useful in the prevention of pancreatitis?

ZIMMON: That is a very hard question to answer because the incidence of pancreatitis associated with this procedure is so low. I am not impressed with Trasylol. However I am impressed with the procedure of putting antibiotics in the dye, a procedure which has reduced the incidence of biliary tract infection to 0.2 - 0.3% of cases.

ARIAS: Would Dr. Lavoie like to comment on the overall success of the minilap technique. In countries where the burden of cost of these procedures falls upon the patient their value in terms of diagnosis becomes of great importance. In our institution the first 100 minilaps were undertaken entirely by the Department of Surgery. Only 55 were done in patients who actually had surgical disease. The second 100 patients were evaluated in collaboration with the Department of Medicine and almost 90 turned out to have surgical disease. These are complex invasive procedures and I think that we need a better evaluation of when they should actually be performed.

LAVOIE: In my paper I reported on the advantage of portal catheterization and venography as an adjunct in the management of already proven cases of surgical jaundice. We work closely with our physicians and we do not consider portography particularly useful in problems of intrahepatic cholestasis.

LESTER: You can get a certain amount of portal fibrosis and of bile ductular proliferation with hepatitis and in the neonate I don't think that you find polymorphonuclear leucocytes in extrahepatic biliary obstruction. Could Dr. Thaler give us the precise criteria which he uses in distinguishing between hepatitis and extrahepatic biliary atresia?

THALER: In a typical case of biliary atresia one finds, while scanning on low power, that the abnormalities are confined to the portal regions. On higher power one finds bile ductular proliferation with little disturbance of the parenchyma except cholestasis. If the portal region is relatively obscured by edema, giant cell transformation and inflammation, the average pathologist will hesitate to make a diagnosis of any kind, but it is likely a hepatitis rather than bile duct obstruction.

LESTER: You would say that bile duct proliferation with or without a modest amount of hepatocellular disease leads one to a diagnosis of obstruction?

THALER: Yes, with the possible exception of patients with α_1-antitrypsin deficiency.

GARTNER: We now recognize that the time in the infant's course at which the biopsy is done is extremely important. What may appear initially as giant cell hepatitis may several weeks later appear to be biliary atresia. I think that it is important to get serial biopsies in these infants.

THALER: I have also had the impression that the earlier biopsies show more inflammatory changes.

PHILLIPS: It would be a mistake to end with the view that liver biopsy plays no role in the differential diagnosis of cholestasis. I would be the first to agree that the diagnosis of extrahepatic biliary obstruction by liver biopsy can be extremely difficult. However, I would hasten also to state that liver biopsy can provide definitive diagnostic information in the majority of instances of cholestasis. This is certainly true in adult medicine where a number of disorders such as cholestatic viral hepatitis, cirrhosis, alcoholic hepatitis, and others, which can present an obstructive clinical picture, can be easily recognized by liver biopsy. Further, in biliary tract obstruction, there are many histopathological features, even in early cases, which can suggest the correct diagnosis; for instance, duct ectasia, ductular proliferation, edema of portal connective tissue and leucocytic infiltration in the presence of centrilobular bile stasis should suggest biliary tract obstruction. The size of the biopsy, the stage of the disease and the skill of the pathologist are key factors. Two biopsies separated by three to four weeks are invariably completely diagnostic to experienced pathologists.

SASS-KORTSAK: I think that we all agree that the term "neonatal hepatitis" should be abandoned. I also think that even though it may be difficult it is extremely important to try and establish a definite diagnosis in the young infant with cholestasis. We now realise that hepatitis B virus infection is not an important cause of intrahepatic cholestasis in the infant. On the other hand, α_1-antitrypsin deficiency is an important cause and indeed it accounts for 50% of the cases in our experience. We are very disappointed with the role of needle biopsy in the diagnosis of these cases and if we find a fecal Rose Bengal excretion under 10% and don't have a definite diagnosis, we proceed with surgical exploration and a wedge biopsy. If we find that the Rose Bengal excretion is over 10% then we do a needle biopsy to be sure that we are not dealing with biliary atresia.

[illegible]: Liver biopsy can provide definitive diagnostic information in the majority of instances of cholestasis. This is certainly true in adult medicine where a number of disorders, such as cholestatic viral hepatitis, cirrhosis, alcoholic hepatitis, and others, which can present an obstructive clinical picture, can be easily recognized by liver biopsy. Further, with biliary tract obstruction, there are many histopathological features, even in early cases, which can suggest the correct diagnosis. For instance, the edema, ductular proliferation, streaming of portal connective tissue and leucocytic infiltration in the presence of centrilobular bile casts should suggest biliary tract obstruction. The size of the biopsy, the stage of the disease, and the skill of the pathologist are key factors. Two biopsies separated by three to four weeks are invariably completely diagnostic to the expert pathologist.

[illegible]: I think that we all agree that the term "neonatal hepatitis" should be abandoned. I also think that even though it may be difficult, it is extremely important to try to establish [illegible]

CAUSATION AND CONSEQUENCES OF CHOLESTASIS: AN OVERVIEW

Fenton Schaffner and Hans Popper

Stratton Laboratory for Liver Diseases
Mount Sinai School of Medicine of The City
University of New York, New York, N.Y. 10029

"Intrahepatic cholestasis" was coined in 1952 to describe the morphologic findings in the liver when clinical and laboratory features pointed to biliary obstruction and none was found (1). That the condition could be caused by drugs was recognized more than a decade earlier (2). It was originally called intrahepatic obstructive jaundice and many proposals have been made about the mechanism by which the phenomenon is produced.

MECHANICAL THEORIES OF CHOLESTASIS

Early theories about the pathogenesis of jaundice held that obstruction to the flow of bile led to regurgitation either from ducts or between liver cells. Parenchymal liver disease, by contrast, caused jaundice because bile was not properly secreted by the sick liver or because bile plugs blocked the biliary passages. This theory was refined to the concept of "cholangiolitis" with leakage from or blockage of the connection between the canalicular network and the bile duct system, the canals of Hering or cholangioles later to be called ductules (3,4).

With the advent of more varieties and many more cases of drug induced cholestasis, it became apparent that inflammation around bile ductules is not always present, and that severe inflammation can exist without cholestasis (5). The numerous cases spurred the search for differential diagnostic tools to avoid unnecessary and sometimes harmful surgery. At the same time newly developed histochemical and electron microscopic techniques were applied in the hope of obtaining a better understanding of the condition (6,7,8). As a result of the early ultrastructural observations, attention was shifted to the canalicular network, the anatomical details of which had just been discerned. Rupture of the canaliculus between hepatocytes into the perisinusoidal space had its proponents, and while rupture can be seen (9,10,11) as a consequence of the death of single hepatocytes, it occurs too late in the course of cholestasis to be its cause.

FUNCTIONAL THEORIES OF CHOLESTASIS

A brief "cholestatic period" is normal after birth (12) and the newborn infant, especially if it is fed parenterally (13), or has pyloric stenosis (14), may develop cholestatic jaundice. Some duodenal stimulus, either neural or hormonal, has been held responsible for bile secretion and a lack of this stimulus for cholestasis at least in neonates (15). A comparable circumstance in adults has not been established but some instances of benign postoperative cholestasis may have such a basis.

The finding in adult cholestasis of reduced histochemical activity of canalicular enzymes such as adenosinetriphosphatase (ATPase) (5,16,17), and the dilatation of bile canaliculi with loss of microvilli, indicated that some altered function of the biliary pole of the hepatocyte might be responsible for the development of cholestasis (7,18,19). Indeed, a set of organelles including the canaliculus, the pericanalicular ectoplasm, the Golgi zone, the lysosomes, and other peribiliary bodies were collectively called the bile secretory apparatus, and cholestasis was felt to represent a failure of the apparatus to function properly (20). Still unexplained were the apparent centrilobular localization, the formation of bile plugs, the differences between species with no bile plugs in rats, and the fact that unrelated chemicals and mechanical obstruction produced the same picture. It was apparent that simple mechanistic or functional explanations would not help in differential diagnosis nor would they provide answers to the questions. One attempt to explain these features was that the centrilobular cells had to push the bile further to get it to the collecting system. This required more energy and the central cells did not have it available because they had less oxygen and were also more vulnerable to toxic injury (21). These factors acting in concert caused bile to accumulate in the canaliculi of the central zone because the bile simply could not be secreted. The lack of uniform distribution of both the histochemical (17) and electron microscopic changes (22) did not support this concept nor did the findings of identical changes in intrahepatic cholestasis and extrahepatic biliary obstruction.

CHOLESTASIS AS A PHENOMENON OF ORGANELLE PATHOLOGY

The observation that taurolithocholate injected intravenously produces all the features of intrahepatic cholestasis in rats and in hamsters, led to the development of the hypothesis that monohydroxy bile salts, formed in excess as a result of altered cholesterol metabolism, are responsible for cholestasis (23,24). Although newer concepts concerning altered cellular metabolism have not provided much help in terms of differential diagnosis or treatment, exploration of the various theories of the causation of cholestasis may lead to a unified concept about the condition and point the way to better diagnosis and rational therapy.

Theory of Hypoactive Endoplasmic Reticulum. Experiments with the pesticide, dieldrin, showed that it initially causes hypertrophy of the hepatocellular smooth endoplasmic reticulum (SER), with a parallel increase in the enzymes involved in microsomal biotransformation, including the terminal oxidase of the xenobiotic system, cytochrome P-450 (25). When the dose of dieldrin is raised beyond the capacity of the system to adapt to the large load, the enzyme activity in the system decreases, while the amount of SER and cytochrome P-450 remains at the induced level. Since the SER is the site of the 7α-hydroxylation of cholesterol (26), the rate-limiting step in the formation of bile salts, it was postulated that cholestasis involves an enzymatic defect in this step with resulting mitochondrial side chain oxidation of incompletely metabolized cholesterol to form monohydroxy bile salts, instead of the usual dihydroxy or trihydroxy bile salts which are the prime movers of bile in the fed state (27). The monohydroxy bile salts are poor micelle formers and liquid crystals of phospholipids (and probably bile salts) form inside the cell and in the bile canaliculi (Figs. 1 and 2). Some support for this hypothesis is provided by the finding of lithocholate and 5β-cholanoic acid in various cholestatic conditions (28,29). Furthermore, the SER is enzymatically hypoactive (30). However, the hypoactivity is mainly the result of the detergent action of chenodeoxycholic acid that also can produce cholestasis, at least in the isolated perfused liver (31). In vitro this substance competitively inhibits microsomal biotransformation at lower concentrations, while at higher concentrations it acts noncompetitively first by removing the lipid binding sites, then the cytochrome P-450 reductase, and finally disassembling the cytochrome itself and stripping it from the membrane (32). Biliary obstruction in the rat (33) as well as in man (34), leads to concentrations of chenodeoxycholic acid that inhibit biotransformation, and quite likely the concentrations are high enough in some cells to disrupt the enzyme complex. The course of events following experimental bile duct ligation indicates that cytochrome P-450 declines after bile duct ligation, while the activity of enzymes acting on

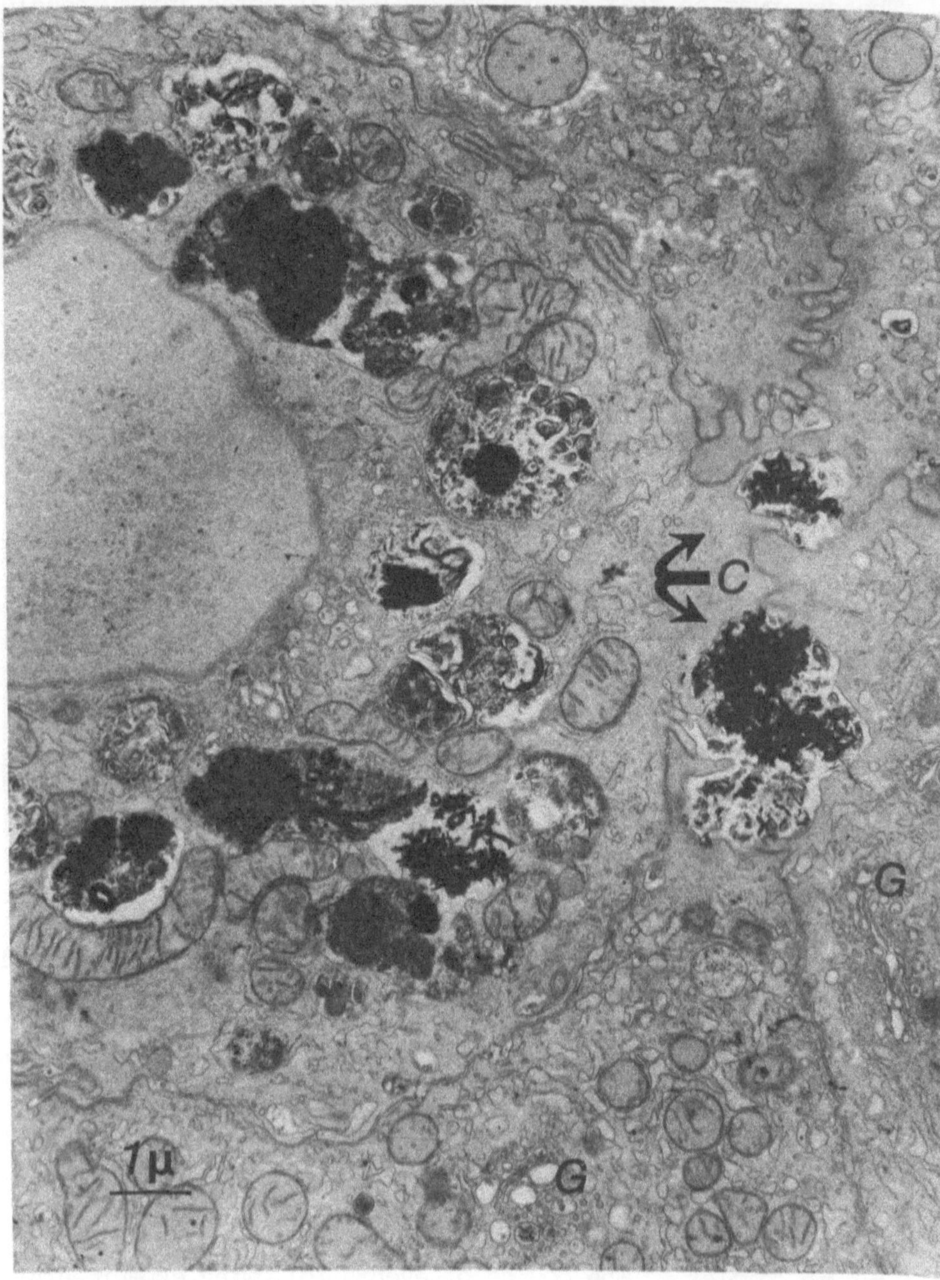
C
G
G
1μ

substrates attached to lipid binding sites decreases even more, although the SER appears hypertrophied (35). The decrease in cytochrome P-450 results from increased synthesis of microsomes that are deficient in enzyme protein. The rate of synthesis of the heme-protein was found to be normal in one study (36) and reduced in another (37), but its rate of degradation was unchanged (36,37). The progressive decrease in microsomal concentration of cytochrome P-450 is exaggerated as more but "empty" SER forms. These studies confirm that the SER is abnormal in cholestasis but the abnormalities found are largely the result rather than the cause of cholestasis. Nevertheless, abnormal metabolism of bile salts in the SER remains as a plausible explanation of the development of cholestasis (38).

The rough endoplasmic reticulum also is affected in cholestasis in that protein synthesis is increased, including lipoprotein synthesis (39). However, the latter is not normal and an abnormal low density lipoprotein, LP-X, is found in cholestasis (40). This substance has a high content of cholesterol, the hepatic synthesis of which is also stimulated by cholestasis (41), either because of loss of feedback control of the rate of synthesis (42), or more likely because of interruption of the enterolymphatic circulation of cholesterol (43).

Theory of Impaired Energy Release. Early electron microscopic studies revealed curling of mitochondrial cristae in cholestasis (44), (Fig. 3). This membrane is the site at which oxidative phosphorylation occurs. Substances that decrease bile flow in vivo like sulfobromophthalein (BSP) interfere with transport of inorganic phosphate across the inner mitochondrial membrane in vitro (45). Furthermore, in both human and experimental cholestasis, a progressive decrease in mitochondrial cytochromes was demonstrated (46). Some of these alterations are probably also the result of the detergent action of bile salts on the mitochondrial membrane (47), although the exact site of this effect remains unknown. Cholate overload (48) and lithocholate administration (23,49), cause curling of mitochondrial cristae before jaundice develops. Bilirubin, too, in concentrations found in the cholestatic liver uncouples oxidative phosphorylation and decreases oxygen uptake by hepatic mitochondria (39). The pigment also can enhance the severity of cholestasis in experimental animals

Fig. 1: Protracted chlorpromazine jaundice showing dilated bile canaliculi (C) containing bile plugs and surrounded by a widened zone of ectoplasm. The cytoplasm in the cell on the left contains vacuoles filled with material that may be in the form of liquid crystals, similar to that in the bile plugs. The Golgi zone (G) in the portion of the cell at the bottom and the one in the lower right are large with dilated vesicles (x 9,000).

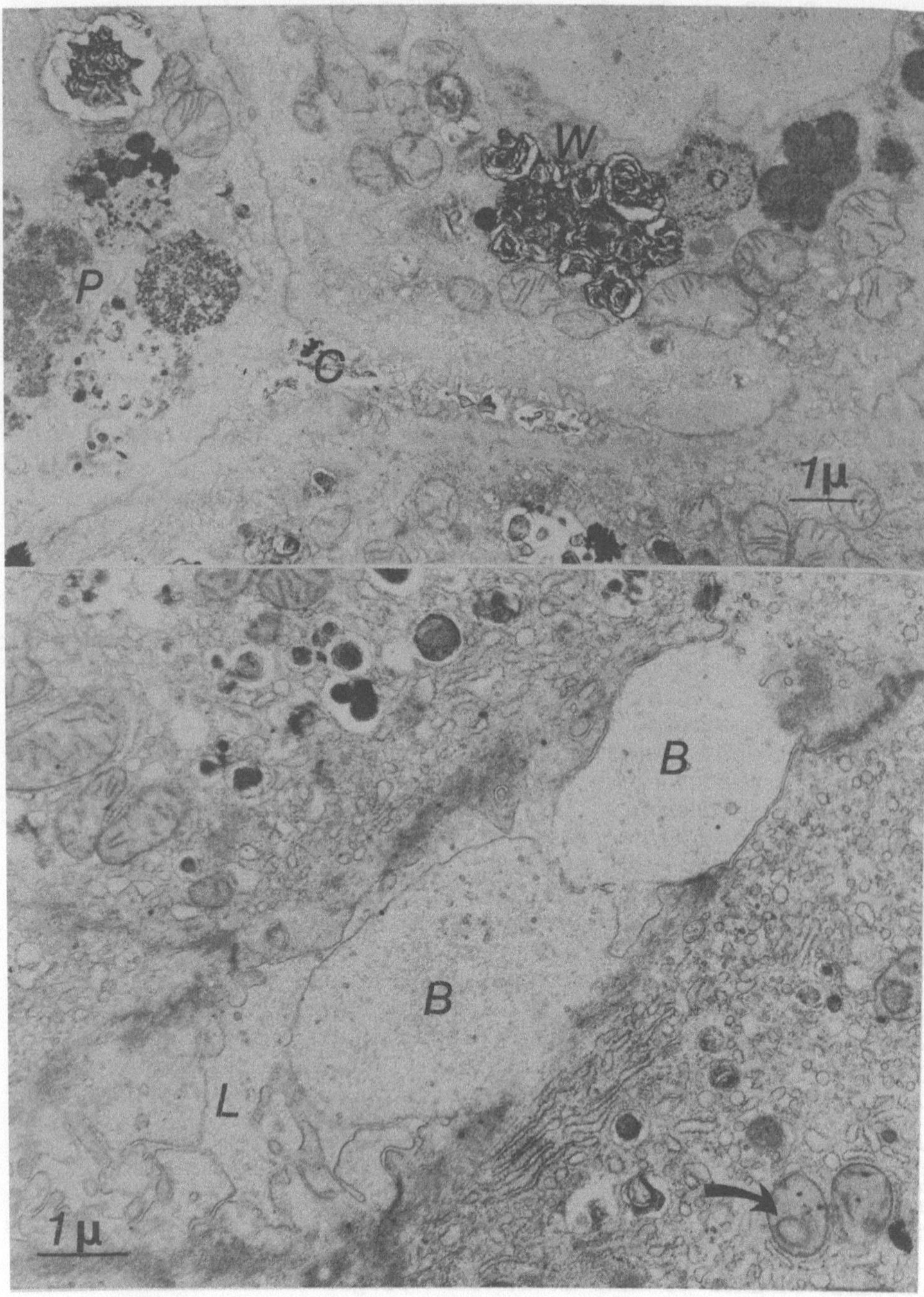
W
P
C
1μ
B
B
L
1μ

(50), just as it does in severe hemolysis in man (51). These changes in mitochondria are, at least in part, the result of cholestasis, although selective failure to provide energy for secretion remains a possible explanation of the genesis of cholestasis.

Theory of Impaired Canalicular Membrane Transport. The rate limiting step in the secretion of at least several of the constituents of bile is the transfer across the membrane into the canalicular lumen (52). Although the basis for this energy dependent process is unknown, there are at least three concurrently operating transport mechanisms involved: 1) inorganic cation (sodium) transport, 2) bile salt transport which also appears to be responsible for the transport of other lipids, and 3) organic anion transport for cholephilic substances other than bile salts (53).

While the histochemically demonstrable activities of canalicular ATPase and 5'-nucleotidase decrease in cholestasis, alkaline phosphatase increases (17). These phenomena have been confirmed in isolated liver plasma membrane fractions rich in canalicular membranes (54). Furthermore, in these preparations the actual content of ATPase and 5'-nucleotidase is reduced while sialic acid is increased in both intrahepatic and extrahepatic biliary obstruction. Synthesis and degradation rates of membrane proteins, cholesterol, phospholipids and neutral sugars are unchanged. This suggests that a change in the composition of the canalicular membrane is associated with cholestasis, perhaps causally.

ATPase is localized on the canalicular membrane, as well as on other surface membranes (17,55). ATPase appears during development when bile flow begins, usually at term or shortly thereafter (14,56). It disappears when bile flow stops, more rapidly as a result of liver cell injury (intrahepatic cholestasis) than of biliary obstruction (17,57). However, the disappearance is not uniform throughout the liver lobule. Concomitant with the

←

Fig. 2 (Top): Same as Fig. 1, showing whorls (W) (liquid crystals of phospholipids possibly with bile salts) in vacuoles presumably lyosome pigment (P) not surrounded by a membrane. The canaliculus (C) is normal in appearance but it contains a few strands of material similar to that in the whorls (x 10,800).

Fig. 3 (Bottom): Late stage of primary biliary cirrhosis showing dilated bile canaliculus filled with large blebs (B) from the canalicular surface greatly reducing the lumen (L). The mitochondrion (arrow) in the lower right-hand corner has a curled crista (x 12,600).

disappearance of canalicular ATPase, sinusoidal membrane ATPase increases (16,17). The loss of ATPase activity may be related to a decrease in the rate of secretion of the bile salt independent fraction of bile which is Na^{+}-K^{+} ATPase dependent (58). This inorganic cation pump which can be stimulated by adrenal steroids (59), is responsible for much of the fasting bile secretion and its function is decreased by inhibitors of sodium transport, by low concentrations of monohydroxy bile salts, and by various other organic anions. These substances, except for lithocholate in higher concentrations, do not produce cholestasis, yet the first event in the intrahepatic cholestasis may be a shutting down of sodium transport.

The trihydroxy and dihydroxy bile salts, cholate, chenodeoxycholate and deoxycholate, are the main determinants of postprandial bile flow (58,60), although they, too, can under certain circumstances diminish bile production in isolated perfused livers (49,58). Several possibilities may explain how cholestasis results from impaired transmembrane transport of these substances. First, cations probably have to be in the canalicular lumen in order for secretion to begin. Therefore, impaired cholate transport and impaired sodium excretion may be linked to one another (58). Secondly, bile salts may be precipitated with drugs like chlorpromazine or other amines, or may be in the form of nontransportable liquid crystals in the pericanalicular ectoplasm because of the presence of steroids with configurations that alter micelle forming ability, thus preventing transmembrane transport. Examples are the C-17 alpha alkylated anabolic or contraceptive steroids, and some of the steroids found during pregnancy. Thirdly, the detergent action of excess bile salts, particularly the dihydroxy ones, may alter the composition of the membrane to form bile salt-membrane complexes in the canalicular lumen (61). The altered membranes then cannot excrete bile normally. Regardless of the exact mechanism, impaired bile salt secretion across the canalicular membrane appears to be an important factor, perhaps the main factor, in the development of cholestasis (38, 62). One clinical consequence of this retention of bile salts is the pruritus which characterizes cholestasis (63).

A defect in the mechanism for secreting organic anions other than bile salts has been responsible for such conditions as the Dubin-Johnson syndrome. This selective secretory failure by itself is not cholestasis, but when cholestasis is present the organic anions are not secreted. Therefore, while this defect cannot be held responsible for cholestasis, it is present during cholestasis and is responsible for jaundice.

Canalicular membrane changes were held responsible for cholestasis on the basis of early electron microscopic studies in which they were the most prominent abnormality noted (7). This concept has only lately received the biochemical support already described. Yet time studies suggest that canalicular membrane changes are the result of events occurring within the hepatocyte. Following the intravenous administration of lithocholate, bile flow ceases in minutes (24). After four hours canalicular microvilli have disappeared (23). Scanning electron microscopic studies suggest that the microvilli retract into the canalicular cell membrane after secretion has stopped (64). Thus, abnormal structure results from reduced function, namely decreased bile secretion. The uneven distribution of the histochemical and elctron microscopic changes described suggests that the loss of secretory function is spotty even in the same cell, which may have a dilated canaliculus on one side and a normal one on another side (22). This observation favors the concept of a bile secretory apparatus for each canaliculus with failure of some but not others in cholestasis. Nevertheless, decrease in canalicular transport must remain a possible explanation of cholestasis.

CHOLESTASIS AS A RESULT OF MALFUNCTION OF OTHER ORGANELLES

The Golgi apparatus, by virtue of its proximity to the bile canaliculus, is thought to play a role in bile secretion. Impairment of this secretion either by biliary obstruction or by lithocholate administration is associated with enlargement of the Golgi system (23). The lamellae become dilated and the vesicles and vacuoles enlarged (Fig. 1). The Golgi apparatus also enlarges in uninvolved portions of the liver when a bile duct is ligated in another portion of the organ (65). Thus, reduced function and increased function have similar effects. Serum low density lipoproteins are assembled in the hepatocellular Golgi zone (66,67). However, the role of the Golgi apparatus in bile secretion and what the dilated portions are filled with remain unknown. The question of a role for the Golgi apparatus in the genesis of cholestasis must therefore remain unanswered.

Lysosomes increase in number in cholestasis and some peribiliary vacuoles contain acid phosphatase and material that resembles phospholipid (and possibly bile salt) liquid crystals (17,39), (Fig. 2). Lysosomes also contain glucuronidase which can liberate free bilirubin and other possibly cytotoxic substances. Some of the products of lysosomal digestion and, indeed, entire lysosomes are excreted into the bile. Whether lysosomes have any place in the development of cholestasis, however, remains to be established.

The hyaloplasm contains two proteins, Y and Z, that bind organic anions. Both intrahepatic cholestasis and biliary obstruction reduce Y and Z (68). However, a defect in either of these two proteins does not seem to be responsible for cholestasis because acute bile duct ligation has no effect on the amount present.

ROLE OF THE DUCTULE IN CHOLESTASIS

The "cholangiolitic" theory of cholestasis described previously has long been largely abandoned. Yet ductules and ducts have a role in bile secretion in that they can add bicarbonate (and perhaps calcium) to bile, and they can reabsorb water, bile salts and to some extent bile pigment, at least under certain circumstances like cholestasis (69,70). Ductular secretion is in part controlled by gastrointestinal hormones like secretin. It probably is also regulated by a countercurrent mechanism created by the slow flow of the bile toward the porta hepatis, and the rapid flow of blood in closely proximated vessels in the other direction. The exchange involves inorganic ions and water. In cholestasis, ductules proliferate, the ductular basement membrane is duplicated and often surrounded by inflammatory cells and collagen bundles, the lateral cell borders of ductules are straightened, the ductular cell cytoplasm contains vacuoles with liquid crystals, and presumably bile pigment in vacuoles and free in the cytoplasm, and the microvilli are shortened, missing or replaced by large blebs (69, 70,71,72). Thus, in cholestasis the reabsorptive role of the ductule appears to be enhanced. This increased reabsorption coupled with the appearance of many normal canaliculi in long standing complete biliary obstruction, suggests that there is a hepatocellular-ductular cell circulation in cholestasis. This circulation also is operative for glucose in the absence of cholestasis (73), but how much of the biliary solids can be reabsorbed under normal circumstances is unknown.

Thus, reabsorption from ductules (regurgitation) does occur in cholestasis and presumably as a result of it. However, it may be the primary event in early primary biliary cirrhosis that produces a syndrome resembling cholestasis. It also is one factor among several responsible for jaundice in experimental intoxication with alpha-naphthylisothiocyanate (ANIT) (74). Both in primary biliary cirrhosis (75) and in ANIT intoxication (74), bleb formation in ductules is striking. Many lumens are filled with ballooned ductular cell surfaces. Whether this adds an obstructive component early is unknown but unlikely. In long standing cholestasis, periductular inflammation and fibrosis are probably responsible for compressing the ductule and separating it from its blood supply and from the canalicular network (38). The result is mechanical obstruction of the flow of bile which in turn leads to cholestasis (see below). Long term administration of lithocholate produces ductular proliferation and periductal fibrosis in several species (76,77). These observations suggest a relationship between the altered bile salt metabolism and the ductular cell reaction in cholestasis.

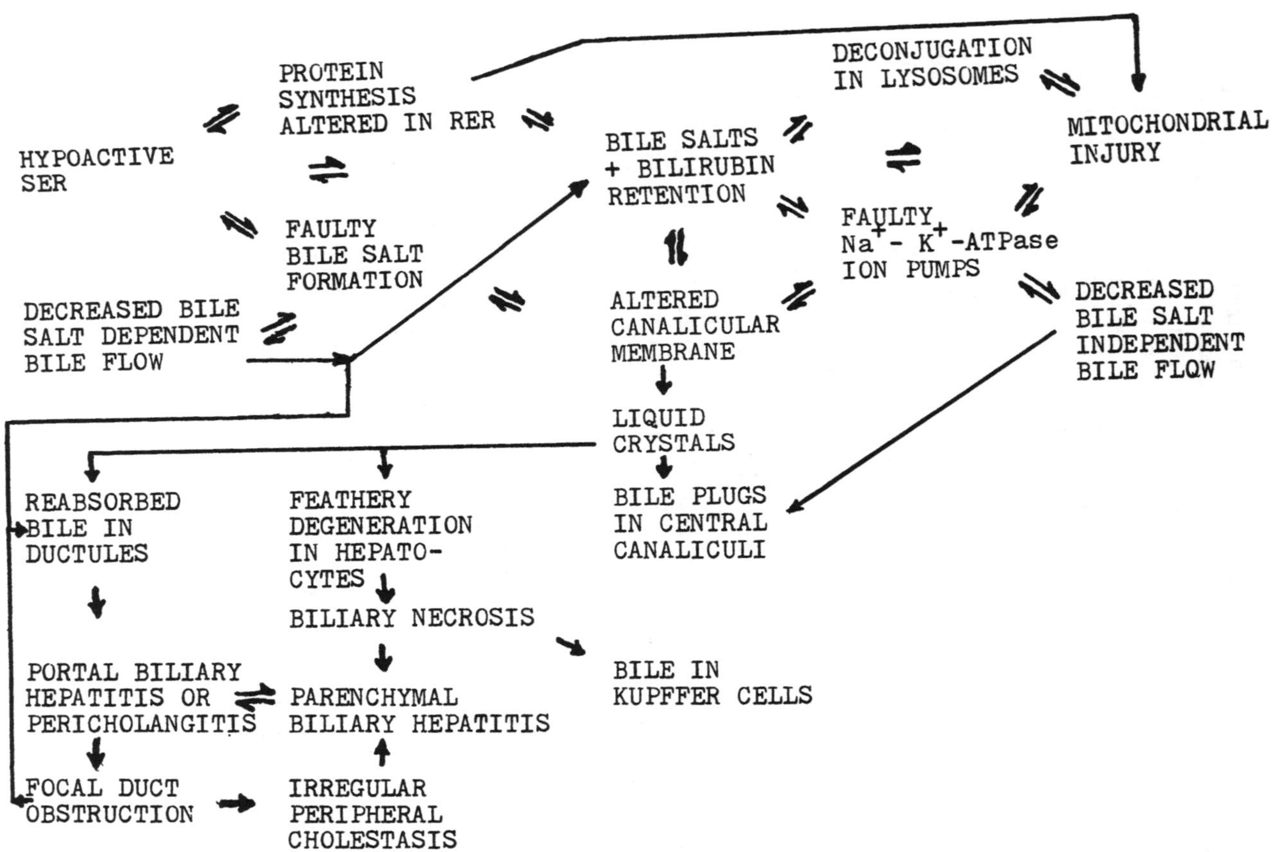

Fig. 4: Vicious circles operative in cholestasis; the one in the upper half is at the organelle level while the one in the left lower portion is at the lobular level.

EXPLANATION OF CENTRAL AND PERIPHERAL CHOLESTASIS

The main factor for the centrilobular accumulation of bile in cholestasis is the generally decreased secretion of bile water, probably because of faulty bile salt secretion. In addition there may be enhanced bile water reabsorption from the canaliculus itself. The concentration of cholesterol, lecithin and bilirubin increases either because the concentration of bile salts is too low to keep the lipids in suspension, or there is too little water to keep them in the form of micelles and not liquid crystals. Both amorphous material like bile pigment and lamellated material like phospholipid liquid crystals are found in the bile plugs (78). Closer to the ductular collecting system, the rate of flow is more rapid because more cells are contributing their bile even though the total amount of bile secreted by the liver is decreased. Furthermore, ductular absorption may exert a sucking effect. Therefore, near the ductular collecting system, bile plugs are not seen early in cholestasis. Later periductular fibrosis obstructs some of the ductules and then canaliculi nearest the obstruction dilate (38,79). This is analogous to dilatation of the extrahepatic bile ducts proximal to an obstruction at the papilla of Vater. Therefore, initially central cholestasis becomes irregularly peripheral if it lasts long enough. This nonuniform peripheral cholestasis is noted in late primary biliary cirrhosis and in the portal fibrosis that develops in biliary atresia or after long standing extrahepatic biliary obstruction (38). Associated with long standing cholestasis from any cause is the appearance of hepatocellular and ductular cell hyalin identical to that seen in alcoholic liver disease. But the hyalin is in the lobular periphery not in the center as it is in alcoholics (80).

A UNIFIED CONCEPT

Many ultrastructural and biochemical features of cholestasis have been reviewed. Most are the result of cholestasis and some, like the relative amounts of dihydroxy and trihydroxy bile salts, may be of diagnostic importance (81). Some may in some circumstances initiate cholestasis as well as result from it, thereby prolonging it. This combination seems to be especially true for hypoactive smooth endoplasmic reticulum. Membrane changes in canaliculi and mitochondrial injury also result from cholestasis and possibly can cause cholestasis. Probably under different circumstances, one or another serves as a cause while the others are effects. This implies that cholestasis is a single nosologic entity but one that can be initiated in different ways.

Cholestasis can be looked upon as two vicious circles, interrelated but operating at different levels; one is at the organelle level and the other at the lobular level (Fig. 4). The main biochemical phenomenon is retention of the two main solids of bile, bilirubin and bile salts. Primary involvement of different organelles may explain the failure of phenobarbital or other inducers of the SER to reinstitute bile flow and lower serum bilirubin and stop pruritus in some instances, and its success in doing so in others (82,83,84). This concept also means that the differential diagnosis of cholestasis ultimately may have to include the differential diagnosis of organelle pathology.

On the lobular level, the circle involves hepatocytes and bile ductules or small ducts. Injury to either of these structures leads to injury of the other, with the end result being mechanical obstruction at the small portal tracts. This obstruction causes retention of bile salts and bilirubin that in turn feed back both into the organelle cycle and into the lobular cycle by causing peripheral cholestasis and more biliary hepatitis. Once the lobular cycle is set in motion, even surgery may not interrupt it.

SUMMARY

Intrahepatic cholestasis can be explained by several hypotheses involving malfunction of various organelles in the hepatocyte. One theory involves injury to the smooth endoplasmic reticulum with altered microsomal metabolism of cholesterol and formation of monohydroxy bile salts. Another theory involves alteration of the bile canalicular membrane and still another holds that defective energy metabolism in mitochondria is responsible. Examination of several theories as well as the role of the bile ductules leads to the suggestion that alterations in different organelles may initiate cholestasis under different circumstances. The cholestasis in turn causes alterations in the other organelles and changes in the liver lobule visible with the light microscope. These then can lead to further morphologic changes on one hand and to more organelle changes on the other. Thus cause and result are not the same in each instance although the cholestasis is the same in all the circumstances. Once it begins, two vicious circles are set in motion, one at the organelle level and one at the light microscopic level.

ACKNOWLEDGEMENT

The original observations quoted were made with the help of USPHS Grant AM 03846, National Institutes of Health.

REFERENCES

1. POPPER H, SCHAFFNER F: Laboratory diagnosis of liver disease. Coordinated use of histological and biochemical observations. JAMA 150: 1367-1372, 1952.

2. HANGER FM, GUTMAN AB: Postarsphenamine jaundice apparently due to obstruction of intrahepatic biliary tract. JAMA 115: 263-271, 1940.

3. RÖSSLE R: Die cholangiolitische Zirrhose. In Entzündungen der Leber, vol. 5, no. 1, of Handbuch der speziellen pathologischen Anatomie und Histologie. Ed. F Henke, O Lubarsch. Berlin, Springer, 1939, pp 448-452.

4. WATSON CJ, HOFFBAUER FW: Problem of prolonged hepatitis with particular reference to cholangiolitic type and to development of cholangiolitic cirrhosis of liver. Ann Intern Med 25: 195-227, 1946.

5. POPPER H, SZATO PB: Intrahepatic cholestasis ("cholangiolitis"). Gastroenterology 31: 683-699, 1956.

6. WACHSTEIN M, MEISEL E: Histochemistry of hepatic phosphatase at a physiologic pH. With special reference to the demonstration of bile canaliculi. Am J Clin Pathol 27: 13-23, 1957.

7. ROUILLER C: Les canalicules biliares. Etude au microscope electronique. Acta Anat (Basel) 26: 94-109, 1956.

8. SCHAFFNER F, POPPER H: Morphologic studies of cholestasis. Gastroenterology 37: 565-573, 1959.

9. STEINER JW, JEZEQUEL AM, PHILLIPS MJ, et al: Some aspects of the ultrastructural pathology of the liver. In Progress in Liver Diseases, vol. 2. Ed. H. Popper, F. Schaffner. New York, Grune and Stratton, 1965. pp. 303-372.

10. ZAKI FG: Ultrastructure of hepatic cholestasis. Medicine 45: 537-545, 1966.

11. SCHATZKI P: The passage of radioactive lanthanum from the biliary to the vascular system. An electron microscopic and radioactive tracer study. Z Zellforsch 119: 451-459, 1971.

12. DEWOLF-PEETERS C, DEVOS R, DESMET V: Histochemical evidence of a cholestatic period in neonatal rats. Pediatr Res 5: 704-709, 1971.

13. TOULOUKIAN RJ, DOWNING SE: Cholestasis associated with long-term parenteral hyperalimentation. Arch Surg 106: 58-62, 1973.

14. LEVINE G, FAVARA BE, MIERAU G, BAILEY WC: Jaundice, liver ultrastructure, and congenital pyloric stenosis. Arch Pathol 95: 267-270, 1973.

15. RAGER R, FINEGOLD MJ: Cholestasis in low birth weight prematures: is parenteral alimentation the cause? Am J Pathol 74: 6a-7a, 1974.

16. WILLS EJ, EPSTEIN ME: Subcellular changes in surface adenosine triphosphatase activity of human liver in extrahepatic obstructive jaundice. Am J Pathol 49: 605-635, 1966.

17. DESMET VJ: Morphologic and histochemical aspects of cholestasis. In Progress in Liver Diseases, vol. 4. Ed. H. Popper, F. Schaffner. New York, Grune and Stratton, 1972. pp. 97-132.

18. STEINER JW, CARRUTHERS JS: Studies on the fine structure of the terminal branches of the biliary tree. II. Observations of pathologically altered bile canaliculi. Am J Pathol 39: 41-63, 1961.

19. HAMPTON JC: Electron microscopic study of extrahepatic biliary obstruction in the mouse. Lab Invest 10: 502-513, 1961.

20. POPPER H: Cholestasis. Ann Rev Med 19: 39-56, 1968.

21. DUBIN IN, PETERSON LH: An explanation for the centrolobular localization of intrahepatic bile stasis in acute liver diseases. Am J Med Sci 236: 45-52, 1958.

22. SCHAFFNER F, KNIFFEN JC: Electron microscopy as related to hepatotoxicity. Ann NY Acad Sci 104: 847-857, 1963.

23. SCHAFFNER F, JAVITT NB: Morphologic changes in hamster liver during intrahepatic cholestasis induced by taurolithocholate. Lab Invest 15: 1783-1792, 1966.

24. JAVITT NB, EMERMAN S: Effect of sodium taurolithocholate on bile flow and bile acid excretion. J Clin Invest 47: 1002-1014, 1968.

25. HUTTERER F, KLION FM, WENGRAF A, et al: Hepatocellular adaptation and injury. Structural and biochemical changes following dieldrin and methyl butter yellow. Lab Invest 20: 455-464, 1969.

26. BOYD GS, PERCY-ROBB IW: Enzymatic regulation of bile acid synthesis. Am J Med 51: 580-587, 1971.

27. SCHAFFNER F, POPPER H: Hypothesis: cholestasis is the result of hypoactive hypertrophic smooth endoplasmic reticulum in the hepatocyte. Lancet 2: 355-359, 1969.

28. MAKINO I, SJOVALL J, NORMAN A, et al: Excretion of 3β-hydroxy-5-cholanoic and 3α-hydroxy-5α-cholanoic acids in urine of infants with biliary atresia. FEBS Letters 15: 161-164, 1971.

29. BACK P: Identification and quantitative determination of urinary bile acids excreted in cholestasis. Clin Chim Acta 44: 199-207, 1973.

30. HUTTERER F, BACCHIN PG, RAISFELD IH, et al: Alteration of microsomal biotransformation in the liver in cholestasis. Proc Soc Exp Biol Med 133: 702-706, 1970.

31. FISHER MM, MAGNUSSON R, MIYAI K: Bile acid metabolism in mammals. I. Bile acid-induced intrahepatic cholestasis. Lab Invest 25: 88-91, 1971.

32. HUTTERER F, DENK H, BACCHIN PG, et al: Mechanism of cholestasis. I. Effect of bile acids on microsomal cytochrome P-450 dependent biotransformation system in vitro. Life Sci 9: 877-887, 1970.

33. GREIM H, TRULZSCH D, ROBOZ J, et al: Mechanism of cholestasis. 5. Bile acids in normal rat livers and in those after bile duct ligation. Gastroenterology 63: 837-845, 1972.

34. GREIM H, TRULZSCH D, CZYGAN P, et al: Mechanism of cholestasis. 6. Bile acids in human livers with or without biliary obstruction. Gastroenterology 63: 846-850, 1972.

35. SCHAFFNER F, BACCHIN PG, HUTTERER F, et al: Mechanism of cholestasis. 4. Structural and biochemical changes in the liver and serum in rats after bile duct ligation. Gastroenterology 60: 888-897, 1971.

36. DENK H, GREIM H, HUTTERER F, et al: Turnover of hepatic cytochrome P-450 in experimental cholestasis. Exp Mol Pathol 19: 241-247, 1973.

37. MACKINNON AM, SIMON FR: Reduced synthesis of hepatic microsomal cytochrome P-450 in the bile duct ligated rat. Biochem Biophys Res Commun 56: 437-443, 1974.

38. POPPER H, SCHAFFNER F: Pathophysiology of cholestasis. Hum Pathol 1: 1-24, 1970.

39. SCHERSTEN T: Metabolic differences between hepatitis and cholestasis in human liver. In Progress in Liver Diseases, vol. 4. Ed. H. Popper, F. Schaffner. New York, Grune and Stratton, 1972. pp. 133-150.

40. SEIDEL D, ALAUPOVIC P, FURMAN RH: A lipoprotein characterizing obstructive jaundice. I. Method for quantitative separation and identification of lipoproteins in jaundiced subjects. J Clin Invest 48: 1211-1223, 1969.

41. HARRY DS, DINI M, McINTYRE N: Effect of cholesterol feeding and biliary obstruction on hepatic cholesterol biosynthesis in the rat. Biochim Biophys Acta 296: 209-220, 1973.

42. KATTERMAN R, CREUTZFELDT W: The effect of experimental cholestasis on the negative feedback regulation of cholesterol in rat liver. Scand J Gastroenterol 5: 337-342, 1970.

43. WEIS JH, DIETSCHY JM: Presence of an intact cholesterol feedback mechanism in the liver in biliary stasis. Gastroenterology 61: 77-84, 1971.

44. CARRUTHERS JS, STEINER JW: Experimental extrahepatic biliary obstruction: fine structural changes of liver cell mitochondria. Gastroenterology 42: 419-430, 1962.

45. KILLENBERG PG, HOPPEL CL: Inhibition of rat liver mitochondrial oxidative phosphorylation by sulfobromophthalein. Mol Pharmacol 10: 108-118, 1974.

46. OZAWA K, TAKASAN H, KITAMURA O, et al: Alteration in liver mitochondrial metabolism in a patient with biliary obstruction due to liver carcinoma. Am J Surg 126: 653-657, 1973.

47. LEE MJ, WHITEHOUSE MW: Inhibition of electron transport and coupled phosphorylation in liver mitochondria by cholanic (bile) acids and their conjugates. Biochim Biophys Acta 100: 317-328, 1965.

48. WITZLEBEN CL: Hepatic ultrastructural effects of cholic acid overload. Exp Mol Pathol 16: 47-53, 1972.

49. MIYAI K, PRICE VM, FISHER MM: Bile acid metabolism in mammals. Ultrastructural studies on the intrahepatic cholestasis induced by lithocholic and chenodeoxycholic acids in the rat. Lab Invest 24: 292-302, 1971.

50. BOYCE W, WITZLEBEN CL: Bilirubin as a cholestatic agent. II.Effect of variable doses of bilirubin on the severity of manganese-bilirubin cholestasis. Am J Pathol 72: 427-431, 1973.

51. FULOP M, KATZ S, LAWRENCE C: Extreme hyperbilirubinemia. Arch Int Med 127: 254-258, 1971.

52. MULDER GJ: The rate limiting step in the biliary elimination of some substrates of uridine diphosphate glucuronyl transferase in the rat. Biochem Pharmacol 22: 1751-1763, 1973.

53. ALPERT S, MOSHER M, SHANSKE A et al: Multiplicity of hepatic excretory mechanisms for organic anions. J Gen Physiol 53: 238-247, 1969.

54. SIMON FR, ARIAS IM: Alteration of bile canalicular enzymes in cholestasis. A possible cause of bile secretory failure. J Clin Invest 52: 765-775, 1973.

55. ESSNER E, NOVIKOFF A, MASEK B: Adenosinetriphosphatase activities in the plasma membrane of liver cells as revealed by electron microscopy. J Biochem Biophys Cytol 4: 711-716, 1958.

56. SANDSTROM B: The functional significance of bile canalicular nucleoside phosphatase activity. Histochemie 25: 9-14, 1971.

57. HOLZNER J: Fermenthistochemische Untersuchungen au Leberbiopsien. Verh Dtsch Ged Pathol 44: 233-237, 1960.

58. ERLINGER S, DHUMEAUX D: Mechanisms and control of secretion of bile water and electrolytes. Gastroenterology 66: 281-304, 1974.

59. DUMONT M, ERLINGER S: Influence of hydrocortisone on bile formation in the rat. Biol Gastroenterol (Paris) 6: 197-203, 1973.

60. SPERBER I: Biliary secretion of organic anions and its influence on bile flow. In The Biliary System. A Symposium of the NATO Advanced Study Institute. Ed. W. Taylor, Philadelphia, F.A. Davis, 1965. pp. 457-467.

61. SIMON FR, ARIAS IM: Alterations in liver plasma membranes and their possible role in cholestasis. Gastroenterology 62: 342-345, 1972.

62. JAVITT NB: The cholestatic syndrome - 1971. Am J Med 51: 637-641, 1971.

63. HERNDON JH Jr: Pathophysiology of pruritus associated with elevated bile acids in serum. Arch Intern Med 130: 632-637, 1972.

64. MIYAI K, MAYR W, RICHARDSON A: Freeze fracture study of bile canalicular changes induced by lithocholic acid. Lab Invest 30: 384, 1974.

65. COOPER AD, JONES AL, KOLDINGER RE, et al: Selective biliary obstruction: a model for the study of lipid metabolism in cholestasis. Gastroenterology 66: 574-585, 1974.

66. CLAUDE A: Growth and differentiation of cytoplasmic membranes in the course of lipoprotein granule synthesis in the hepatic cell. I.Elaboration of elements of the Golgi complex. J Cell Biol 47: 745-766, 1970.

67. STEIN O, BAR-ON H, STEIN Y: Lipoproteins and the liver. In Progress in Liver Diseases, vol. 4. Ed. H. Popper, F. Schaffner. New York, Grune and Stratton, 1972. pp. 45-62.

68. REYES H, LEVI AJ, GATMAITAN Z, et al: Studies of Y and Z, two hepatic cytoplasmic anion-binding proteins: effect of drugs, chemicals, hormones, and cholestasis. J Clin Invest 50: 2242-2252, 1971.

69. STEINER JW, CARRUTHERS JS: Experimental extrahepatic biliary obstruction. Some aspects of the fine sturctural changes of bile ductules and pre-ductules (Ducts of Hering). Am J Pathol 40: 253-270, 1962.

70. SASAKI H, SCHAFFNER F, POPPER H: Bile ductules in cholestasis. Morphologic evidence for secretion and absorption in man. Lab Invest 16: 84-95, 1967.

71. SCHAFFNER F, POPPER H: Electron microscopic studies of normal and proliferated bile ductules. Am J Pathol 38: 393-410, 1961.

72. STEINER JW, CARRUTHERS JS, KALIFAT SR: The ductular cell reaction of rat liver in extrahepatic cholestasis. I. Proliferated biliary epithelial cells. Exp Mol Pathol 1: 162-185, 1962.

73. GUZELIAN P, BOYER JL: Glucose reabsorption from bile. Evidence for a biliohepatic circulation. J Clin Invest 53: 526-535, 1974.

74. SCHAFFNER F, SCHARNBECK HH, HUTTERER F, et al: Mechanism of cholestasis. VII: α-naphthylisothiocyanate induced jaundice. Lab Invest 28: 321-331, 1973.

75. KLION FM, SCHAFFNER F: Electron microscopic observations in primary biliary cirrhosis. Arch Pathol (Chicago) 81: 152-161, 1966.

76. HUNT R, LEVEILLE G, SAUBERLICH H: Dietary bile acids and lipid metabolism. Effects of lithocholic acid in mammalian species. Proc Soc Exp Biol Med 115: 277-280, 1964.

77. PALMER RH, HRUBAN Z: Production of bile duct hyperplasia and gallstones by lithocholic acid. J Clin Invest 45: 1255-1267, 1966.

78. BIAVA C: Studies on cholestasis. The fine structure and morphogenesis of hepatocellular and canalicular bile pigment. Lab Invest 13: 1099-1123, 1964.

79. HOLLANDER M, SCHAFFNER F: Electron microscopic studies in biliary atresia. I. Bile ductular proliferation. Am J Dis Child 116: 49-56, 1968.

80. GERBER MA, ORR W, DENK H, et al: Hepatocellular hyalin in cholestasis and cirrhosis: its diagnostic significance. Gastroenterology 64: 89-98, 1973.

81. JAVITT NB, MORRISSEY KP, SIEGEL E, et al: Cholestatic syndromes in infancy: diagnostic value of serum bile acid pattern and cholestyramine administration. Pediatr. Res 7: 119-125, 1973.

82. SHARP HL, MIRKIN BL: Effect of phenobarbital on hyperbilirubinemia, bile acid metabolism and microsomal enzyme activity in chronic intrahepatic cholestasis of childhood. J Pediatr 81: 116-126, 1972.

83. BRAUN W, WOCKEL W, GIERTLER U, et al: Phenobarbital behandlung der benignen rezidivierenden intrahepatischen Cholestase. Schweiz Med Wochenschr 102: 1769-1772, 1972.

84. STIEHL A, THALER MM, ADMIRAND WH: Effects of phenobarbital on bile salt metabolism in cholestasis due to bile duct hypoplasia. Pediatrics 51: 992-997, 1973.

NONSTEROID DRUG-INDUCED CHOLESTASIS AND EXPERIMENTAL CHOLESTASIS

Gabriel L. Plaa

Université de Montréal

Montréal, Québec

While chemically induced hepatotoxic reactions appeared in the medical literature of the early 1900's, it can be said that the problem of drug-induced cholestasis is a relatively recent occurrence. Its emergence as a distinct clinical problem arises from the time of the introduction of chlorpromazine as a therapeutic agent. Since this time, a number of other nonsteroid drugs have been shown to possess this property (Table I). It can be seen that while certain classes of pharmacologic agents have been associated with this adverse response, chemical similarities between all of the substances are really lacking. In addition to the drugs listed in Table I, certain steroids have been associated with cholestatic reactions in man; among these drugs one finds several anabolic steroids and the oral contraceptives. While the production of liver injury in man by drugs or other chemicals is not a new phenomenon, one can say that the cholestatic reactions produced by these drugs were largely unexpected and unpredictable from their known effects in laboratory animals.

DRUG-INDUCED CHOLESTASIS VERSUS TOXIC HEPATITIS

One could ask how these substances differ from those that produce toxic hepatitis. Table II lists the characteristics of toxic hepatitis as produced by known hepatotoxic agents. These criteria are those which have been observed with agents (carbon tetrachloride, chloroform, bromobenzene, acetaminophen, etc.) which produce necrosis of the hepatic parenchyma. How well do the cholestatic reactions associated with drug usage compare when matched against the criteria of these known hepatotoxic agents? Generally speaking, those substances associated with the production

TABLE I

SOME NON-STEROID DRUGS THAT HAVE BEEN ASSOCIATED WITH CHOLESTATIC REACTIONS IN MAN

CHLORPROMAZINE	PROPYLTHIOURACIL
PROCHLORPERAZINE	CHLORPROPAMIDE
PROMAZINE	METAHEXAMIDE
TRIFLUOPERAZINE	CARBUTAMIDE
THIORIDAZINE	ACETOHEXAMIDE
MEPAZINE	SULFANILAMIDE
CARBAMAZEPINE	SULFADIAZINE
AMITRYPTYLINE	ERYTHROMYCIN ESTOLATE
ECTYLUREA	SODIUM OXACILLIN
p-AMINOSALICYLIC ACID	TRIACETYLOLEANDOMYCIN
CHLORTHIAZIDE	NITROFURANTOIN
THIOURACIL	PHENINDONE
METHIMAZOLE	ARSPHENAMINE
	CARBARSONE

of cholestasis do produce distinct, histologic lesions, or at least hepatic ultrastructural changes in those individuals which show this adverse reaction. However, generally they fail to exhibit a well defined dose-related effect. While carbon tetrachloride does exhibit a dose-response relationship, chlorpromazine, for example, does not, nor do the other nonsteroid compounds associated with cholestasis. This means that predictability on the basis of therapeutic dosage is risky with those substances associated with cholestasis. With carbon tetrachloride it is possible to predetermine the environmental concentrations that are highly unlikely to produce acute liver injury and those that will. However, with chlorpromazine, cholestatic reactions have been reported to occur with extremely small therapeutic doses while patients have also been known to withstand extremely large therapeutic doses without exhibiting cholestasis.

The incidence of the toxic reaction is also different when one compares potential cholestatic drugs to those chemicals that produce toxic hepatitis. With carbon tetrachloride it is possible

TABLE II

CHARACTERISTICS OF TOXIC HEPATITIS

1. Distinctive histologic lesion
2. Presence of a dose-response relationship
3. High incidence
4. Reproducible in experimental animals
5. Predictable latent period

to determine a dose that will produce centrilobular necrosis in virtually 100% of the population (animal or human) at risk. However, with the drugs listed in Table I the reported incidence of cholestatic reactions is well below 1%, regardless of the doses employed. Therefore, while it might be possible to demonstrate alterations in hepatic function (BSP retention after treatment with anabolic steroids) the incidence of jaundice is very small.

The fourth important characteristic difference between necrogenic substances and cholestatic drugs is the fact that the former can produce necrotic lesions in most experimental animals whereas with the nonsteroid drugs listed in Table I, it has been virtually impossible to reproduce in animals the cholestatic lesion found in man. This factor is an extremely important one. It is the major reason for the lack of predictability of the cholestatic potential of drugs currently on the market. In addition, it has been a major stumbling block in the determination of the etiology and pathogenesis of these drug-induced reactions.

Some have used the lack of reproducibility in experimental animals as being an indication that allergic reactions in man are the cause of the cholestasis. It certainly is possible that allergic reactions can lead to cholestasis in man, but it appears that in most situations in which this mechanism has been invoked, it has been arrived at only indirectly. The number of clearly established allergic drug reactions leading to cholestasis is quite small.

A predictable latent period does not seem to exist for the cholestatic responses associated with the drugs listed in Table I. Such reactions have been reported in some cases shortly upon initiation of therapy whereas in other cases these reactions have occurred only after a number of weeks of treatment have passed.

PROBLEMS ASSOCIATED WITH LOW-FREQUENCY RESPONSES

One of the tools which is used by the toxicologist to predict the relative hazard involved in the exposure of man to chemicals is the fact that a dose-response relationship exists. The toxicologist has been able to predict the occurrence, or the probability, of toxicity in man in those instances in which he has been able to demonstrate the dose-response relationship in animals and the dose, even if abnormally high, which will eventually produce the lesion in most of the test population at risk. Unfortunately with drug-induced cholestasis, this has not been possible. Does this mean that no dose-response relationship exists? Or does it mean that the overall incidence is so low in the population at risk that the dose-response relationship is not discernible? The second possibility appears more likely.

Can we expect a better degree of predictability from the current tests that are utilized for the evaluation of safety regarding new drugs and their potential for the production of cholestasis? If one assumes that the cholestatic reaction produced in man by certain drugs is also reproducible in experimental animals but that only a small percentage of the animals, or the human population, at risk will present the cholestatic lesions, it is possible to begin to comprehend the problem the toxicologist has in uncovering this kind of reaction. Table III lists the minimal number of animals required on test to put into evidence the toxic reaction in at least one animal, for the various expected frequencies in man (1). If the expected frequency in man and animals is 1%, it would take about 300 animals on test to be able to produce the cholestatic reaction in at least one single animal with a 95% probability of success. However a 1% incidence of cholestasis is relatively high when one considers the incidence associated with those drugs listed in Table I. If the true incidence of the cholestatic reaction in man were only 0.1%, it would require about 3,000 animals on test in order to be able to produce this experimental lesion at least once with a 95% probability. If the incidence in man were 0.01%, one would have to test about 30,000 animals in order to pick up at least one animal. These types of calculations demonstrate why it is essentially impractical to expect that normal occurrences which have a very low incidence can be picked up in laboratory animals. Now this does not mean that the animal tests are insufficient or insensitive for the production of the toxic reaction; it merely means that if the incidence in the animal population is similar to the incidence in the human population, and if the reaction occurs with an extremely low frequency in both populations, it is virtually impossible to organize an animal test system which would detect the injury before the drug can be given to hundreds of thousands and maybe millions of individuals. While

TABLE III

NUMBERS OF ANIMALS REQUIRED IN LIVER STUDY TO SHOW CHOLESTASIS[a]

Expected Frequency in man (%)	Number of animals to be tested
1	299
0.1	2,995
0.01	29,956
0.001	299,572

[a] Number required to find at least 1 animal that develops cholestasis, with 0.95% probability. It is assumed that man and animals exhibit the same incidence of cholestasis. Data adapted from (1).

some could interpret this situation as a failing of our experimental assessment of toxicity, this type of calculation really demonstrates that it is asking too much of our current testing methods to be able to uncover and to study in depth all types of low-frequency toxic reactions.

The solution to this problem is not self evident. Obviously the mere increase in the numbers of animals to be tested is not a fruitful solution. The use of less commonly available species or strains of animals for test purposes may be one approach. Imai and Hayashi (2) reported that certain inbred species of mice develop morphologic signs of cholestasis and jaundice, in a dose-related manner, when given large doses of certain steroids. However, the choice of the species or strain remains empirical. In vitro test systems might be envisioned, but how can their predictability be assessed without an experimental in vivo response on which to make such a comparison? Unfortunately our current knowledge regarding cholestatic mechanisms is too sparse to permit the rational design of adequate test systems.

CONSIDERATIONS REGARDING MECHANISMS OF ACTION

Now it is time to turn to another aspect of the problem. For the last 40 years, extensive work has been carried out to determine how fatty livers are produced by numerous agents both in man and in animals. Table IV lists five theoretical reactions which can lead to the production of a fatty liver. It has been demonstrated in animals with known hepatotoxic agents that most of these mechanisms can be involved. With some agents, one or two mechanisms may be more important than others; with some agents only one mechanism may be involved. Yet all of these mechanisms can lead to the same final response, that is the production of a fatty liver. With cholestasis, that is the diminution or the complete cessation of bile flow accompanied by hyperbilirubinemia and jaundice, is it really inconceivable that more than one mechanism can be involved? Have we not been rather simplistic when we expect to be able to uncover the one mechanism for the production of cholestasis? To further illustrate the complexity of the situation, let us consider the ways in which hepatic triglyceride secretion can be affected (Table V). At least three mechanisms can lead to diminution of triglyceride secretion and thus triglyceride accumulation in the liver. All of these mechanisms have been shown to be affected in laboratory animals by various hepatotoxic agents that lead to the production of fatty liver. This further illustrates that it is inconceivable at this point in time to consider that as experimentalists we can uncover only one mechanism for the production of cholestasis. When one views the problem of cholestasis in this light, it then appears quite reasonable why chemically unrelated drugs, like those in Table I, can be associated with cholestatic reactions in man.

TABLE IV

THEORETICAL MECHANISMS INVOLVED IN THE

PRODUCTION OF FATTY LIVER

1. Increased mobilization of fatty acids

2. Decreased oxidation of fatty acids

3. Increased synthesis of fatty acids

4. Increased conversion to triglycerides

5. Decreased hepatic secretion of triglycerides

TABLE V

FACTORS INVOLVED IN HEPATIC

TRIGLYCERIDE SECRETION

1. Synthesis of protein

2. Coupling of apoprotein and triglyceride

3. Secretion of lipoprotein

α-NAPHTHYLISOTHIOCYANATE-INDUCED CHOLESTASIS

However, all is not black in the area of experimental cholestasis. Although it is relatively difficult to demonstrate cholestatic reactions with drugs in animals under the usual laboratory conditions, there are chemicals which are known to produce cholestatic reactions in laboratory animals. For the last 15 years, considerable experimental work has been carried out with a few of these agents. This type of work should continue and should be encouraged in order to uncover the various means by which chemical substances can produce cholestatic reactions in mammalian systems. This is not to say that these chemical substances reproduce in animals lesions which are entirely similar to those that are observed in man with drugs. However, they do lead to the cessation of bile flow, the accumulation of bile acids and the retention of bilirubin in the plasma. It is these experimental substances which have to be studied in order to uncover the various mechanisms involved in the production of cholestasis. It is only by such studies that one can eventually arrive at test systems, in vivo or in vitro, which may afford the index of predictability necessary for the screening of new drugs with cholestatic potential.

α-Naphthylisothiocyanate (ANIT) produces cholestasis and hyperbilirubinemia in several rodent species (3). In mice and rats it is possible to show that this substance exhibits a reproducible dose-response relationship. Figure 1 shows the effects of an acute administration of ANIT in the rat. Cholestasis, hyperbilirubinemia and bilirubinuria are all demonstrable in this species (4). Bilirubin retention reaches a peak at about 5 days. With time the animals recover their normal hepatic excretory function. ANIT can affect various hepatic parameters of bilirubin metabolism (5). Within a few hours after its administration, and before complete cessation of bile flow has occurred, ANIT decreases bilirubin uptake by the liver and the

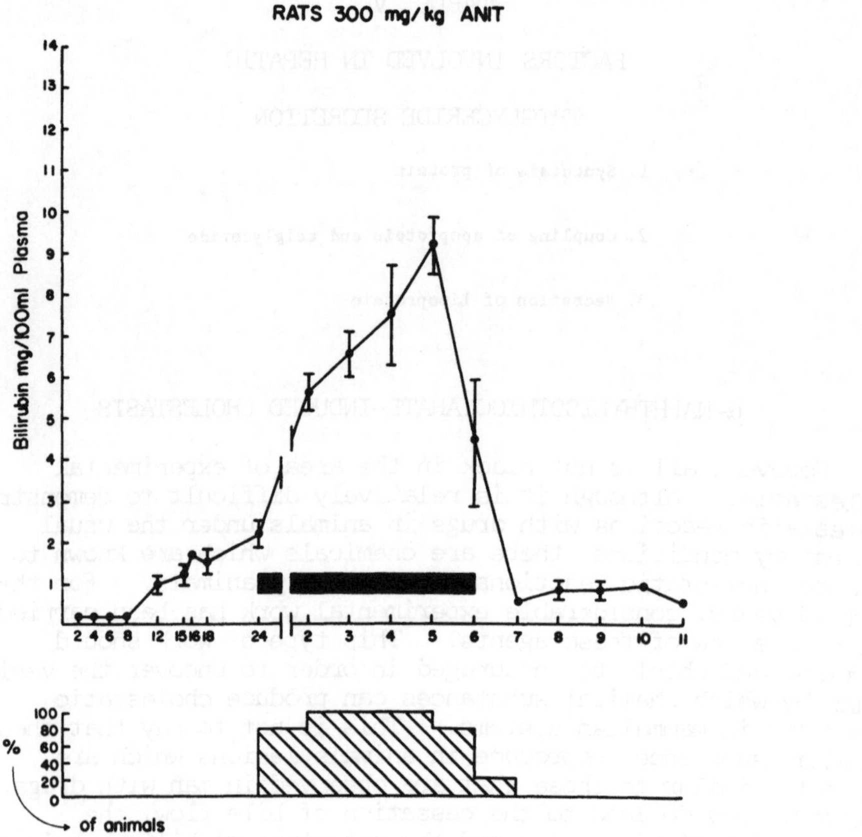

Fig. 1: ANIT-induced hyperbilirubinemia, bilirubinuria and cholestasis in rats. The upper portion of the figure denotes plasma bilirubin concentrations; the black horizontal bar indicates the period when bilirubinuria occurred. The lower portion of the figure indicates the percentage of animals which exhibited cholestasis. The time after the administration of ANIT is given in hours (2-24) and in days (2-11). From (4). Reproduced with the permission of Academic Press, Inc.

biliary excretory maximum for bilirubin (Table VI). ANIT also causes BSP retention 2 hours after its administration (6). Therefore we see that ANIT can cause bilirubin retention either by a diminution of the amount of bilirubin excreted into the bile, or by a failure of the liver to take up and store bilirubin from the circulatory compartment.

ANIT has a marked effect on the hepatic parenchyma although it does not produce necrosis. Table VII shows the inhibition

TABLE VI

EFFECT OF ANIT ON PLASMA BILIRUBIN DISAPPEARANCE AND BILIARY EXCRETION IN MICE AND RATS[a]

	CONTROL	ANIT
Plasma Bilirubin Half-life (min) (2 hours after ANIT)	12	18
Plasma Bilirubin Half-life (min) (24 hours after ANIT)	14	135
Plasma Bilirubin Half-life (min) (24 hours after ANIT in bile duct-ligated animals)	39	182
Liver Bilirubin Concentration (μg/g) (24 hours after ANIT)	158 ± 6	113 ± 7
Bilirubin Excretory Maximum (μg/100 g/min) (12 hours after ANIT)	56	19
Biliary Bilirubin Concentration (μg/μl) (12 hours after ANIT)	10	7

[a] From (5). Mice were used to calculate plasma bilirubin half-life and liver bilirubin concentration; rats were used for bilirubin excretory maximum.

of ANIT on the function of the endoplasmic reticulum as measured by the ability of this organelle to metabolize drugs in vitro. Two hours after the in vivo administration of ANIT it was possible to show a profound inhibition of drug metabolizing enzymes in vitro; this effect lasts for days (7).

ANIT also increases bilirubin synthesis from nonerythroid sources (8). Table VIII shows how ANIT can increase the incorporation of delta-aminolevulinic acid into bilirubin two hours after the administration of ANIT.

Therefore with this chemical, one is able to show that bilirubin excretion, bilirubin uptake, BSP retention, nonerythropoietic bilirubin synthesis and endoplasmic reticulum activity are all affected. Can all of these parameters contribute to the

TABLE VII

EFFECT OF ANIT ON HEPATIC MICROSOMAL ACTIVITY IN MICE[a]

	Percent of Control Activity		
Time after ANIT	Hexobarbital Oxidase	Aniline Hydroxylase	Chlorpromazine Sulfoxidase
2 hours	27	32	108
1 day	29	40	95
5 days	65	65	98
9 days	70	68	90

[a] From (7).

TABLE VIII

EFFECT OF ANIT ON NONERYTHROPOIETICALLY DERIVED BILIRUBIN IN RATS[a]

Parameter	Control	ANIT
Bile flow (ml/100 g/hr)	0.39 ± 0.01	0.33 ± 0.01
Biliary bilirubin conc. (μg/ml)	49 ± 2	109 ± 9
Biliary bilirubin excretion (μg/100 g/hr)	18.3 ± 0.7	34.5 ± 1.9
Total bilirubin ^{14}C (dpm/100 g x 10^{-3})	17.9 ± 0.5	30.4 ± 0.5
Incorporation of ^{14}C-ALA (%)	13.2 ± 0.5	21.7 ± 0.3

[a] From (8).

TABLE IX

EFFECT OF CYCLOHEXIMIDE ON ANIT-INDUCED HYPERBILIRUBINEMIA CHOLESTASIS AND EARLY BSP RETENTION IN RATS[a]

Group	Hyperbilirubinemia (mg/100 ml)	Cholestasis (No. blocked/No. tested)	BSP Retention (mg/100 ml)
Control	0.55 ± 0.03	0/6	4.0 ± 1.6
ANIT	3.9 ± 0.35	6/6	8.9 ± 0.7
Cycloheximide + ANIT	0.52 ± 0.03	1/6	12.9 ± 3.2

[a] From (6, 9). Bilirubinemia and bile flow were determined 24 hours after ANIT. BSP was determined 2 hours after ANIT.

hyperbilirubinemia and cholestasis produced by ANIT? In a recent series of experiments, we have used inhibitors of protein synthesis like cycloheximide, actinomycin D, ethionine and puromycin in an attempt to unravel the various mechanisms involved in the ANIT response (6,9). Pretreatment of the animals with inhibitors of protein synthesis can markedly protect the animals against the production of hyperbilirubinemia. Those animals treated with cycloheximide are completely protected against a hyperbilirubinemic and cholestatic dose of ANIT (Table IX). Pretreatment with cycloheximide has been shown (10) to block the production of bilirubin from nonerythroid sources induced by ANIT (Table X). However, cycloheximide pretreatment does not affect the inhibition of microsomal enzymes produced by ANIT and surprisingly does not affect the early BSP retention (Table IX) observed after administration of ANIT (6). Consequently, experimentally it can be shown that of the four major hepatic responses to ANIT, only two can be blocked by the administration of an inhibitor of protein synthesis. This would suggest very strongly that the effect of ANIT on endoplasmic reticulum function related to the microsomal drug metabolizing enzymes has little to do with the cholestatic or hyperbilirubinemic response and that the BSP retention observed early after ANIT administration is also unrelated to the hyperbilirubinemia one sees eventually. However, the factors which do seem to be involved in the ANIT hyperbilirubinemic response include the diminution in bilirubin excretion and the increased production of bilirubin from nonerythroid sources. Thus it can be seen that with this cholestatic reaction in experimental animals, it is possible to gain information about possible functional mechanisms of action.

TABLE X

EFFECT OF CYCLOHEXIMIDE ON ANIT-INDUCED NONERYTHROPOIETICALLY DERIVED BILIRUBIN IN RATS[a]

Parameter	Control	ANIT	Cycloheximide + ANIT
Total Bilirubin excreted (μg/100 g)	73.6 ± 4.0	15.8 ± 32.1	54.4 ± 4.3
Total bilibubin - ^{14}C (dpm/100 g x 10^{-3})	13.2 ± 1.3	23.7 ± 1.5	13.5 ± 1.2
Incorporation of ^{14}C-ALA (%)	8.2 ± 0.8	14.8 ± 0.9	8.4 ± 0.9

[a] From (10).

The ANIT model is interesting from another point of view. ANIT-induced hyperbilirubinemia in the mouse can be potentiated by the pretreatment of the animals with inducers of microsomal enzymes (11,12). Table XI illustrates a study which was carried out in the mouse. A threshold dose of ANIT was administered to animals which had been pretreated with saline or pretreated with enzyme-inducing doses of phenobarbital, chlorpromazine, norethandrolone or Enovid. It is evident that the magnitude of the hyperbilirubinemia after this threshold dose of ANIT was enhanced in animals which had been pretreated with microsomal enzyme inducers; the duration of the hyperbilirubinemia was also prolonged. The same phenomenon was demonstrated when bile flow was used as the end point; those animals treated with the inducers exhibited more positive cholestatic responses. From these experiments one could conclude that inducing agents or substances which enhance microsomal enzyme activity will lead to an enhanced hyperbilirubinemic response to ANIT. However, such a generalization is a hazardous one to make. Selye (13) has shown that catatoxic steroids, which possess little or no mineralo- or glucocorticoid activity, can protect animals from a number of various toxic agents. They have been shown to produce induction of microsomal enzymes leading to end results which are very similar to those observed with phenobarbital. We tested one of the steroids in our laboratory against ANIT and we expected that like phenobarbital it should enhance the toxicity produced by ANIT. However this was not the case at all; pretreatment of animals with doses of 16-α-pregnenolone carbonitrile (PEN) which are known to produce microsomal enzyme induction did not lead to enhanced ANIT hepatotoxicity; in fact, they protected against the hyperbilirubinemic response (14).

TABLE XI

EFFECT OF INDUCERS OF MICROSOMAL ENZYMES ON ANIT-INDUCED HYPERBILIRUBINEMIA AND CHOLESTASIS IN MICE[a]

Treatment	Plasma Bilirubin Concentration (mg/100 ml)	No. with Cholestasis / No. treated
ANIT	1.3 ± 0.3	3/10
Phenobarbital + ANIT	4.5 ± 0.6	9/10
Chlorpromazine + ANIT	5.9 ± 0.3	10/10
ANIT	1.1 ± 0.3	5/20
Norethandrolone + ANIT	4.9 ± 0.6	10/10
Enovid + ANIT	2.4 ± 0.3	8/10

[a] From (11, 12). Bilirubin concentrations were determined 24 hours after ANIT; the presence of cholestasis was assessed 10 hours after ANIT.

Therefore, unfortunately, we cannot make generalizations about drug interactions merely on the basis of the microsomal enzyme inducing properties of one of the interacting pairs. It appears that while there is a number of microsomal enzyme inducing agents, these substances have to be treated as individual entities or classes of inducers before one can make generalizations regarding their possible effects on hepatotoxic agents.

ANIT-induced hyperbilirubinemia can be enhanced by other substances which are not known to be potent inducers. It has been shown that isopropanol and acetone will potentiate the necrogenic effects of carbon tetrachloride in rats (15,16).

In Table XII it is seen that isopropanol and acetone pretreatment will also potentiate the hyperbilirubinemic response produced by ANIT (17). This enhanced response to ANIT does not seem to be due to an effect of isopropanol or acetone on bilirubin metabolism disposition; the hyperbilirubinemia caused by bile duct ligation is not affected by isopropanol or acetone.

Another experimental non-steroid model has been described. Witzleben et al (18) reported that the acute administration of manganese results in morphologic signs of intrahepatic cholestasis;

TABLE XII

EFFECT OF ISOPROPANOL AND ACETONE ON ANIT-INDUCED HYPERBILIRUBINEMIA IN RATS[a]

Treatment	Plasma Bilirubin Concentration (mg/100 ml)
Control	0.2 ± 0.0
ANIT	2.6 ± 0.3
Isopropanol + ANIT	4.2 ± 0.2
Control	0.4 ± 0.1
ANIT	1.5 ± 0.3
Acetone + ANIT	3.1 ± 0.2

[a] From (17).

the biliary bilirubin excretory maximum is markedly reduced. The infusion of bilirubin enhances the cholestatic response to manganese in a dose-related manner (19). Nothing is known about the possible mechanisms of action involved in this interesting model, but it affords another approach for the study of cholestasis.

SUMMARY

The nonsteroid drugs that have been associated with cholestatic reactions in man do not produce similar responses in animals under the usual laboratory conditions. These drug reactions in man also seem to be unrelated to the dose ingested. The cholestatic reaction in man occurs with a low frequency.

The induction of cholestasis and hyperbilirubinemia in animals by α-naphthylisothiocyanate (ANIT), however, has been achieved and this model allows one to study various mechanisms of action. Cycloheximide protects rats against ANIT-induced cholestasis and hyperbilirubinemia. However, cycloheximide does not affect the depressant effect of ANIT on microsomal enzymes nor its stimulatory effect on nonerythropoietically derived bilirubin. Phenobarbital, chlorpromazine, norethandrolone, Enovid, isopropanol and acetone enhance the hepatotoxic response to ANIT.

REFERENCES

1. ZBINDEN G: Progress in Toxicology. Special Topics. New York, Springer-Verlag, 1974. p. 18.

2. IMAI K, HAYASHI Y: Steroid-induced intrahepatic cholestasis in mice. Japan J Pharmacol 20: 473-481, 1970.

3. PLAA GL: Hyperbilirubinemia and cholestasis, a different form of liver injury produced in animals. In Essays in Toxicology, vol. 2. Edited by Blood, F. New York, Academic Press, 1970. pp. 137-154.

4. INDACOCHEA-REDMOND N, PLAA GL: Functional effects of α-naphthylisothiocyanate in various species. Toxicol Appl Pharmacol 19: 71-80, 1971.

5. ROBERTS RJ, PLAA GL: Alteration of the plasma disappearance and biliary excretion patterns of exogenously administered bilirubin by α-naphthylisothiocyanate. J Pharmacol Exp Ther 155: 330-336, 1967.

6. INDACOCHEA-REDMOND N, WITSCHI HP, PLAA GL: Effects of inhibitors of protein and ribonucleic acid synthesis on α-naphthylisothiocyanate-induced hyperbilirubinemia, sulfobromophthalein retention and prolongation of pentobarbital hypnosis. J Pharmacol Exp Ther 189: 278-284, 1974.

7. PLAA GL, ROGERS LA, FOUTS JR: Effect of acute alpha-naphthylisothiocyanate administration on hepatic microsomal drug metabolism in the mouse. Proc Soc Exp Biol Med 119: 1045-1048, 1965.

8. ROBERTS RJ, PLAA GL: Alteration in biliary bilirubin content and nonerythropoietically derived bilirubin synthesis in rats after α-naphthylisothiocyanate administration. J Pharmacol Exp Ther 161: 382-388, 1968.

9. INDACOCHEA-REDMOND N, WITSCHI HP, PLAA GL: Effect of inhibitors of protein and ribonucleic acid synthesis on the hyperbilirubinemia and cholestasis produced by α-naphthylisothiocyanate. J Pharmacol Exp Ther 184: 780-786, 1973.

10. TRAIGER GJ, DE REPENTIGNY L, PLAA GL: Effect of inhibitors of protein and ribonucleic acid synthesis on the alteration in biliary bilirubin excretion and non-erythropoietically derived bilirubin synthesis in rats after

α-naphthylisothiocyanate administration. Biochem Pharmacol (in press)

11. ROBERTS RJ, PLAA GL: Potentiation and inhibition of α-naphthylisothiocyanate-induced hyperbilirubinemia and cholestasis. J Pharmacol Exp Ther 150: 499-506, 1965.

12. ROBERTS RJ, PLAA GL: Effect of norethandrolone, acetohexamide, and Enovid on α-naphthylisothiocyanate-induced hyperbilirubinemia and cholestasis. Biochem Pharmacol 15: 333-341, 1966.

13. SELYE H: Hormones and Resistance, vol. 1. New York, Springer-Verlag, 1974. p 273.

14. INDACOCHEA-REDMOND N, PLAA GL: Effect of 16-α-pregnenolone carbonitrile (PCN) on α-naphthylisothiocyanate (ANIT)-induced hepatotoxicity. Proc Can Fed Biol Soc 17: 53, 1974.

15. TRAIGER GJ, PLAA GL: Differences in the potentiation of carbon tetrachloride in rats by ethanol and isopropanol pretreatment. Toxicol Appl Pharmacol 20: 105-112, 1971.

16. TRAIGER GJ, PLAA GL: Relationship of alcohol metabolism to the potentiation of CCl_4 hepatotoxicity induced by aliphatic alcohols. J Pharmacol Exp Ther 183: 481-488, 1972.

17. PLAA GL, TRAIGER GJ, HANASONO GK, WITSCHI HP: Effect of alcohols on various forms of chemically induced liver injury. In Alcholic Liver Pathology, edited by Israel Y, Khanna J, Kalant H. Toronto, Addiction Research Foundation (in press).

18. WITZLEBEN CL, PITLICK P, BERGMEYER J, et al. Acute manganese overload. A new experimental model of intrahepatic cholestasis. Amer J Pathol 53: 409-423, 1968.

19. BOYCE W, WITZLEBEN CL: Bilirubin as a cholestatic agent. II. Effect of variable doses of bilirubin on the severity of manganese-bilirubin cholestasis. Amer J Pathol 72: 427-432, 1973.

BILE CANALICULAR STRUCTURE AND FUNCTION

M.James Phillips, Masaya Oda, Ellen Mak & M.M. Fisher

Banting Institute, University of Toronto

100 College Street, Toronto, Ontario M5G 1L5

INTRODUCTION

Bile canaliculi from normal and cholestatic liver have been extensively studied using conventional electron microscopic techniques (1-8). Other studies have dealt with the relationships of the bile canaliculi to the sinusoids and the space of Disse (9-11). It is now well established that bile canaliculi are formed by two or three hepatocytes , are closed by junctional complexes, and are surrounded by an organelle-free ectoplasmic zone. It has been suggested that the pericanalicular ectoplasmic layer is composed of filamentous structures in human (1) and in calf liver (12), but the filamentous structures were not distinctly defined.

This report deals with further ultrastructural characterization of the bile canaliculus and with preliminary results on the effects of cytochalasin B on bile canalicular structure and function.

MATERIAL AND METHODS

Male Wistar strain rats (High Oak Ranch, Toronto, Canada) weighing 150-200 g were used. The rats used in the in vivo experiments were maintained on a commercial diet (Rockland mouse and rat diet) and were fasted overnight. The rats used in the in vitro studies were maintained on a semi-synthetic diet (General Biochemicals Basal Diet, TD-72460) and 2 hours before sacrifice were given a 1 g supplement of the diet by stomach tube.

Isolated bile canaliculi, partially disrupted hepatocytes, isolated hepatocytes and in vivo liver

The isolation of bile canalicular fractions from rat liver was carried out according to a modification of the method of Song et al (13). The liver was perfused in situ with NaCl (0.15 M) at 4°C, homogenized whole using a Willems Polytron for 5 - 10 seconds and centrifuged at 500 x g for 5 minutes and then at 1000 x g for 10 minutes. Using a discontinuous sucrose gradient centrifugation at 66,000 x g for 60 minutes, an upper membrane fraction present between the sucrose solutions of density 1.16 and 1.18 was obtained. It was composed mainly of isolated bile canaliculi and was designated the BC fraction. The pellet (P) contained partially disrupted hepatocytes. These fractions were fixed for 10 minutes at 0°C in cacodylate buffered 1.2% gluteraldehyde (pH 7.4), containing 1,000 ppm ruthenium red (RR). The blocks were post fixed in 2% osmium tetroxide buffered in 0.06 M sodium cacodylate at pH 7.4 containing 1,000 ppm RR. Other samples from both P and BC fractions were fixed in gluteraldehyde and osmium tetroxide, as above, but without the addition of RR. Other samples were stained using 4% aqueous uranyl acetate for 1 hour at room temperature after exposure to osmium tetroxide but before dehydration.

Isolated hepatocytes from rat liver obtained by the method of Berry and Friend (14) and cultured in vitro in a horse serum enriched medium according to the method of Jeejeebhoy et al (15) were prepared for electrom microscopic study using the same techniques.

Liver samples from normal anaesthetized rats were fixed for 3 to 5 minutes with 1.2% gluteraldehyde in 0.06 M sodium cacodylate buffer, pH 7.4, containing 1,000 ppm RR. Small blocks were made and subjected to further fixation for 30 minutes at 0°C in the same aldehyde-RR mixture. The blocks were then rinsed in buffer and post fixed for 3 hours in the osmium tetroxide-RR solution mentioned above.

After osmification, all specimens were dehydrated in a graded series of ethanol solutions and embedded in an Epon-Araldite mixture. The adequacy of the RR staining was assessed in 1 μ sections. Ultra-thin sections were cut on an LKB ultramicrotome with a diamond knife. They were mounted on uncoated copper grids, stained with lead citrate or unstained and examined in a Philips EM-300 electron microscope with a 60KV acceleration voltage.

Heavy Meromyosin (HMM)

Bile canalicular fractions were also treated with heavy meromyosin (HMM). The HMM was prepared by the method of Lowey and Cohen (16) using myosin obtained from rabbit muscle by the method of Mommaert and Parrish (17). The concentration was 0.8 mg protein/ml. It was dialyzed against 0.5M KCl in 0.03 M potassium phosphate buffer (pH 7.0); the purity of the HMM was checked using alkaline gel electrophoresis. A modification of the non-glycerinated technique of Pollard and Korn (18) or the glycerinated technique described by Ishikawa et al (19) was used. Control specimens were treated in identical manner but without HMM. Subsequently, the HMM treated and control specimens were processed and stained by the RR techniques described above.

Mg^{++} activated adenosine triphosphatase (ATPase)

Some samples of the isolated bile canaliculi, partially disrupted hepatocytes and intact liver were stained with RR after incubation in a Wachstein-Meisel type medium for Mg^{++} activated adenosine triphosphatase (ATPase) (20,21) in order to distinguish the bile canaliculi from other membranes. Controls were incubated in an identical manner but in medium lacking the substrate.

Cytochalasin B

Cytochalasin B (CB, Aldrich Chemical Company Inc. USA) solution was prepared immediately before use by diluting a stock solution containing 10 mg/ml of cytochalasin B in dimethyl sulfoxide (DMSO) with 0.006 M phosphate buffer, pH 7.4, to a concentration of 80 μg/ml. Cultured hepatocytes obtained as previously cited, were used in the cytochalasin B experiments. The culture medium containing hepatocytes was divided into the following three groups. Group A: 0.006 M phosphate buffer was added to the culture medium at a final concentration of 0.0015 M. Group B: the cytochalasin B solution described above was added to the culture medium at the final concentration of 20 μg/ml CB and 0.2% DMSO. Group C: 0.8% DMSO solution diluted with 0.006 M phosphate buffer was added to the culture medium at the final concentration of 0.2%. Samples for light and electron microscopy were obtained respectively after one, three and six hours incubation at 37°C.

RESULTS

The Bile Canalicular Web

The bile canalicular fraction consisted almost exclusively of intact bile canaliculi complete with their junctional complexes and segments of the contiguous plasma membrane (Fig. 1). In lead citrate stained specimens, the pericanalicular ectoplasm

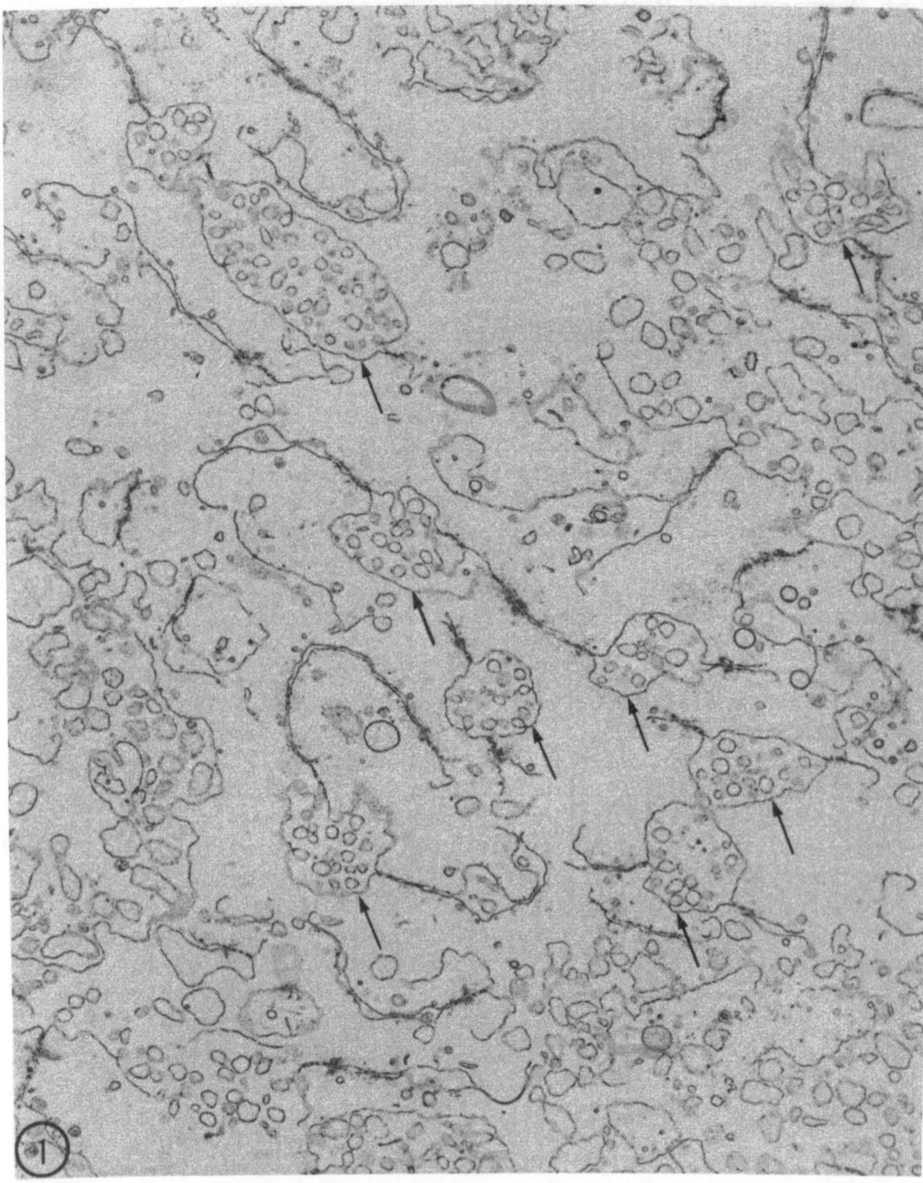

Fig. 1: Bile canaliculus fraction. This fraction is clean and extremely rich in intact bile canaliculi (unlabelled arrows). Canalicular microvilli, the contiguous lateral cell membranes, and the junctional complexes can be seen. A scanty amount of fuzzy material is present at the margins of some canaliculi. Lead citrate x 9,360.

appeared finely granular but was ill-defined. In the uranyl-acetate preparations, the pericanalicular filamentous structures were more sharply stained. Microfilaments of two sizes were easily recognized and were approximately 50 Å and 100 Å in diameter. The RR stain demonstrated a rich network of microfilaments around the entire bile canaliculus (Fig. 2). The thin microfilament component measured 70-85 Å using this staining technique, and the thick filaments 100-150 Å. The plasma membranes and bile canalicular membranes were also well stained. An RR positive surface coat was present over both the canalicular membranes and the plasma membranes. The four components of the junctional complex: zonula occludens (tight junction), zonula adherens (intermediate junction), macula adherens (desmosome) and gap junction (nexus) were easily recognized (Fig. 2). Many of the pericanalicular microfilaments inserted into the zonula adherens and macula adherens portions of the junctional complex. A few smooth surfaced vesicles were associated with the pericanalicular web and appeared entrapped within the network of filaments.

In the partially disrupted hepatocyte preparations, the inner compartment of the liver cell was exposed to the RR staining procedure. In these cells, a very rich network of microfilaments was found within the cytoplasm, and these filaments were particularly numerous near the bile canaliculi. The ATPase reaction was useful in localizing the bile canaliculus region in the partially disrupted hepatocytes. An intimate association between pericanalicular microfilaments and intracytoplasmic vesicles was again shown.

In the in vivo liver preparations the pericanalicular network of microfilaments was not evident since the RR did not penetrate the intact cell membranes. In some instances, however, the surface coat on the bile canalicular membrane of intact liver cells was demonstrable.

In the cultured hepatocytes, the surface coat was always stained intensely, and the microfilamentous structures were sometimes visualized in the canalicular microvilli and in the pericanalicular ectoplasmic region. The bile canaliculi of single cultured hepatocytes were intracellular. Approximately 20% of the isolated cells were joined together in pairs and they were always joined at their canalicular regions. In such cell pairs, the bile canaliculus was tightly closed with no demonstrable canalicular lumen evident.

The heavy meromyosin experiment was carried out on the isolated bile canalicular fractions since these showed the microfilaments to best advantage. In these preparations, the thin microfilaments (50 Å in uranyl acetate stain) were distinctly

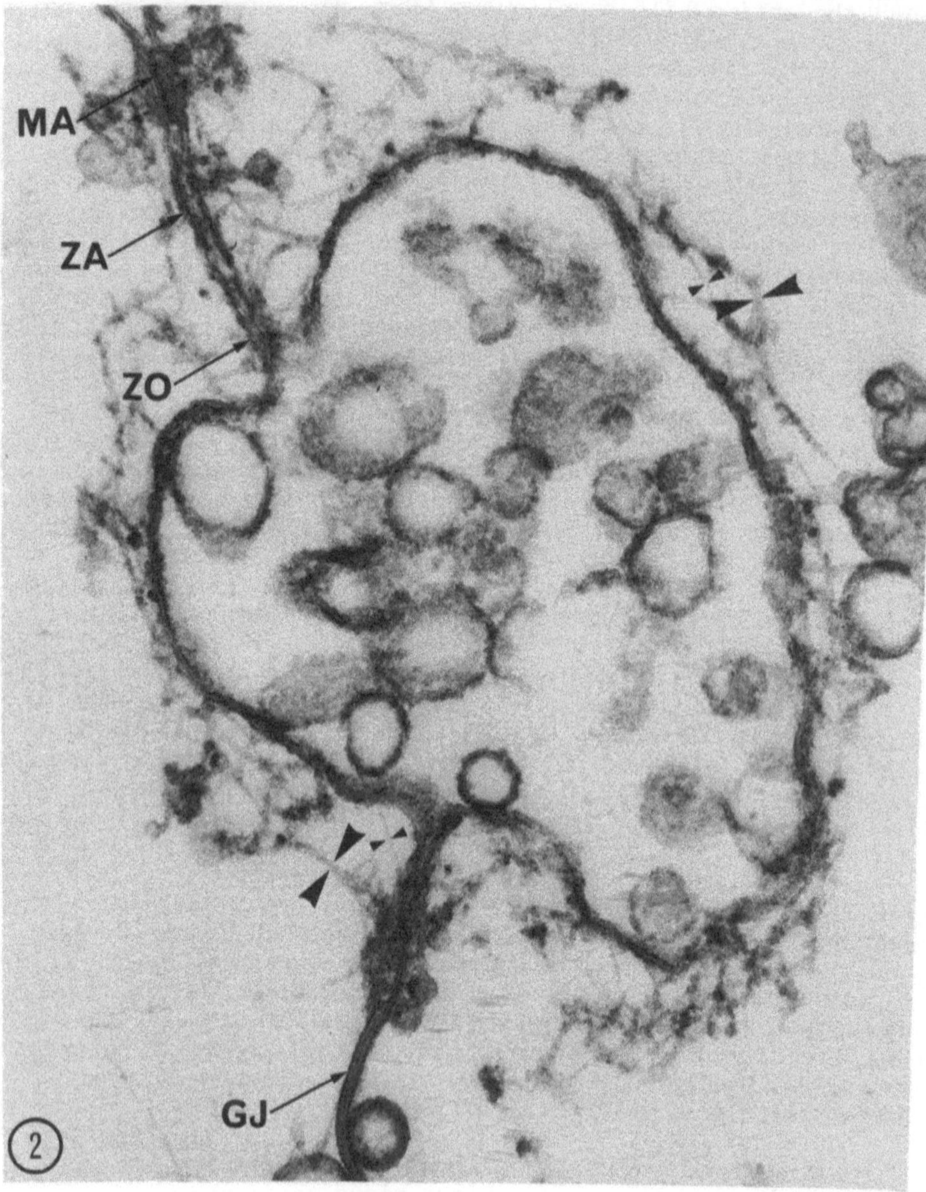
MA
ZA
ZO
GJ
2

decorated indicating binding of HMM (Fig. 4). In places, the decorations suggested a regularity in the binding pattern. Control specimens treated with buffer solution only showed no reaction and the microfilaments remained smooth (Fig. 3).

Effects of cytochalasin B on bile canalicular structure and function

In the isolated liver cell preparations in which cytochalasin B was added to the culture medium, the bile canaliculi were all widely patent. The dilatation was marked and easily seen in the 1 micron sections by light microscopy. In single cells, the intracytoplasmic canaliculi were distended resembling a large empty vacuole within the hepatocyte. In those instances in which the hepatocytes were paired, the dilated bile canaliculus was very obvious because of its location at the junction between the two cells. By electron microscopy, the hepatocytes appeared normal aside from the bile canalicular region. Some of the dilated bile canaliculi had no microvilli, and in the others all were reduced in number, shortened and had no RR positive surface coat (Fig. 8). In high resolution pictures, the pericanalicular ectoplasmic zone was also shown to be altered. Microfilaments were not present and in their place was granular material (Fig. 6). Microtubules were noted in the region of the pericanalicular granules. In control preparations treated only with DMSO or buffer, the bile canaliculi were normally stained and tightly closed (Fig. 7) and bundles of microfilaments were present in the pericanalicular ectoplasm and microvillous cores (Fig. 5).

DISCUSSION

The bile canalicular web

Filamentous structures in the pericanalicular ectoplasm have been demonstrated previously in in vivo whole liver (1,12), in isolated bile canaliculi (9), and in association with junctional complexes (22), but in all these instances they were poorly

Fig. 2: Bile canaliculus fraction. This preparation has been stained by the ruthenium red technique. Note the network of microfilaments around the canaliculus. The various components of the junctional complex (ZO, zonula occludens; ZA, zonula adherens; MA, macula adherens; GJ, gap junction) are well seen. Many of the microfilaments insert into the zonula adherens (intermediate junction) and macula adherens (desmosome) regions of the junctional complex. Note also that the microfilaments are of two sizes; thin microfilaments (small arrow heads) and thick microfilaments (large arrow heads).
Ruthenium red, lead citrate counterstain, x 72,000.

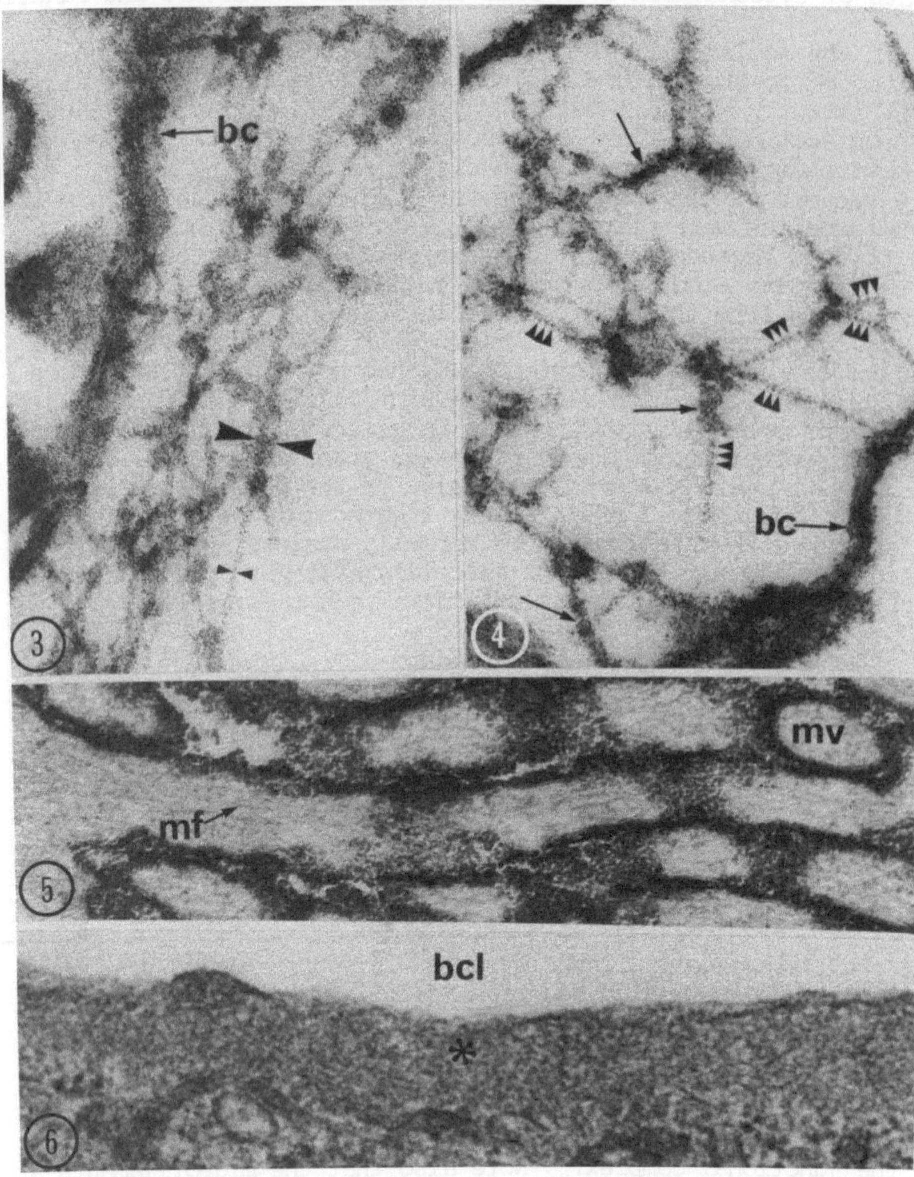
bc
3
bc
4
mv
mf
5
bcl
*
6

visualized. The microfilaments described in this report and in an accompanying paper (23), demonstrate for the first time that they form a pericanalicular network, and that they are of two sizes. The thin microfilaments measure approximately 50 Å in diameter and the thick microfilaments 100 Å, in preparations stained with uranyl acetate. The slightly larger size observed in the RR stained preparations compared to the uranyl acetate-en bloc specimens, is presumably due to the staining of materials coating the filaments in the RR method. An appreciation of the importance of microfilaments has come from a variety of recent studies. Microfilaments have been described in a wide variety of cell types and suggestions have been made that bundles or meshworks of these filaments represent the contractile machinery of such cells (24). For instance, Cloney (25) found that the microfilament system was responsible for the rapid shortening of ascidian tadpole tails during metamorphosis. Baker and Schroeder (26) explained the sinking of the amphibian embryonic plate to form the neural groove on a purse-string type of contraction by microfilaments. As a result of such studies, it

<u>Fig. 3:</u> Bile canalicular fraction, from a control specimen (HMM omitted). The edge of the bile canaliculus is marked bc. The pericanalicular network of microfilaments is easily discerned. Thin (small arrow heads) and thick microfilaments (large arrow heads) are evident.
Ruthenium red x 108,000

<u>Fig. 4:</u> Bile canalicular fraction treated by the non-glycerinated HMM technique. Note the HMM binding to thin microfilaments (arrows). Note also the regularity and apparent periodicity to the decorations (arrowheads). The edge of the bile canaliculus is marked bc.
Ruthenium red x 108,000.

<u>Fig. 5:</u> Higher magnification of bile canaliculus of DMSO treated cultured hepatocyte (cytochalasin B control). Note the microfilaments (mf) in bundles in the pericanalicular ectoplasm and in microvillous cores (mv). The black staining material is the surface coat.
Ruthenium red x 98,100.

<u>Fig. 6:</u> Higher magnification of bile canaliculus region of cytochalasin B treated cultured hepatocyte. The edge of a dilated canaliculus is shown; its lumen is marked bcl. Note that microvilli are absent. The surface coat is also absent. The region of the microfilaments is occupied by amorphous granular material (*).
Ruthenium red x 98,100.

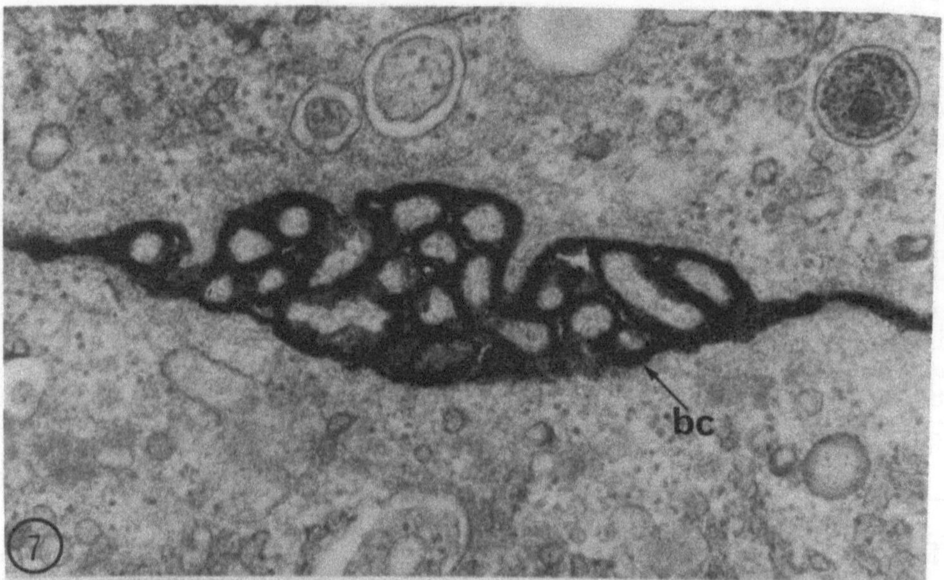
bc
7

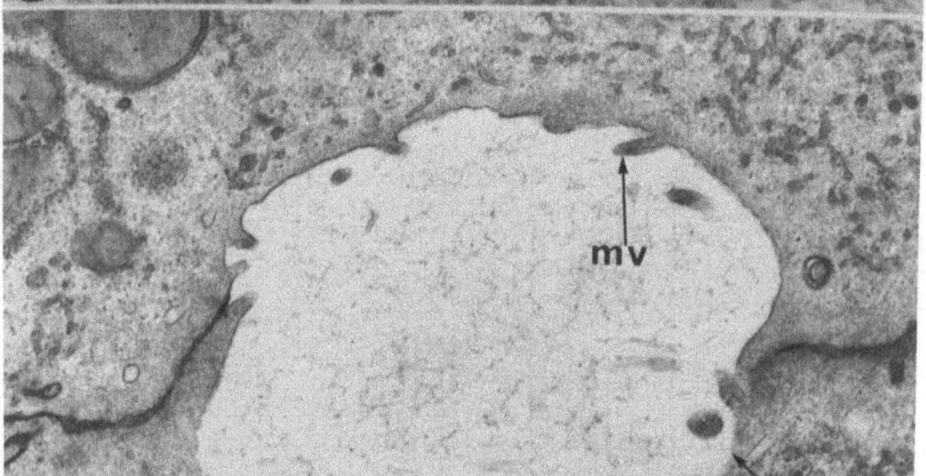
mv
bc
8

has become evident that the 50-70 Å microfilaments are very similar to actin filaments from muscle in size, in their contractile function and in their content of actin or actin-like protein (27). It has been shown that even primitive cells such as slime-molds contain actin-like protein which interacts with muscle HMM to form arrowhead complexes (28). The formation of arrowhead complexes is characteristic of muscle acto-HMM (29). Moreover it has been shown by a number of investigators that microfilaments react with HMM to form arrowhead complexes (19,30). In the present study, the thin microfilament component of the pericanalicular web showed HMM binding. It is noted that rather than arrowhead complexes, decoration with HMM was found: this was an expected variation and is the result of prior fixation as previously pointed out by Spooner et al (31). Indeed the decoration with HMM observed in our study was similar to that observed by Spooner et al (31) since there was an overall impression of regularity in the HMM-binding pattern. Since the present evidence is overwhelming that microfilaments of 50 Å diameter which show HMM binding have a contractile function, we suggest that the thin microfilament component of the pericanalicular web maintains the bile canaliculus in a contracted or partly contracted state.

Effects of cytochalasin B on bile canalicular structure

The experiment with cytochalasin B provides strong support for the above hypothesis. Cytochalasin B, a fungal alkaloid, disrupts microfilaments and inhibits their contractile function. Cytochalasin B has been shown to inhibit diverse contractile movements including cardiac muscle contraction (32), cytoplasmic streaming (24), phagocytosis (33), hormone secretion (34), platelet activation (35), and clot retraction (36). The microfilaments in all these various cell types are very similar

Fig. 7: Cultured hepatocyte preparation treated with 0.2% DMSO for 3 hours (cytochalasin B control) stained by ruthenium red. The bile canalicular zone (bc) between two contiguous hepatocytes is shown. No canalicular lumen is evident, the microvilli are tightly opposed. The black material is the RR positive surface coat.
Ruthenium red x 54,000.

Fig. 8: Cultured hepatocyte preparation following 3 hours cytochalasin B (20 μg/ml) treatment. Note the extreme bile canalicular (bc) dilatation. Note also that microvilli (mv) are short and absent from much of its circumference. The RR positive surface coat is absent over the canalicular membrane but is present over other portions of the plasma membrane.
Ruthenium red x 28,800.

to muscle actin filaments in their size (50-70 Å in diameter) and their binding with HMM. It has also been noted that cytochalasin B alters the structural conformation of the microfilaments in that they lose their filamentous structure and become granular and amorphous (24,27). In the present study, cytochalasin B administration resulted in marked ectasia of the bile canaliculi. Moreover, the microfilamentous zone became granular and amorphous. These observations suggest that in hepatocytes, cytochalasin B alters the structural conformation of the pericanalicular microfilaments with consequent dilatation of the bile canaliculi. The reduction in canalicular microvilli may be related to the marked ectasia with ironing out of the microvilli, or may be the result of an effect on the microvilli per se since it is known that the microfilaments extend into the canalicular microvilli (23). Marked dilation of bile canaliculi and loss of microvilli are common ultrastructural findings in cholestasis (6-8). The relationships of microfilament structure and function to bile flow and to the pathogenesis of cholestasis are presently under study.

SUMMARY

A rich network of microfilaments is present around the bile canaliculi. This network corresponds to the ectoplasmic zone observed in conventional electron micrographs of normal liver. The thin microfilaments of the network have all the ultrastructural characteristics of actin-containing microfilaments including their size, configuration, heavy meromyosin binding and altered structural conformation with cytochalasin B. In view of these findings, it is reasonable to suggest that these microfilaments may have a contractile function. Their location and disposition are such that they may provide a system for the contraction and dilation of bile canaliculi depending on the functional state of the liver. Because the canaliculi were closed in the control isolated hepatocytes but widely dilated in those hepatocytes treated with cytochalasin B it is suggested that under normal circumstances, the microfilaments maintain the canalicular system in a closed or partially closed state. This leads to the conclusion that the microfilaments are not just a means of mechanical support but also provide tone to the bile canalicular system. Hence, normal pericanalicular microfilament function would tend to reduce stagnation of bile and facilitate the flow of bile from the canaliculi to the bile ducts; conversely, altered microfilament function would be expected to result in intrahepatic cholestasis.

ACKNOWLEDGEMENTS

This research was supported by a Grant-in-Aid of the Medical Research Council of Canada (MT-785). Mrs. Ellen Mak, 2nd year Medical Student, University of Toronto, was supported by a Summer Student Scholarship of the Canadian Hepatic Foundation. The authors also wish to thank Dr. S. French, Department of Pathology, University of British Columbia, for the heavy meromyosin, and for his helpful comments. We also thank Miss Valerie Price and Mrs. Janet Rowley for excellent technical assistance.

REFERENCES

1. BIAVA CG: Studies on cholestasis. A re-evaluation of the fine structure of normal human bile canaliculi. Lab Invest 13: 840-864, 1964.

2. FAWCETT DW: Observations on the cytology and electron microscopy of hepatic cells. J Natl Cancer Inst (suppl) 15: 1475-1503, 1955.

3. ROUILLER C: Les canalicules biliares. Etude au microscope electronique. C.R.Soc Biol(Paris) 148: 2008-2011, 1954.

4. ROUILLER C: Les canalicules biliares. Etude au microscope electronique. Acta Anat 26: 94-109, 1956.

5. STEINER JW, CARRUTHERS JS: Studies on the fine structure of the terminal branches of the biliary tree. I. The morphology of normal bile canaliculi, bile pre-ductules (ducts of Hering) and bile ductules. Amer J Pathol 38: 639-661, 1961.

6. STEINER JW, CARRUTHERS JS: Studies on the fine structure of the terminal branches of the biliary tree. II Observations of pathologically altered bile canaliculi. Amer J Pathol 39: 41-63, 1961.

7. STEINER JW, PHILLIPS MJ, BAGLIO CM: Electron microscopy of the excretory pathways in the liver in alpha-naphthyl isothiocyanate intoxication. A study of intrahepatic cholestasis. Amer J Pathol 43: 677-696, 1963.

8. POPPER H, SCHAFFNER F: Pathophysiology of cholestasis. Human Pathol 1: 1-24, 1970.

9. GOODENOUGH DA, REVEL JP: A fine structural analysis of intracellular junctions in the mouse liver. J Cell Biol 45: 272-290, 1970.

10. MATTER A, ORCI L, ROUILLER C: A study on the permeability barriers between Disse's space and the bile canaliculus. J Ultrastruct Res (suppl) 11: 5, Oct. 1969.

11. SCHATZKI PF: Bile canaliculus and space of Disse. Electron microscopic relationships as delineated by lanthanum. Lab Invest 20: 87-93, 1969.

12. WOOD RL: Some structural features of the bile canaliculus in calf liver. Anat Rec 140: 207-215, 1961.

13. SONG CS, RUBIN W, RIFKIND AB, KAPPAS A: Plasma membranes of the rat liver. Isolation and enzymatic characterization of a fraction rich in bile canaliculi. J Cell Biol 41: 124-132, 1969.

14. BERRY MN, FRIEND DS: High-yield preparation of isolated rat liver parenchymal cells. A biochemical and fine structural study. J Cell Biol 43: 506-520, 1969.

15. JEEJEEBHOY KN, HO J, GREENBERG GR, PHILLIPS MJ, BRUCE-ROBERTSON A, SODTKE U: Albumin and fibrinogen synthesis in isolated rat hepatocyte suspensions. A model for the study of plasma protein synthesis. J Clin Invest 1975 (in press).

16. LOWEY S, COHEN C: Studies on the structures of myosin. J Molec Biol 4: 293-308, 1962.

17. MOMMAERTS WFHM, PARRISH RG: Studies on myosin. I. Preparation and criteria of purity. J Biol Chem 188: 545-552, 1951.

18. POLLARD RD, KORN ED: Electron microscopic identification of actin associated with isolated amoeba plasma membranes. J Biol Chem 248: 448-450, 1973.

19. ISHIKAWA H, BISHOFF R, HOLTZER H: Formation of arrowhead complexes with heavy meromyosin in a variety of cell types. J Cell Biol 43: 312-328, 1969.

20. ESSNER E, NOVIKOFF AB, MASEK B: Adenosine triphosphatase and 5-nucleotidase activities in the plasma membrane of liver cells as revealed by electron microscopy. J Biophys Biochem Cytol 4: 711-716, 1958.

21. WACHSTEIN M, MEISEL E: Histochemistry of hepatic phosphatases at a physiological pH. With special reference to the demonstration of bile canaliculi. Am J Clin Path 27: 13-23, 1957.

22. FARQUHAR MG, PALADE GE: Junctional complexes in various epithelia. J Cell Biol 17: 375-412, 1963.

23. ODA M, PRICE VM, FISHER MM, PHILLIPS MJ: Ultrastructure of bile canaliculi with special reference to the surface coat and the pericanalicular web. Lab Invest 31: 314-323, 1974.

24. WESSELLS NK, SPOONER BS, ASH JF, BRADLEY MO, LUDVENA MA, TAYLOR EL, WRENN JR, YAMADA KM: Microfilaments in cellular and developmental processes. Science 171: 135-143, 1971.

25. CLONEY RA: Cytoplasmic filaments and morphogenesis: the role of the notochord in ascidian metamorphosis. Z Zellforsch 100: 31-53, 1969.

26. BAKER P, SCHROEDER RE: Cytoplasmic filaments and morphogenetic movement in amphibian neural tube. Devel Biol 15: 432-450, 1967.

27. SPUDICH JA: Effects of cytochalasin B on actin filaments. Cold Spring Harbor Symposia on Quantitative Biology 37: 585-593, 1972.

28. NACHMIAS VT, HUXLEY HE, KESSLER D: Electron microscope observations on actomyosin and actin preparations from physarum polycephalum and on their interaction with heavy meromyosin subfragment I from muscle myosin. J Molec Biol 50: 83-90, 1970.

29. HUXLEY HE: Electron microscope studies on the structure of natural and synthetic protein filaments from striated muscle. J Molec Biol 7: 281-308, 1963.

30. POLLARD TD, SHELTON E, WEIHING RR, KORN ED: Ultrastructural characterization of F-actin isolated from Acanthamoeba castellanii and identification of cytoplasmic filaments as F-actin by reaction with rabbit heavy meromyosin. J Molec Biol 50: 91-97, 1970.

31. SPOONER BS, ASH JF, WRENN JT, FRATER RB, WESSELLS NK: Heavy meromyosin binding to microfilaments involved in cell and morphogenetic movements. Tissue and Cell 5: 37-46, 1973.

32. MANASEK FJ, BURNSIDE B, STROMAN J: The sensitivity of developing cardiac myofibrils to cytochalasin-B. Proc Nat Acad Sci 69: 308-312, 1972.

33. ALLISON AC, DAVIES P, DE PETRIS S: Role of contractile microfilaments in macrophage movement and endocytosis. Nature New Biol 232: 153-155, 1971.

34. ORCI L, GABBAY KH, MALAISSE WJ: Pancreatic beta-cell web: its possible role in insulin secretion. Science 175: 1128-1130, 1972.

35. BOYLE KAY MM, FUDENBERG HH: Inhibition and reversal of platelet activation by cytochalasin B or colcemid. Nature 244: 288-289, 1973.

36. SHEPRO D, BELAMARICH FA, ROBBLEE L, CHAO FC: Antimotility effect of cytochalasin B observed in mammalian clot retraction. J Cell Biol 47: 544-547, 1970.

AN ULTRASTRUCTURAL LOOK AT INTRAHEPATIC CHOLESTASIS

K. Miyai, W. Mayr, A. Richardson, and M.M. Fisher

University of California at San Diego
La Jolla, California 92037
and University of Toronto, Toronto, Ontario

Ultrastructural studies of the cholestatic liver in man and experimental animals have indicated that the subcellular changes are most frequently localized to the bile canaliculus and the immediately adjacent structures in the liver cell (1,2,5,22, 24,30). The mechanisms causing these localized hepatocellular changes have yet to be established but one of the experimental models most intensively studied in this regard has been the cholestasis induced by the monohydroxy bile acid, lithocholic acid (LCA) (4,10,11,12,14,29,31).

Currently LCA is thought to cause cholestasis through one or more of the following mechanisms: (i) Suppression of the bile acid-dependent fraction of canalicular flow through a reduction in the relative amount of choleretic bile acid delivered to the canaliculi (12), (ii) Inhibition of the active transport of inorganic ions (the bile acid-independent fraction of canalicular flow (3,8),) and (iii) mechanical obstruction following its precipitation within the bile canaliculi (12). In addition, LCA may affect the function of the endoplasmic reticulum with consequent impairment of bile acid hydroxylation and micelle formation (21).

Schaffner and Javitt (23) induced cholestasis in the hamster liver by taurolithocholate and showed that the initial changes were localized to the bile canaliculi and pericanalicular structures. Using the isolated perfused rat liver we demonstrated that LCA produced a characteristic 'lamellar' transformation of the bile canalicular wall in addition to the localization of major changes to the bile canaliculi (15,18). In order to further characterize the morphogenesis of this type of cholestasis we induced acute cholestasis in the rat with a bile fistula by the continuous intravenous infusion of LCA (16,17). Ultrastructural changes identical to those noted in the isolated perfused rat liver were reproduced and they have been examined by transmission and scanning electron microscopy including the freeze-fracture replica technique.

MATERIALS AND METHODS

Isolated perfused rat liver

Female Wistar rats weighing approximately 250 g were used as liver and perfusion medium donors. The isolated liver was perfused with whole rat blood for up to 5 hours. In the experimental group, LCA was added at a concentration of 0.3 micromoles per ml at the end of 2 hours and the perfusion was continued for 3 hours thereafter. Details of this technique have been described in other communications (9).

Bile fistula rat

Female Wistar rats weighing approximately 250 g were used. After cannulating the common bile duct and femoral vein with polyethylene tubing, each animal was placed in a restraining cage. After a stable secretion of bile had been present for 2 hours, sodium lithocholate (NaLCA) (grade A, Calbiochem) was infused at a constant rate of 0.1 or 0.2 micromoles per minute per 100 g of body weight through the femoral vein catheter. The NaLCA was dissolved in 0.45% saline containing serum albumin at a concentration of 7.5%. Controls were infused with the same solution without NaLCA at the rate equivalent to that of the experimental group. Hepatic tissue for morphological studies was obtained at the end of the 2nd, 3rd and 4th hour after the onset of NaLCA infusion and at the end of the 3rd or 4th hour of control infusion. After perfusion-fixation through the portal vein with 1 or 2% gluteraldehyde in 0.1 M Sorenson's buffer (pH 7.4), the tissue was processed as follows: (i) embedding in Epon after postfixation in buffered 2% osmium tetroxide for conventional transmission electron microscopy (TEM); (ii) for freeze-fracture, tissue blocks were immersed in 25% glycerol in 0.1 M cacodylate buffer (pH 7.4) overnight, dipped briefly in Freon 22 and quickly frozen in liquid nitrogen. The specimens were then fractured and coated with platinum and carbon which were evaporated in a high vacuum (10^{-5} Torr) at -120°C. After removal from the tissue blocks, the metal replicas were examined in the transmission microscope (17). (iii) For scanning electron microscopy (SEM), tissue blocks were further fixed overnight followed by postfixation in buffered 2% OsO_4.

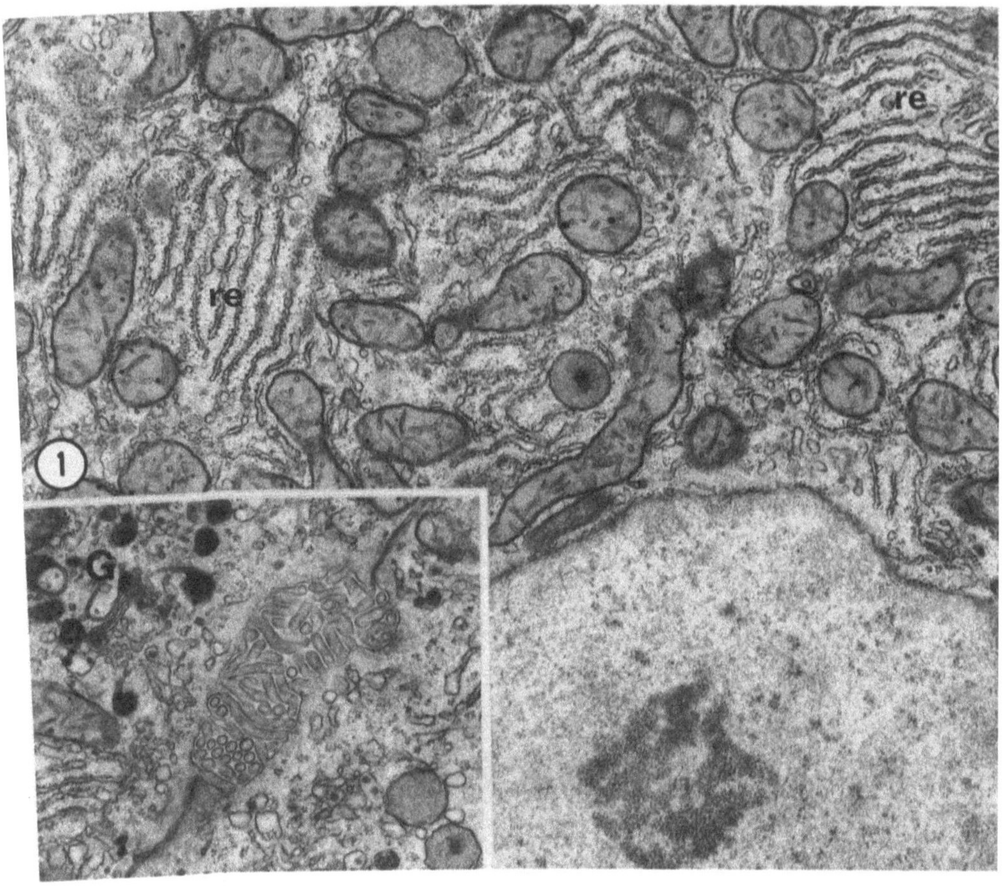

Fig. 1: Control liver after 5 hours of isolated perfusion. Hepatic ultrastructure is well preserved and virtually indistinguishable from that of the in situ liver. Rough endoplasmic reticulum (re) is well organized. Inset: Control liver after 5 hours of isolated perfusion. No significant alteration is seen in the bile canaliculus. G, Golgi complex.
Fig. 1: x 15,550. Inset: x 14,450.

The specimens were then either (a) freeze-fractured in Freon followed by critical point drying, or (b) freeze-fractured in water followed by freeze-drying. Details of these techniques have been reported elsewhere (19).

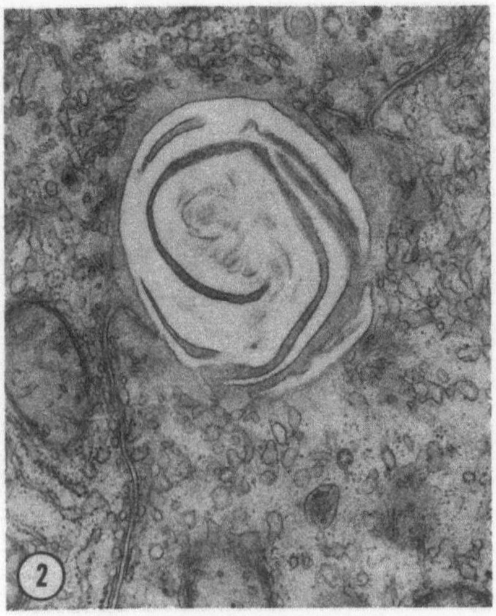

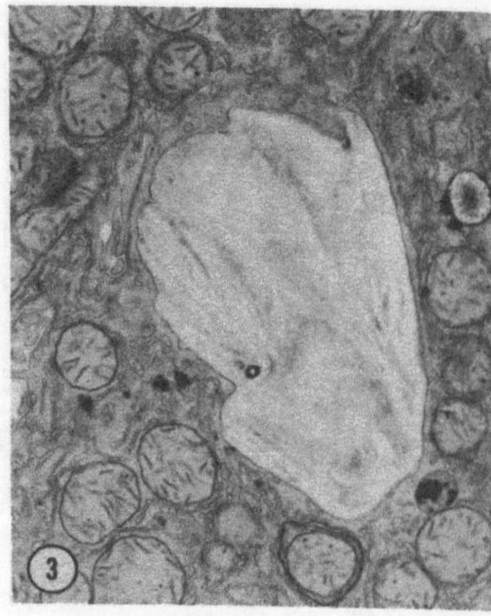

Fig. 2: A bile canaliculus of the isolated liver after 3 hours of perfusion with lithocholic acid. Canalicular wall is transformed into thin lamellar projections. Pericanalicular ectoplasm is prominent. x 17,990.

Fig. 3: An electron lucent material in a dilated bile canaliculus. Streaks of moderate density in this material and angulated contour of the canaliculus suggest a crystalline nature of the canalicular content. x 11,200.

RESULTS

Isolated perfused rat liver

In control experiments bile output remained relatively constant throughout the course of 5 hours of perfusion (9). The hepatic ultrastructure was well preserved and after 5 hours of perfusion was virtually indistinguishable from that of in situ liver (Fig. 1).

Addition of LCA to the perfusion medium at a concentration of 0.3 micromoles per ml, after 2 hours of baseline perfusion induced early and total cholestasis with no significant secretion of bile occurring after 1 hour of adding the bile acid to the perfusion medium (9). Study of the hepatic ultrastructure showed significant changes after 3 hours of perfusion with LCA. These changes involved primarily the bile canaliculi. Many canaliculi were dilated with partial or total loss of microvilli. A bizarre transformation of the canalicular membrane was noted frequently. This consisted of multiple projections of the canalicular membranes which overlapped one another to produce a lamellar pattern (Fig. 2). The pericanalicular ectoplasm had an increased density. In a few hepatocytes an electron lucent material with streaks of moderate density filled the bile canalicular lumen or single membrane-bound vacuoles in the pericanalicular zone. These canaliculi and vacuoles often had an angulated contour (Fig. 3). Some minor changes noted in the rough and smooth endoplasmic reticulum (RER and SER), mitochondria and Golgi complex are tabulated in Table 2.

Rats with a bile fistula

The rate of bile secretion in the control animals remained nearly constant (Table 1). No significant ultrastructural changes were noted in the control livers either by transmission or scanning electron microscopy (Fig. 4). TEM examination of the tissue which had been prepared for SEM by critical point drying and subsequently embedded in Epon revealed that the ultrastructural preservation was virtually indistinguishable from that of the tissue processed for TEM (Fig. 5). Freeze-fracture replica studies revealed that the fractured surface of the microvilli of the bile canaliculi were studded diffusely with granules which measured 60-100 Å in diameter (Fig. 6).

With the infusion of NaLCA at the higher rate, biliary secretion decreased rapidly during the first hour and virtually stopped during the second hour and thereafter (Table 1). With the lower dose, bile flow decreased to less than 10% of pre-infusion level within 2 hours (Table 1).

Hepatic ultrastructural changes were similar but more advanced and widespread with the higher infusion rate. TEM examination at the end of the second hour of infusion revealed frequent dilatation of the canaliculi. Microvilli were less numerous and often irregular in size and shape. Canalicular diverticuli were seen frequently (Fig. 8) and SEM showed that they were outpouchings of the bile canaliculi (Fig. 9). There was significant variation in the degree of the bile canalicular changes even in that segment of the canaliculus involving a single hepatocyte (Fig. 9). The peculiar, lamellar transformation of the bile canalicular membrane was also seen (Fig. 10). By the third hour and thereafter, bile canalicular changes, especially the lamellar transformation of the canalicular wall, were prominent and seen more extensively. Examination of freeze-fracture

TABLE 1

EFFECT OF SODIUM LITHOCHOLATE INFUSION
ON BILE FLOW OF WISTAR RATS (mg/hr)

Type of experiments	hours					
	0-1	1-2	2-3	3-4	4-5	5-6
Controls						
	520.1	565.8	534.5	509.5	518.8	520.0
	787.8	797.8	786.3	810.2	706.1	691.6
	526.7	540.9	528.3	467.5	454.1	
	526.9	724.6	709.4	690.6	681.3	
NaLCA 0.1 µM/min/100g body wt*						
	505.4	452.1	130.7	26.3	38.1	
	597.8	656.1	569.7	375.6	34.7	
	390.8	331.1	122.4	22.6	20.7	
NaLCA 0.2 µM/min/100g body wt*						
	598.9	618.8	271.2	10.3	4.2	0
	749.6	748.0	288.8	2.1	7.9	0
	517.4	670.9	173.2	4.3	0	
	565.5	590.6	203.1	40.5	3.2	

* Infusion was started at the end of the 2nd hour and maintained continuously until the end of the experiments.

TABLE 2

ULTRASTRUCTURAL CHANGES OF LIVER IN CHOLESTASIS INDUCED BY LITHOCHOLATE

	LCA induced cholestasis*				
	Isolated Perfused Rat Liver	Rat with Bile Fistula		Hamster**	
Bile canaliculi	3 hr	2 hr	4 hr	1 hr	4 hr
Dilation	++	+	++	0	++
Diverticuli	+	0/+	+		
Microvilli					
loss	++	+	++	++	++
bleb-like change	0	0	0	0	0
lamellar transformation	++	+	++	0	0
Bile plug	0	0	0	0	0
Electron lucent material with laminar structure (? crystal)	+	0/+	+	0	0
Pericanalicular zone					
ectoplasm widened	+	0/+	+	++	++
Golgi prominent	0/+	0/+	0/+	++	+
autophagic vacuoles increased	+	0/+	0/+	+	++
SER					
proliferation	0/+	0	0/+	0	+
RER					
fragmentation	0/+	0/+	0/+	+	++
Mitochondria					
fission	0/+	0/+	0/+	+	++
cristae, elongated/curled	0/+	0/+	0/+	+	++

0 = no change; 0/+ = change may be present;
+ = change present; ++ = severe change.

* ref: 1,2,5,21,23,30
** ref: 23.

SER = smooth endoplasmic reticulum
RER = rough endoplasmic reticulum

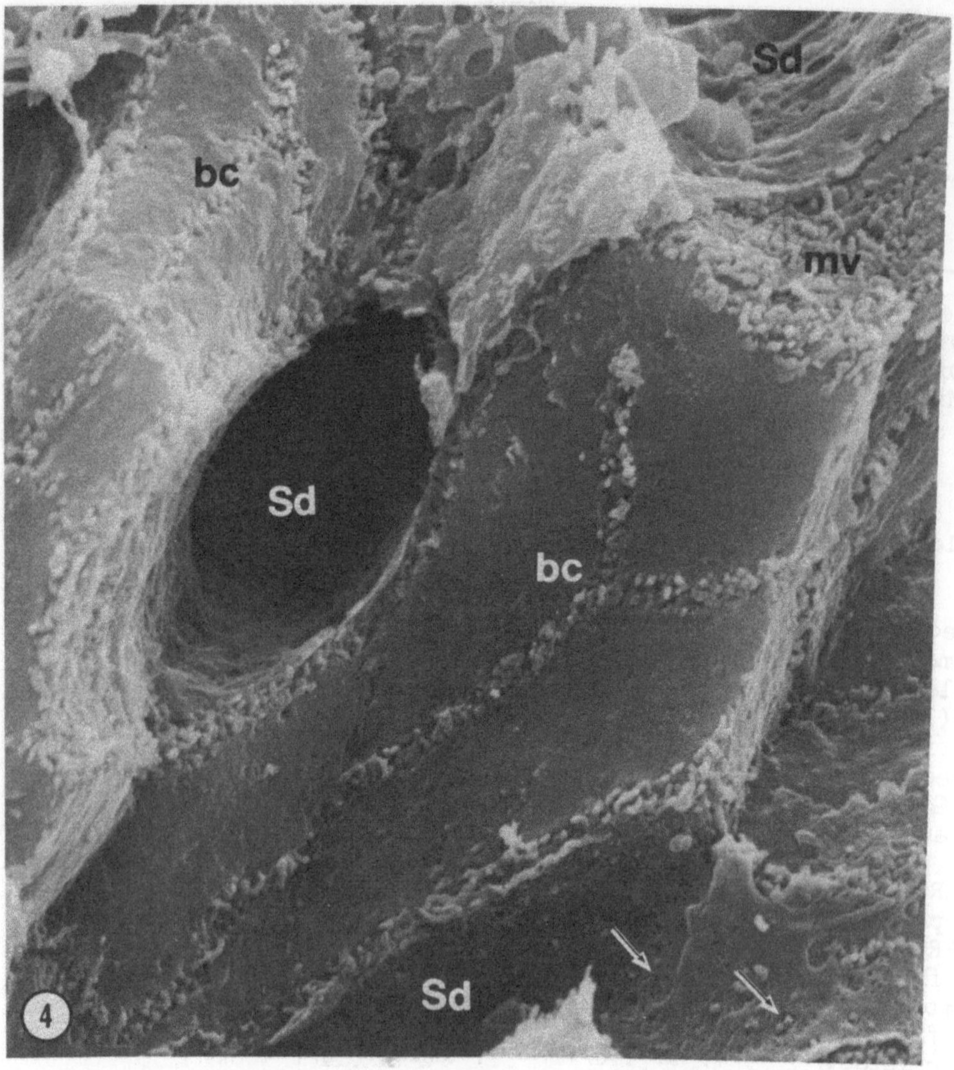

Fig. 4: SEM of the liver of a control rat prepared by freeze-fracture followed by critical point drying. Longitudinal profiles of bile canaliculi (bc) are seen on the intercellular surface of hepatocytes. Note branching of bile canaliculi and numerous microvilli projecting into the canalicular lumen. Sinusoid lining cells have fenestrations in their cytoplasm (arrows). Sinusoidal surface of hepatocytes is studded with microvilli (mv). Sd, sinusoid. x 5,950.

NOTE: Figs. 4-11 are taken from the liver of rats with a bile fistula. Figs. 4,5,6 are taken from the control rats.

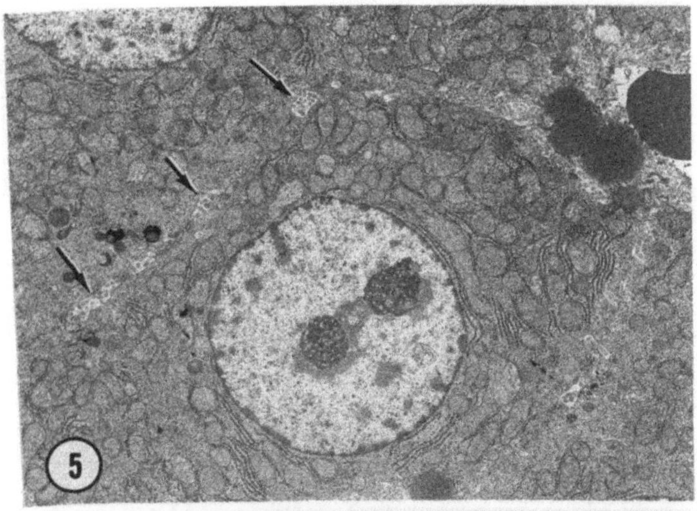

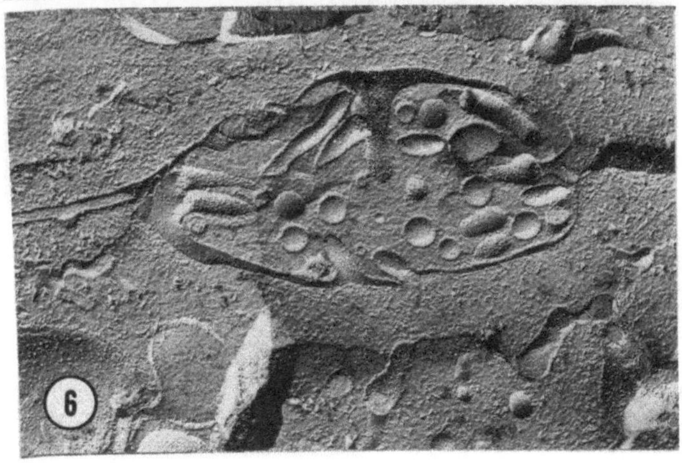

Fig. 5: TEM of the control liver which had been prepared for SEM by freeze-fracture followed by critical point drying and subsequently embedded in Epon. Ultrastructure is well preserved and nearly indistinguishable from that prepared by the conventional method for TEM. Arrows point to bile canaliculi. x 4,500.

Fig. 6: Freeze-fracture replica of a bile canaliculus in the control rat. Fractured surfaces of microvilli are diffusely studded with fine granules. x 20,700.

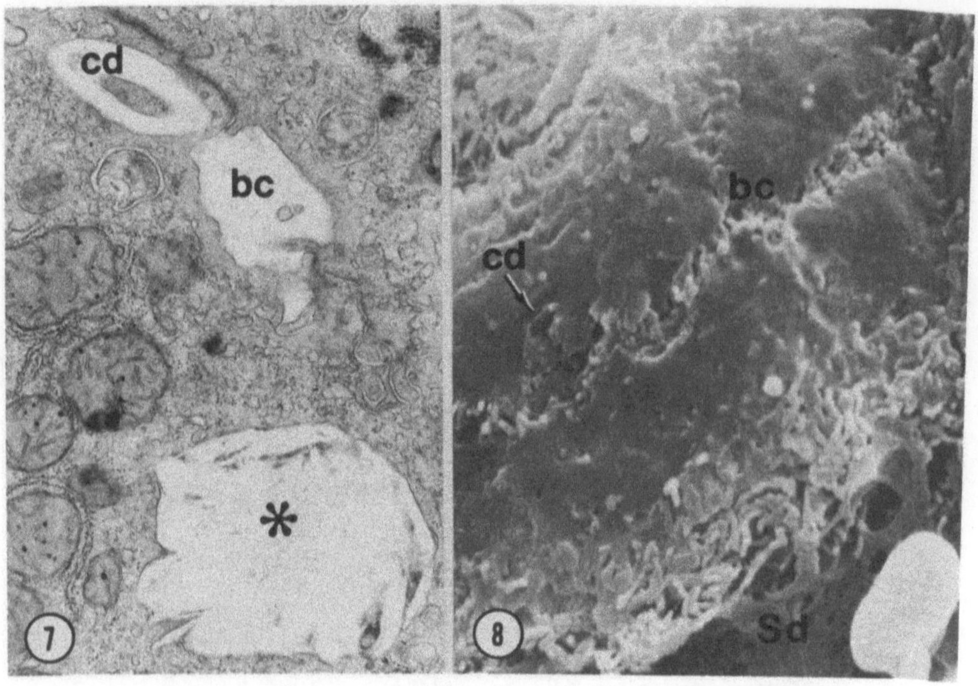

Fig. 7: Dilated bile canaliculi (bc) and canalicular diverticuli (cd) after 2 hours of infusion with lithocholic acid. A pericanalicular vacuole (asterisk) which may be a canalicular diverticulum is apparently filled with an electron lucent material. Streaks in the vacuolar content and angulated contour of the vacuole suggest a crystalline nature of the vacuolar content. x 16,400.

Fig. 8: SEM of the liver prepared by freeze-fracture followed by critical point drying. Bile canaliculus (bc) is dilated segmentally with loss of microvilli and formation of canalicular diverticuli (cd) while normal morphology is retained in adjacent segments of canaliculi. x 5,740.

NOTE: Figs. 7 - 11 are from the livers of rats infused with lithocholic acid.

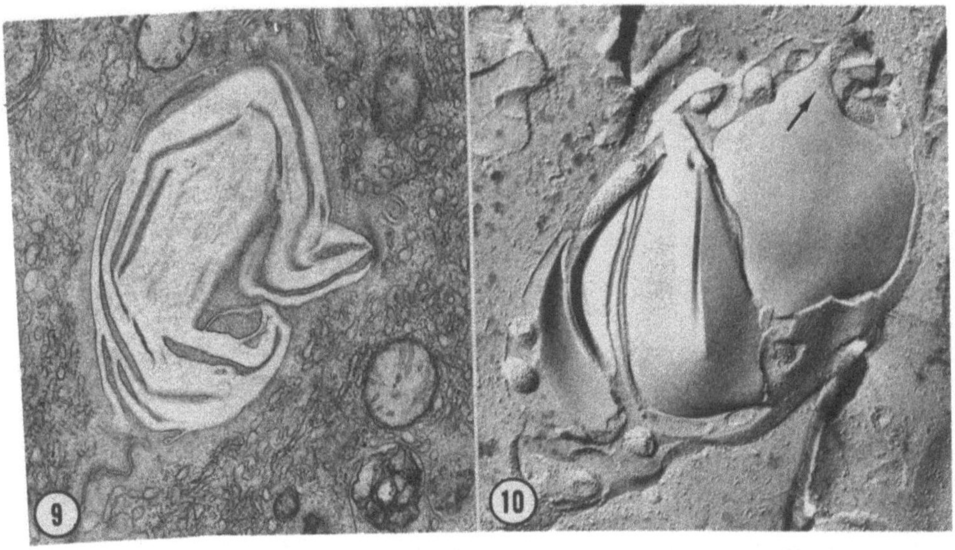

Fig. 9: Lamellar transformation of the wall of a bile canaliculus. Two hours of infusion with lithocholic acid. x 20,770.

Fig. 10: Freeze-fracture replica of a bile canaliculus after 3 hours of lithocholate infusion. There is a marked variation in the morphology of microvilli. Some of them apparently have been transformed into wide and thin lamellae. This is indicated by the partial presence of intramembranous granules (arrow) near the stalk of the lamellae. x 37,125.

replicas after the second and third hours of infusion revealed a spectrum of changes in the canalicular microvilli which indicated that the microvilli transformed through widening and flattening into lamellar ridges which often overlapped each other closely (Fig. 11). There were marked variations in the distribution of the intra-membranous granules on the fractured surface of the bile canalicular membrane. The granules were sparsely scattered or absent in the areas which were transformed into lamellar ridges, while their distribution was not altered in the microvilli which retained their normal configuration (Fig. 11). There were occasional bile canaliculi and vacuoles in the pericanalicular region which contained a material of low electron opacity with thin streaks of moderate density, a change identical to that seen in the isolated perfused liver (Fig. 7). Freeze-fracture replica study revealed sharply angulated, crystalline material in the lumen of the bile canaliculi (Fig. 11) and in pericanalicular vacuoles. Occasionally, the crystalline material filled the canaliculi or pericanalicular vacuoles. Minor changes similar

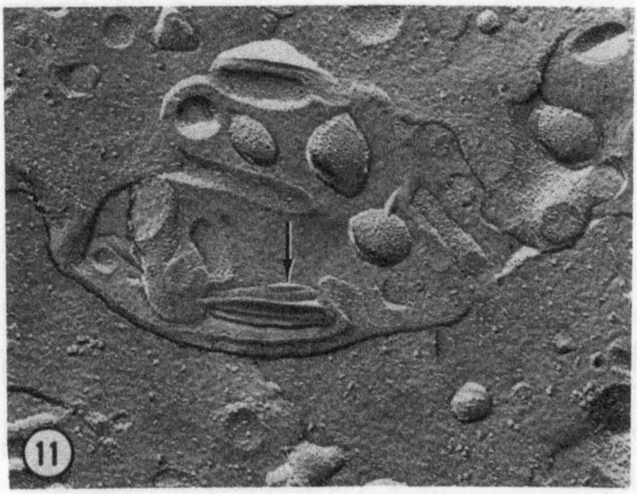

Fig. 11: Freeze-fracture replica of a bile canaliculus. A sharply angulated crystalline material (arrow) is seen within the canalicular lumen. Fractured surface of microvilli is studded with intramembranous granules. x 43,350.

to those seen in the isolated perfused rat liver were also noted in several other organelles (Table 2). Ultrastructural changes noted in this study are tabulated in Table 2.

DISCUSSION

This study has demonstrated: (i) the acute ultrastructural changes induced by lithocholate are nearly identical in the isolated perfused rat liver and in the liver of the rat with a bile fistula; (ii) the principal changes are localized to the biliary region of the hepatocyte and especially to the bile canaliculus, and (iii) the ultrastructural changes are more prominent with larger doses of lithocholate and with the progression of time.

The above findings suggest that the lesions of the bile canaliculus are primarily responsible for the acute cholestasis induced by lithocholate. Most noteworthy among the ultrastructural changes are distortions of the bile canalicular wall, including its transformation into thin, lamellar folds. Our freeze-fracture replica study has indicated that the canalicular microvilli undergo widening and flattening to become lamellar ridges.

These changes may be similar to the crenation of the erythrocyte membrane induced by a variety of amphipathic substances. Anionic or non-ionized compounds transform the erythrocytes into crenated forms whereas cationic compounds induce cuplike invaginations of the cell membrane (6,25,26). These changes are thought to represent an asymmetrical expansion of the lipid bilayer of the cell membrane through a nonspecific physical effect of the amphipathic compounds (25). Although the above concept has been derived from studies on the erythrocyte, the study by Deuticke (6) includes bile acids among the agents which induce crenation.

Our freeze-fracture studies have also demonstrated that the intramembranous granules are absent or only sparsely scattered on the cleaved surfaces of the transformed regions of the canalicular membrane. According to recent studies (19,26,27), the intramembranous granules are thought to correspond to protein globules which are intercalated in the lipid bilayer and considered to be involved in a variety of functions of the membrane. It is also known that the frequency of these granules is greatest in functionally specialized membranes whereas they are absent in myelin (20). In our study we were unable to determine whether the paucity of the granules mentioned above was relative or absolute. However, it is conceivable that the transformed portion of the canalicular membrane is deficient with respect to its fluid transport function.

One of the hypotheses which has been proposed to explain the pathogenesis of the cholestasis induced by lithocholate is that lithocholate precipitates within the canalicular lumen because of its low solubility in aqueous solution (12,28). The crystalline structures within the bile canaliculi which were revealed in our freeze-fracture studies and the negative images of sharply angulated material in the canaliculi which were revealed by transmission electron microscopy add support to this concept. Since lithocholate is readily extracted by the ethanol and acetone used for dehydration of the tissue (28), precipitates containing lithocholate would appear as a negative image. Although the incidence of the 'precipitates' seems to be related to the amount of lithocholate administered, it remains difficult to assess the extent to which they contribute to the cholestasis.

Schaffner and Javitt did not observe the lamellar transformation of the canalicular membrane or the 'crystalline precipitates' in the bile canaliculi in their studies with the hamster (23). Although the influence of other factors such as bile fistula, species difference, conjugation of lithocholate, cannot be excluded, these discrepancies are probably attributable to differences in the dose of lithocholate. In our study with rats with a bile fistula, the amount of lithocholate infused during the first hour (12 μM at a rate of 0.2 μM/min/100 g body weight) was alone nearly equal to the total dose of taurolithocholate administered to the hamsters in a single injection (13.5 μM/100 g body weight). It should be noted also that the doses used in our study are within the range used by Javitt and Emerman (12) in a study from which they derived a hypothesis regarding the intracanalicular precipitation of lithocholate.

Application of scanning electron microscopy to this study has shown (i) that this technique is useful to examine longitudinal profiles of the bile canaliculi, and (ii) that structural changes in the canaliculi develop focally, leaving segments of morphologically intact canaliculi between them. At present we are unable to offer any plausible interpretation for the segmental development of the canalicular changes.

In the present study we have examined the ultrastructural changes in a severe, acute cholestasis induced by high doses of lithocholate and have speculated that the structural alterations of the bile canalicular membrane are related to the failure of the canalicular secretion of bile. We have also suggested that the intracanalicular precipitates probably contribute to the acute cholestasis.

According to King and Schoenfield (13), low doses of lithocholate selectively inhibit the bile acid-independent fraction of bile secretion without inducing any morphological changes recognizable by light microscopy. Further study using such experimental models may help to clarify the relationship between the subcellular structure of the liver and cholestasis.

SUMMARY

Acute cholestasis induced by lithocholic acid (LCA) was studied (i) in the isolated perfused rat liver, and (ii) in rats with a bile fistula. In the former LCA rapidly induced cholestasis with marked structural changes primarily in the bile canaliculi and pericanalicular zones. These changes included a lamellar folding of the canalicular membrane and deposition of a crystalline material in the bile canaliculi. In rats with a bile fistula, LCA was continuously infused intravenously (0.1 or 0.2 μM/min/100 g body weight). The high dose induced complete cholestasis while cholestasis was partial with the low dose. Ultrastructural changes were identical to those found in the isolated perfused liver. Freeze-fracture replica studies showed transformation of the microvilli into lamellar folds, crystalline material in the bile canaliculi and a paucity of the intramembranous granules in the transformed region of the canalicular membrane. It appears that the structural changes of the canalicular membrane are related to the failure of the canalicular secretion of bile. The intracanalicular precipitates probably contribute to the acute cholestasis.

ACKNOWLEDGEMENTS

Dr. Miyai is supported by USPHS Contracts SP 17HL 14169 and HL-123-73 and Grant R01 AM16110.

REFERENCES

1. BIAVA CG: Studies on cholestasis. A re-evaluation of the fine structure of normal human bile canaliculi. Lab Invest 13: 840-864, 1964.

2. BIAVA CG: Studies on cholestasis. The fine structure and morphogenesis of hepatocellular and canalicular bile pigment. Lab Invest 13: 1099-1123, 1964.

3. BOYER JL, KLATSKIN G: Canalicular bile flow and bile secretory pressure. Evidence for a non-bile salt dependent fraction in the isolated perfused rat liver. Gastroenterology 59: 853-859, 1970.

4. CAREY JB: Bile salts and hepatobiliary disease. In Diseases of the Liver. Edited by Schiff, L. Philadelphia and Toronto. JB Lippincott Co. 1969. pp. 103-146.

5. DESMET VJ: Morphologic and histochemical aspects of cholestasis. In Progress in Liver Diseases. Edited by Popper, H, Schaffner F. New York, Grune & Stratton, 1972. vol 4: 97-132.

6. DEUTICKE B: Transformation and restoration of biconcave shape of human erythrocytes induced by amphipathic agents and changes of ionic environment. Biochim Biophys Acta 163: 494-500, 1968.

7. ERLINGER S: Physiology of bile flow. In Progress in Liver Diseases, vol. 4. Edited by Popper H, Schaffner F. New York, Grune & Stratton, 1972. pp 63-82.

8. ERLINGER S, DHUMEAUX D: Mechanisms and control of secretion of bile water and electrolytes. Gastroenterology 66: 281-304, 1974.

9. FISHER MM, MAGNUSSON R, MIYAI K: Bile acid metabolism in mammals. I. Bile acid induced intrahepatic cholestasis. Lab Invest 25: 88-91, 1971.

10. HEATON KW: Bile salts in health and disease. Edinburgh and London, Churchill Livingstone, 1972. pp. 98-172.

11. HOLSTI P: Cirrhosis of the liver induced in rabbits by gastric instillation of 3-monohydroxy-cholanic acid. Nature (Lond) 186: 250, 1960.

12. JAVITT NB, EMERMAN S: Effect of sodium taurolithocholate on bile flow and bile acid excretion. J. Clin Invest 47: 1002-1014, 1968.

13. KING JE, SCHOENFIELD LJ: Cholestasis induced by sodium taurolithocholate in isolated hamster liver. J Clin Invest 50: 2305-2312, 1971.

14. MIETTINEN TA: Clinical implications of bile acid metabolism in man. In The Bile Acids. Edited by Nair PN, and Kritchevsky D, New York, Plenum Press, 1973. vol. 2, pp 191-247.

15. MIYAI K, FISHER MM: Influence of bile acids on biliary secretion. (Abstract). In Proceedings 7th International Congress on Electron Microscopy. Edited by Favard P. Societe Francaise de Microscopie Electronique, Paris, 1970. Vol. 3, pp 495-496.

16. MIYAI K, MAYR W, RICHARDSON A: Freeze-fracture study of bile canalicular changes induced by lithocholic acid (abstract). Lab Invest 30: 16, 1974.

17. MIYAI K, MAYR WW, RICHARDSON A: Acute cholestasis induced by lithocholic acid in the rat: A freeze-fracture replica and thin section study. Lab Invest (in press)

18. MIYAI K, PRICE VM, FISHER MM: Bile acid metabolism in mammals. Ultrastructural studies on the intrahepatic cholestasis induced by lithocholic and chenodeoxycholic acids in the rat. Lab Invest 24: 292-302, 1971.

19. MIYAI K, WAGNER RM, RICHARDSON AL: Preparation of liver for combined SEM and TEM study. Scanning Electron Microscopy/1974 (part 1). In Proceedings of 7th Annual Scanning Electron Microscopy Symposium. Edited by Johari O, IIT Research Institute, Chicago. pp 282-289.

20. OSEROF AR, ROBBINS PW, BURGER MM: The cell surface membrane: biochemical aspects and biophysical probes. Ann Rev Biochem 42: 647-682, 1973.

21. POPPER H, SCHAFFNER F: Pathophysiology of cholestasis. Hum Pathol 1: 1-24, 1970.

22. SCHAFFNER F: Ultrastructure of liver in intrahepatic and extrahepatic cholestasis. In Ikterus, International Symposium. Edited by Beck K, Freiburg, Stuttgart, New York, Schattauer Verlag. pp. 143-149, 1968.

23. SCHAFFNER F, JAVITT NB: Morphologic changes in hamster liver during intrahepatic cholestasis induced by taurolithocholate. Lab Invest 15: 1783-1792, 1966.

24. SCHAFFNER F, POPPER H: Cholestasis is the result of hypoactive hypertrophic smooth endoplasmic reticulum in the hepatocyte. Lancet II: 355-359, 1969.

25. SEEMAN P, ROTH S: General anesthetics expand cell membranes at surgical concentrations. Biochim Biophys Acta 225: 171-177, 1972.

26. SINGER SJ: The molecular organization of membranes. Ann Rev Biochem 43: 805-833, 1974.

27. SINGER SJ, NICOLSON GL: The fluid mosaic model of the structure of cell membranes. Cell membranes are viewed as two-dimensional solutions of oriented globular proteins and lipids. Science 175: 720-731, 1972.

28. SMALL DM: The physical chemistry of cholanic acids. In The Bile Acids, vol. 1. Edited by Nair PP, Kritchevsky D. New York, Plenum Press, 1971. pp. 249-356.

29. SPERBER I: Secretion of organic anions in the formation of urine and bile. Pharmacol Rev 11: 109-134, 1959.

30. STEINER JR, JEZEQUEL AM, PHILLIPS MJ, et al: Some aspects of the ultrastructural pathology of the liver. In

Progress in Liver Diseases. Edited by Popper H, Schaffner F. New York, Grune & Stratton, 1965. vol 2. pp 303-372.

31. WHEELER HO: Secretion of bile acids by the liver and their role in the formation of hepatic bile. Arch Intern Med 130: 533-541, 1972.

CURRENT STATUS OF CHOLESTASIS INDUCED BY MONOHYDROXY BILE ACIDS

Norman B. Javitt

New York Hospital - Cornell Medical Center

New York, New York 10021

The development of an experimental model for the induction of cholestasis (1) has led to further exploration of the pathophysiological mechanism and to a search for evidence that monohydroxy bile acids may be a cause of cholestasis in man.

Several studies in both the isolated perfused rat and hamster liver and in the intact animal (2,3,4) have demonstrated that addition of sodium taurolithocholate to the fluid perfusing the liver causes a rapid, but reversible reduction in bile flow.

Further, it is believed that the cholestatic effect is directed at canalicular rather than ductular bile flow. However, if one tries to dissect between effects on bile salt dependent canalicular bile flow and bile salt independent canalicular bile flow, certain problems arise. Schoenfield and King (3) concluded that the major mechanism of taurolithocholate induced cholestasis in the isolated perfused hamster liver was on bile salt independent canalicular flow and/or ductular flow.

In their studies the changes in bile flow following the infusion of taurolithocholate were compared to changes in bile flow following taurocholate administration. In most studies total bile flow was less after taurolithocholate administration compared to taurocholate. This difference in flow response was considered a cholestatic event, although total bile acid excretion remained the same or even increased. Thus the most striking event in their model was the increase in bile acid concentration that occurred during the administration of taurolithocholate. The reduced response in bile flow compared to bile acid excretion was attributed to an effect on the bile salt independent fraction of canalicular bile flow. An effect on ductular flow could not be excluded since no marker, such as mannitol, was used. But it was considered on the basis of previous evidence (5) that the contribution of ductular bile flow to total flow was minimal in the isolated perfused liver.

However, if one analyzes the relationship of mannitol excretion to bile acid excretion in response to taurocholate and to taurolithocholate infusions in vivo, a marked change in the slope of the line occurs (Figs. 1 and 2). A reduction in the bile salt independent fraction would have given a reduced excretion rate of mannitol per µmole of bile salt with no change in slope. The change in slope indicates a change in the relationship of canalicular bile flow compared to bile salt excretion. Such an event can occur if there is a change in the relationship of mannitol excretion to canalicular bile flow or if there is a change in the relationship of the osmotic activity of those solutes generating canalicular bile flow.

Examination of the relationship between bile flow and mannitol excretion during taurocholate and taurolithocholate infusions (Fig. 3) indicates that the proportionality between mannitol and water flow has not been altered.

The data therefore do not support the interpretation of Schoenfield and King. Indeed, the most reasonable explanation is that in the hamster, much of the infused taurolithocholate is metabolized to taurochenodeoxycholate (6) and therefore the proportion of this bile salt in bile must increase. It has been shown by Small (7) that at physiological salt concentrations the molecular weight of the chenodeoxycholate micelle is approximately twice that of the cholate micelle. The increased aggregation number reduces the osmotic activity and therefore a reduction in bile salt dependent canalicular bile flow and increase in concentration is predictable.

Thus the findings of Schoenfield and King may be an in vivo confirmation of the in vitro studies on bile salt micelle size and the possible effects of micelle size on bile flow. In retrospect it seems unlikely that they were dealing with the phenomenon of cholestasis. Finally, one should be aware that monohydroxy bile acids are capable of total suppression of bile flow, so that the distinction between the different sources of bile water does not in itself provide a complete explanation.

Further evidence that cholestasis did not occur in the study of Schoenfield and King can be derived from their failure to observe any morphological changes. Since the only fixative was formalin it seems likely that electron microscopic studies were not done. In contrast, electron microscopic evaluation from three separate laboratories (2,4,8) has demonstrated marked changes in hepatic morphology. These studies have confirmed that total cholestasis occurs in association with marked dilatation of canaliculi, loss of microvilli and considerable canalicular debris. When cholestasis is prevented by the simultaneous administration of taurocholate these morphologic changes do not occur.

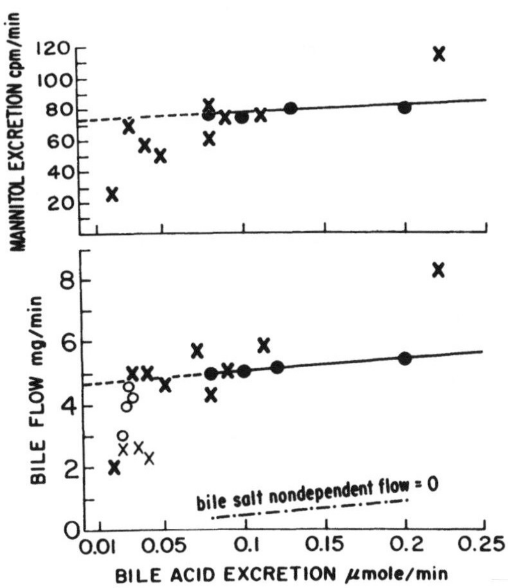

Fig. 1: Analysis of canalicular bile flow in hamster given taurocholate (●) and taurolithocholate (X).
(o,x) L. Schoenfield and J.E. King.
The data of King, J.E. and Schoenfield, L. (3) in the isolated perfused hamster liver are plotted together with those obtained from the intact animal (1). In the in vitro studies, canalicular bile flow failed to increase as expected when taurolithocholate was infused thus giving an increase in bile acid concentration. Since most of the infused taurolithocholate is metabolized to taurochenodeoxycholate, the increase in micelle size can account for the relative reduction in bile flow. In the intact hamster the data obtained following taurolithocholate infusion indicate a change in the slope of the line relating mannitol excretion to canalicular bile flow, a finding that does not support the concept that the effect is on bile salt nondependent canalicular bile flow.

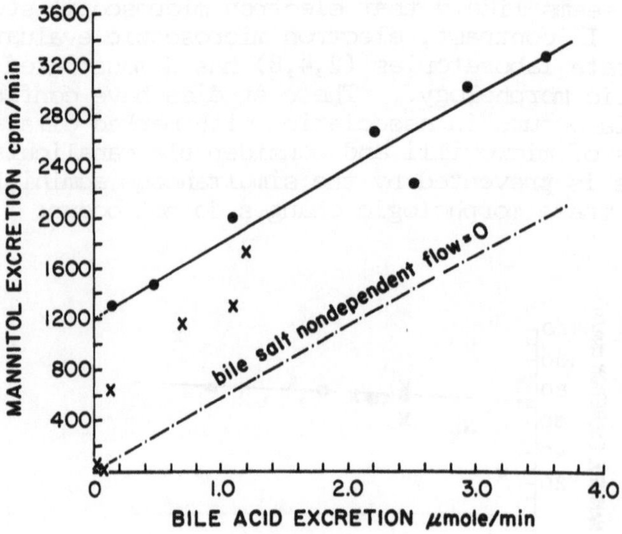

Fig. 2: Analysis of canalicular bile flow in rat given taurocholate (•) and/or taurolithocholate (x)
Administration of taurolithocholate to the rat causes a change in the slope of a line that could be drawn between mannitol excretion and bile acid excretion. The finding is contrary to what would be expected if taurolithocholate was affecting the bile salt nondependent flow.

Of particular interest is that the morphologic appearance of monohydroxy bile acid induced cholestasis is different from that occurring during administration of chenodeoxycholic acid, which affects the hepatocytes primarily. The bile duct alterations caused by monohydroxy bile acids resemble the changes that occur following mechanical obstruction of the biliary tree.

Further support for the concept that the initiation of cholestasis is related to the insolubility of the monohydroxy bile acids can be derived from the knowledge that more polar derivatives of these bile acids do not cause cholestasis (9). Hence, infusion of the 3-sulfate ester of lithocholic acid causes only a transient reduction in bile flow and the 3-sulfate ester of taurolithocholic acid does not have any cholestatic effect. Although it may be argued that these derivatives are less toxic chemically, relatively large amounts of taurolithocholate can be excreted in bile without cholestasis, provided sufficient dihydroxy or trihydroxy bile acids are also being excreted.

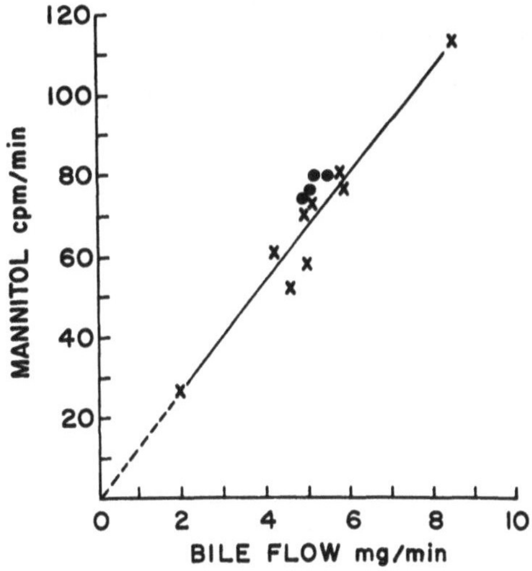

Fig. 3: Relationship of bile flow to mannitol excretion in the hamster. (Infusion of taurocholate (•) or taurolithocholate (x).) The data obtained following administration of both taurocholate and taurolithocholate all fit a single line thus indicating no altered relationship between mannitol excretion and canalicular bile flow.

At present the most attractive hypothesis still appears to be the concept that when relatively large amounts of monohydroxy bile acids are present in bile they precipitate within the canaliculi, thus initiating cholestasis. The high local concentrations of the compound may then cause deleterious effects on the membrane and surrounding subcellular organelles.

We turn now to evaluate the possibility that an event of this type might occur in man. Because monohydroxy bile acids can be synthesized in the liver, and the proportion that is produced compared to di- and tri-hydroxy bile acids is important to the occurrence of cholestasis, we will restrict our interest to the newborn period when metabolic errors in synthesis might be manifest.

The first intermediate in the pathway would be 26-hydroxycholesterol rather than 7α-hydroxycholesterol or its related 4-ene,3-one structure (Fig. 4). In the past few years, it has been established that 26-hydroxycholesterol is a normal constituent of human meconium (10) and therefore is probably synthesized in the liver during fetal life. The compound is not found as the free sterol, but as the ester disulfate. This chemical form

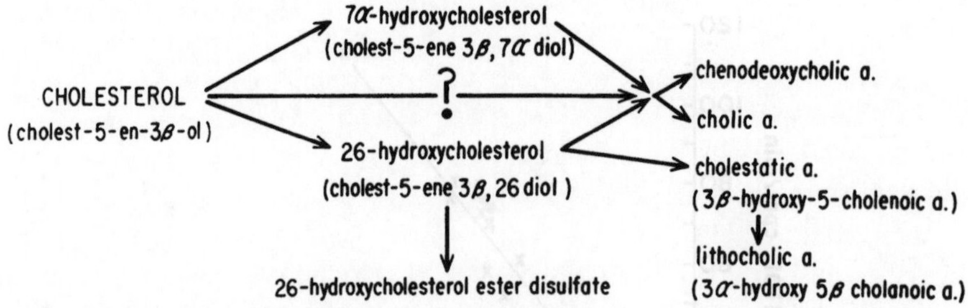

Fig. 4: Bile acid synthesis in neonates.
At the present time it is not known if the pathways for bile acid synthesis in fetal and neonatal life are different from the adult. The role of 26-hydroxycholesterol is undefined.

may imply that it is not an intermediate in bile acid synthesis, but that following its formation it undergoes sulfation rather than oxidation to a bile acid. Perhaps both pathways exist, for another compound present in meconium is 3β-hydroxy-5-cholenoate (11). Although it is possible to construct a pathway going from cholesterol to this bile acid without 26-hydroxycholesterol as an intermediate, no other sterols that would preclude 26-hydroxycholesterol as an intermediate have been identified. If we consider the adult, then we know that man (12) and other species (13,14) can metabolize 26-hydroxycholesterol to both chenodeoxycholic and cholic acids. The picture that emerges therefore is that 26-hydroxycholesterol is synthesized in vivo, that it probably is one of the intermediates in bile acid synthesis and that it can also be metabolized and excreted as an ester sulfate.

The next question I would like to raise is how much monohydroxy bile acid is synthesized in comparison to the di- and tri-hydroxy bile acids.

From the limited information available it appears that the normal infant has no 3β-hydroxy-5-cholenoate in his bile (15) or urine (16). The studies of bile (15) were done without solvolysis, so that if it were present as an ester sulfate it would not have been detected.

When we examine the data from infants with extrahepatic biliary atresia some striking findings have been reported. There is a form of biliary atresia in which no patent bile ducts are found at surgery and the liver has numerous giant cells on biopsy. Although one can find extrahepatic atresia without giant cells and giant cells without atresia, it seems clear that there are some infants considered to have neonatal or giant cell hepatitis who have no patent bile ducts at surgery. In this group we have found a striking elevation of the serum levels of chenodeoxycholate (17) and in one instance this was the only bile acid found in an obstructed duct at the time of surgery.

An infant of this type has been reported with one-third of the total bile acids excreted in the urine per day as the conjugated, sulfated monohydroxy bile acid, 3β-hydroxy-5-cholenoate (16). It seems clear that in this particular group of infants there is a marked alteration in bile acid metabolism early in the course of the disease, and long before cirrhosis occurs. The proportion of monohydroxy bile acid found in urine would be sufficient to cause cholestasis, if, indeed, the non-sulfated compound had been transported into the biliary tree early in life. However, we really have no data on the initial events in this disease and therefore we do not know what role this alteration in bile acid metabolism has in its pathogenesis. Needless to say, these striking findings are worthy of detailed study.

Thus far, infants with cholestatic syndromes but patent bile ducts have not been found to have such high proportions of monohydroxy bile acids in the urine. Bile from one of these infants (17) as well as urine and serum (18) appear to contain almost entirely chenodeoxycholic and cholic acids. The lack of unusual species of bile acids in significant amounts suggests that at least some of these problems may be defects in transport rather than synthesis of bile acids.

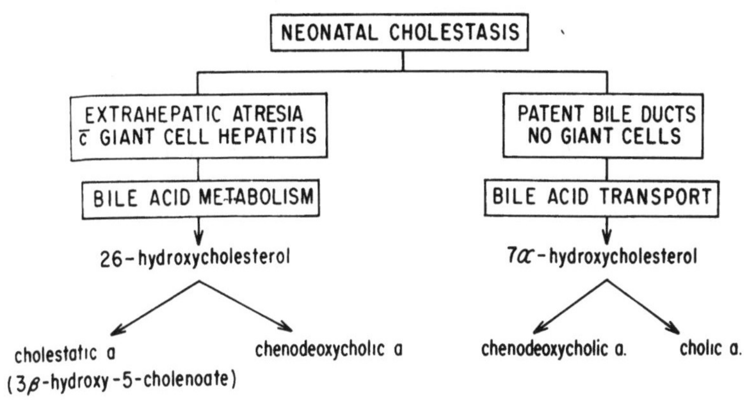

Fig. 5: Abnormalities in bile acid metabolism and excretion in neonatal cholestatic syndromes. This figure is a summary of the abnormalities observed in bile acid metabolism or excretion in various neonatal cholestatic syndromes. The relationship of these alterations to the cause of the cholestasis is unknown. They may be (a) causative (b) contributory or (c) merely the result of some unrelated primary event.

SUMMARY

The induction of cholestasis by infusion of monohydroxy bile acids appears to be a reproducible experimental model with predictable biochemical and morphological events. The occurrence of cholestasis is dependent on the proportion of monohydroxy bile acid transported into the canaliculi and electron microscopic evidence of obstruction of the biliary radicles has been obtained. An abnormality in bile acid metabolism has been identified in extrahepatic biliary atresia associated with giant-cell hepatitis. The role of this change in bile acid metabolism in the pathogenesis of the disease requires further elucidation.

REFERENCES

1. JAVITT N, EMERMAN S: Effect of sodium taurolithocholate on bile flow and bile acid excretion. J Clin Invest 47: 1002-1014, 1968.

2. MIYAI K, PRICE VM, FISHER MM: Bile acid metabolism in mammals. Lab Invest 24: 292-302, 1971.

3. KING JE, SCHOENFIELD L: Cholestasis induced by sodium taurolithocholate in isolated hamster liver. J Clin Invest 50: 2305-2312, 1971.

4. PRIESTLY BG, COTE MG, PLAA GL: Biochemical and morphologic parameters of taurolithcoholate-induced cholestasis. Can J Physiol Pharmacol 49: 1078-1091, 1971.

5. BOYER J: Canalicular bile formation in the isolated perfused rat liver. Amer J Physiol 221: 1156-1163, 1971.

6. EMERMAN S, JAVITT NB: Metabolism of taurolithocholic acid in the hamster. J Biol Chem 242: 661-664, 1967.

7. SMALL DM: Size and structure of bile salt micelles. Influence of structure, concentration, counterion concentration, pH and temperature. Adv Chem Ser 84: 31-52, 1968.

8. SCHAFFNER F, JAVITT NB: Morphological changes in hamster liver during intrahepatic cholestasis induced by taurolithocholate. Lab Invest 15: 1783-1792, 1966.

9. JAVITT NB: Excretion of monohydroxy bile acid ester sulfates in the rat. In The Liver. Quantitative Aspects of Structure and Function. Edited by Paumgartner G and Preisig R. Basel, Karger, 1973. pp. 355-359.

10. LAVY U, BURSTEIN S, JAVITT NB: Fetal bile acid metabolism; quantitation of 26-hydroxycholesterol and 7α-hydroxycholesterol in human meconium. Gastroenterology 65: 556, 1973 (abstract).

11. BACK D, ROSS K: Identification of 3β-hydroxy-5-cholenoic acid in human meconium. Hoppe-Seylers Z. Physiol Chem 354: 83-89, 1973.

12. ANDERSON K, KOK E, JAVITT NB: Bile acid synthesis in man: metabolism of 7α-hydroxycholesterol-^{14}C and 26-hydroxy cholesterol-^{3}H. J Clin Invest 51: 112-117, 1972.

13. WACHTEL N, EMERMAN S, JAVITT NB: Metabolism of cholest-5-ene 3β,26-diol in the rat and hamster. J Biol Chem 243: 5207-5212, 1968.

14. JAVITT NB, EMERMAN S: Metabolic pathways of bile acid formation in the rat. The Mt Sinai J Med 37: 477-481 1970.

15. BONGIOVANNI AM: Bile acid content of gallbladder of infants, children and adults. J Clin Endocr 25: 678-685. 1965.

16. MAKINO I, SJOVALL J, NORMAN A, STANDUIK B: Excretion of 3β-hydroxy-5-cholenoic acid and 3β-hydroxy-5α-cholanoic acids in urine of infants with biliary atresia. FEBS Letters 15: 161-164, 1971.

17. JAVITT NB, MORRISSEY KP, SIEGEL E et al: Cholestatic syndromes in infancy: diagnostic value of serum bile acid patterns and cholestyramine administration. Pediatr Res 7: 119-125, 1973.

18. LAVY U, JAVITT NB: Cholestatic syndromes in childhood: quantitative estimation of bile acid excretion in urine and feces. Gastroenterology 66: 849, 1974 (abstract).

DISCUSSION OF PAPERS ON INTRAHEPATIC CHOLESTASIS

CO-CHAIRMEN: J.W. STEINER AND M.M. FISHER

FISHER: Dr. Schaffner commented on the presence of liquid crystals of monohydroxy bile acids in the canaliculi and within the liver cell cytoplasm in some kinds of cholestasis. Studies by Rouiller suggest that the bile canaliculus has its origin within the liver cell. Might what he has shown us have been canalicular even though it looked as though it was in the cytoplasm?

SCHAFFNER: I don't think that these are intrahepatocytic branches of the bile canaliculi. I think that these are vacuoles. Histochemical studies suggest that they are lysosomes.

MIYAI: Your studies and ours on the isolated perfused rat liver demonstrated that chenodeoxycholic acid can produce liver injury. In view of this what do you think of the current clinical trial of this agent for the treatment of gallstones?

SCHAFFNER: You probably do not get a hepatotoxic concentration of chenodeoxycholic acid in the liver with the administration of a gram of chenodeoxycholic acid a day. In order to competitively inhibit the microsomes you need a concentration of 0.5 to 1 mM and you probably don't get anywhere close to this. The methodology for these measurements is available, we have recently published it, but I don't think that anyone has done the study. (Biochemical Medicine 8: 280-286, 1973.)

FORKER: Dr. Plaa, is anything known about the metabolism of ANIT? The data you have shown suggest that metabolites may be responsible for some of the effects.

PLAA: You are right although the evidence is still indirect. The effects can be potentiated by inducers, and inhibited by SKF-525A. In the cyclohexamide model we have found that the pattern of biliary secretion of tritium and C^{14} material is different in normal animals receiving ANIT than in those protected by cyclohexamide. We are now looking into the whole question of metabolites.

MIYAI: Dr. Phillips, what is the mechanism of action of cytochalasin B, and have you tried this agent on an in vivo system?

PHILLIPS: Cytochalasin B is a fungal alkaloid which has been used as an experimental tool to disrupt microfilaments. Although probably not specific it is an interesting effect which is reversible and appears to wear off in 3 to 4 hours. The mechanism of its action is unknown. It may affect energy metabolism and particularly mitochondrial oxidative phosphorylation. The contractility of microfilaments is an energy requiring function. On the other hand it may affect the magnesium activated ATPase of actomyosin or it may have an effect on the cell membrane itself.

We have studied the effect of cytochalasin B on the isolated perfused rat liver and found a striking dilatation of the bile canaliculi after 3 hours of perfusion. So the agent does appear to have a similar effect in vivo.

Dr. Miyai, did you find any changes in the enzymes of the bile canalicular membranes?

MIYAI: Our preliminary histochemical studies of alkaline phosphatase and ATPase indicate that the reaction is less prominent in the pathologically altered bile canaliculi than in the controls.

PHILLIPS: You get a reduction in bile flow. Have you actually studied the bile?

MIYAI: We examined the bile by negative staining techniques in two experiments but did not find note-worthy differences between the samples taken before and after the onset of lithocholate infusion.

WHEELER: I want to ask Dr. Javitt about his comments concerning taurolithocholate cholestasis in the hamster and specifically about bile acid independent flow. If you plot bile acid output on the horizontal axis and mannitol clearance on the vertical axis, the line has to go through the origin if you do anything which reduces the bile flow to zero, because both of these are quantities which are multiplied by flow. It is no surprise that, in an animal with no bile output at all, the points fall right at the origin and the fact that it extrapolates to the origin does not indicate the elimination of the bile acid independent fraction. You would have to show a perfectly linear relationship which extrapolates through the origin, not one which dips toward the origin as bile flow dips toward zero. Would you admit that this is still an open question?

JAVITT: Yes.

STRASBERG: Did the taurolithocholate have any effect on the feeding pattern of your animals? In partial duct obstruction experiments we obtained a graph similar to yours and I think that the reason for this is that the animals stopped eating. When they did so bile salt independent ductular flow fell and the points fell off the linear regression line.

JAVITT: We cannulated the animals the night before and allowed them to recover. The following day we did not feed them and simply infused bile acids intravenously.

LESTER: The cholestatic effects which you have documented should be tested, as well, on fetal or neonatal liver. The interaction of cholestatic agents with the liver may depend on its stage of maturity. Our results on primate excretion of bile acids tend to show that the mechanism for the excretion develops late in the fetal life of the Rhesus monkey. This species is just beginning to elaborate bile acids toward the end of gestation and it is conceivable that what is not cholestatic in the adult is cholestatic in the fetus and newborn, whose bile mechanisms are immature.

JAVITT: I agree; the model has not been developed.

LESTER: We have looked at the movement of trihydroxy- and dihydroxy- bile acids across the placenta from mother to fetus. The dihydroxy-bile acids seem to go faster than the trihydroxy ones. The monohydroxy-bile acids may be free to go across and this would really multiply the problem.

JAVITT: We don't know what would happen if a pregnant mother was given monohydroxy-bile acids.

FORKER: You expresed the mannitol excretion in terms of mass per unit time, whereas ordinarily one would expect to see mannitol clearance in terms of units of flow. Is this because all the animals have the same plasma concentration?

JAVITT: Yes, it is a single animal and the plasma concentration remains constant throughout the study.

CONTRIBUTORS

Irwin M. Arias, M.D.
Professor of Medicine,
Albert Einstein College of Medicine,
Bronx, N.Y.

Paul D. Berk, M.D.,
Chief, Section on Diseases of the Liver,
Digestive Diseases Branch,
National Institute of Arthritis,
Metabolism and Digestive Diseases,
Bethesda, Maryland

Michael C. Brain, M.D.,
Professor of Medicine,
McMaster University,
Hamilton, Ontario.

Murray M. Fisher, M.D.,
Associate Professor of Medicine and Pathology,
University of Toronto,
Toronto, Ontario.

E. Lee Forker, M.D.,
Professor of Medicine,
University of Iowa,
Iowa City, Iowa.

Lawrence M. Gartner, M.D.,
Professor of Pediatrics,
Albert Einstein College of Medicine,
Bronx, N.Y.

Ellen R. Gordon, Ph.D.,
Assistant Professor of Experimental Medicine,
McGill University,
Montreal, Quebec.

Carl A. Goresky, M.D.,
Professor of Medicine,
McGill University,
Montreal, Quebec.

Lyonel G. Israels, M.D.,
Executive Director,
Manitoba Cancer Treatment and Research Foundation,
700 Bannatyne Avenue,
Winnipeg, Manitoba.

Norman B. Javitt, M.D.,
Professor of Medicine,
New York Hospital - Cornell Medical Center,
New York, N.Y.

Stephen A. Landaw, M.D.,
Associate Chief of Staff, Research,
Veterans Administration Hospital,
Syracuse, N.Y.

Pierre Lavoie, M.D.,
Professeur agrégé de Chirurgie
de l'Université de Montréal,
Montréal, Québec.

Roger Lester, M.D.,
Professor and Chief of Gastroenterology,
University of Pittsburgh School of Medicine,
Pittsburgh, Pennsylvania.

Jerold F. Lucey, M.D.,
Professor of Pediatrics,
University of Vermont,
Burlington, Vermont.

Antony F. McDonagh, Ph.D.,
Assistant Professor of Medicine,
University of California,
San Francisco, California.

Katsumi Miyai, M.D.,
Assistant Professor of Pathology,
University of California, San Diego,
La Jolla, California.

Ursula Muller-Eberhard, M.D.,
Department of Biochemistry,
Scripps Clinic and Research Foundation,
La Jolla, California.

M. James Phillips, M.D.,
Professor of Pathology,
University of Toronto,
Toronto, Ontario.

Gabriel L. Plaa, Ph.D.,
Directeur, Département de pharmacologie,
Université de Montréal,
Montréal, Québec.

Stephen H. Robinson, M.D.,
Associate Professor of Medicine,
Harvard Medical School,
Boston, Massachusetts.

Andrew Sass-Kortsak, M.D.,
Professor of Pediatrics,
Hospital for Sick Children,
Toronto, Ontario.

Brent A. Schacter, M.D.,
Assistant Professor of Internal Medicine,
University of Manitoba,
Winnipeg, Manitoba.

Fenton Schaffner, M.D.,
Professor of Medicine and Pathology,
Mount Sinai School of Medicine,
New York, N.Y.

Rudi Schmid, M.D.,
Professor of Medicine,
University of California,
San Francisco, California.

Jan W. Steiner, M.D.,
Professor of Pathology,
University of Toronto,
Toronto, Ontario.

Steven M. Strasberg, M.D.,
Assistant Professor of Surgery,
University of Toronto,
Toronto, Ontario.

M. Michael Thaler, M.D.,
Associate Professor of Pediatrics,
University of California,
San Francisco, California.

Henry O. Wheeler, M.D.,
Professor of Medicine,
University of California,
San Diego, California.

David S. Zimmon, M.D.,
Chief, Gastroenterology,
Veterans Administration Hospital,
New York, N.Y.

SUBJECT INDEX

MIX
Papier aus verantwortungsvollen Quellen
Paper from responsible sources
FSC® C105338

If you have any concerns about our products,
you can contact us on
ProductSafety@springernature.com

In case Publisher is established outside the EU,
the EU authorized representative is:
Springer Nature Customer Service Center GmbH
Europaplatz 3, 69115 Heidelberg, Germany

Printed by Libri Plureos GmbH
in Hamburg, Germany